Fundamentals of Three-Dimensional Digital Image Processing

Junichiro Toriwaki · Hiroyuki Yoshida

Fundamentals of Three-Dimensional Digital Image Processing

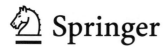 Springer

Professor Junichiro Toriwaki
Chukyo University
Japan

Assoc. Prof. Hiroyuki Yoshida
Harvard Medical School
Massachusetts General Hospital
USA

ISBN 978-1-84800-172-5 e-ISBN 978-1-84800-173-2
DOI 10.1007/978-1-84800-173-2
Springer Dordrecht Heidelberg London New York

British Library Cataloguing in Publication Data
A catalogue record for this book is available from the British Library

Library of Congress Control Number: Applied for

Printed on acid-free paper

Springer is part of Springer Science+Business Media (www.springer.com)

To colleagues in Nagoya University and to my wife
–Junichiro Toriwaki

Preface

This book is a detailed description of the basics of three-dimensional digital image processing. A 3D digital image (abbreviated as "3D image" below) is a digitalized representation of a 3D object or an entire 3D space, stored in a computer as a 3D array. Whereas normal digital image processing is concerned with screens that are a collection of square shapes called "pixels" and their corresponding density levels, the "image plane" in three dimensions is represented by a division into cubical graphical elements (called "voxels") that represent corresponding density levels.

In the context of image processing, in many cases 3D image processing will refer to the input of multiple 2D images and performing processing in order to understand the 3D space (or "scene") that they depict. This is a result of research into how to use input from image sensors such as television cameras as a basis for learning about a 3D scene, thereby replicating the sense of vision for humans or intelligent robots, and this has been the central problem in image processing research since the 1970s.

However, a completely different type of image with its own new problems, the 3D digital image discussed in this book, rapidly took prominence in the 1980s, particularly in the field of medical imaging. These were recordings of human bodies obtained through computed (or "computerized") tomography (CT), images that recorded not only the external, visible surface of the subject but also, to some degree of resolution, its internal structure. This was a type of image that no one had experienced before.

The biggest problem when processing such 3D images is that they include new problems in 3D digital geometry. Examples include surface/axis thinning (equivalent to thinning the lines in a 2D image), topology-preserving processing, calculation of Euler numbers, etc. Another problematic aspect is the limitation of human vision. Humans are not able to directly view a 3D image that includes internal structure. Neither is it a simple task to hold a complex 3D form in one's head. For areas such as these, computer processing is superior to human sight. Another consideration in 3D scene comprehension is "dimensional degeneration" (where it is necessary to recreate a 3D scene based on some small number of images of 2D visible surfaces). For these points to be implemented, however, it is first necessary to establish the fundamentals of handling 3D digital images.

This book describes the geometric properties of 3D images and the fundamentals of 3D image processing. First, Chapter 2 formally defines the concepts and notation used with 3D images and their processing (calculations performed on the image). Next, Chapter 3 introduces localized processing, also known as filtering. This chapter shows how methods of 2D image processing are extended to 3D images, and introduces some localized processes that are frequently used in 3D image processing.

Chapters 4 and 5 are the core portion of the book. Chapter 4 begins with a definition of connectivity and defines some fundamental concepts such as topology preservation conditions, Euler numbers, and path and distance functions, thereby leading to some important properties. Chapter 5 uses the ideas developed in Chapter 4 to present algorithms for processing connected components (for example, labeling, surface/axis thinning, distance transformation, etc.). Algorithms are given as specific examples in a code-like form, and a detailed explanation as to how they were derived is also given.

Chapter 6 is a simple explanation of processing connected components having density values. The book ends with a description of 3D image visualization in Chapter 7. The chapter uses techniques from computer graphics (CG) as typified by volume rendering, but the discussion is limited to those techniques necessary for 3D image visualization, not CG as a whole.

The book has a reference listing at its end. The list is divided by source into those from individual papers, such as from academic journals, and those from technical books. This is done for the benefit of those readers requiring the detailed knowledge available from the technical books. The purpose of the individual papers is of one of three types. The first type is concerned with when and based on what research matters discussed in this book were presented. That is why many of those papers are from when the author was at Nagoya University. The second type indicates when the matters discussed in this book were first presented. These two types taken together indicate the author's desire to record, to the author's knowledge, when and where original results came about. The third type indicates originating research centers from which the algorithms and experimental results included in this book came about. The list includes several papers from Japanese academic journals, each having gone through the academic review processes prescribed by the associated academy. Each should be obtainable from the academy, including those originally written in Japanese. Of course, the English version of each paper is listed where such a version exists. Creating an exhaustive listing of every related paper would be extremely difficult, and so the listing is not claimed as being complete. Hopefully the list will provide a starting point in the pursuit of any further information that may be required.

Acknowledgments

The contents of this book are based on research performed by the author at Nagoya University and Chukyo University, starting in the 1980s. I would like to express my deepest thanks in particular to my fellow researchers at the Nagoya University Faculty of Engineering's Department of Electronics and Department of Information Engineering. Among those members, the research of Tatsuhiro Yonekura (a graduate student at the time, currently a professor at Ibaragi University), Shigeki Yokoi (an associate professor at the time, currently a professor at Nagoya University), Toyofumi Saito (now deceased, a research associate at the time and later a professor at Nagoya University), Yasushi Hirano (a graduate student at the time and now associate professor at Nagoya University), and Kensaku Mori (a graduate student at the time and now associate professor at Nagoya University) were particularly helpful in their contributions to the content of this book.

When creating the manuscript, Nagoya University secretaries Fumiyo Kaba and Hiromi Tanaka were very helpful in their assistance in typing the English version, creating figures, and arranging materials.

Yuichiro Hayashi and Takayuki Kitasaka of Nagoya University aided in creating the TEX version of the document.

Parts of Chapters 4 and 5 of this text are based on papers presented by their authors in the English-language journal FORMA. I would like to thank the Society for Science on Form, Japan, for their permission in using that material.

In 1975, the author had plans for penning an English technical work on 2D image processing, and Ernest L. Hall (currently a professor at the University of Cincinnati) made extensive comments in regard to one part of that manuscript. That project was never completed, but as much of its content is present in Chapter 2, I wish to express my gratitude to him.

I would like to extend my sincerest thanks to Professor Yasuhito Suenaga and Professor Hiroshi Murase of Nagoya University for their accommodations in allowing me use of their laboratories and computers in the creation of this book. I also extend my deepest thanks to Chukyo University's Department of Life System Science and Technology (Toyota City, Aichi Prefecture) for providing me with the opportunity to continue my research and studies from 2003 up to the present.

Last but not least I would like to extend thanks to Professor Hiroyuki Yoshida of Harvard University for all his invaluable assistance from the beginning of this publication project in 2006.

March 2008

Junichiro Toriwaki

Contents

1

INTRODUCTION

1.1 Overview

This book is a systematic and detailed description of the basics of 3D images and their processing. Before beginning with specific details, however, we will discuss an overview of 3D images and their processing, and also will introduce the contents of each chapter in the book.

1.1.1 3D continuous images

Generally, 2D images are printed onto paper or film or displayed on a screen. Therefore, the brightness (luminosity or density), reflectivity, transmissivity, etc. of a given point (x, y) on the screen can be clearly represented by a two-variable real function $f(x, y)$. The value of f is clearly defined physically as the "density" or the "intensity" of the point.

The 3D images (more precisely, the 3D continuous images) covered in this book are formal extension of such 2D images into 3D. In other words, a point (x, y, z) in 3D space is taken as data with a density value function $f(x, y, z)$. The content of the density function f, however, will be completely different. It will change greatly for each individual image, without the high commonality of density as is found in 2D images. For the time being, however, this book will continue to use the term "density." More precise definitions are given in Chapter 2. Specific examples are given in Section 1.2.

1.1.2 3D digital images

This book is concerned with digital image processing; in other words, image processing using computers. In order for such processing to take place, the 3D continuous image must be digitized. By analogy with 2D images, the screen is split up into pixels and the density value of each is represented by a finite number of bits. The pixels themselves also are extended to 3D and are called *voxels*, the 3D equivalent of pixels. An image that has been digitized in such a manner is called a *three-dimensional digital image*, abbreviated as 3D image in this book. Chapter 2 will discuss the details of digitalization and the formal expression of digital images.

Ideally, digital images should be created so that an original continuous image is digitized with the same precision in the x, y, and z axes in 3D space. However, doing so is not always an easy task, given current image acquisition technologies (imaging technologies). A common practice, as we will see in an example below, is to create multiple 2D cross-sectional images that are parallel to a given direction and separated by an appropriate spacing and to create a 3D image by aligning and stacking those images. In such a situation, the size of the pixels in the cross section, that is, the precision of digitalization, and the spacing between cross sections are not necessarily the same. In most cases, the spacing between cross sections will be larger. We will discuss the details in Chapter 2; however, this book will assume that, unless mentioned otherwise, digitalization both between and within cross sections is at the same resolution.

Remark 1.1. Common usage infers that an *image* refers to a 2D representation drawn on a plane. Our use of the term "3D image" probably gives readers an impression somewhat different from the standard meaning of what "image usually means." It is not clear why that word is applied here. The term probably comes from the use in medical imaging and other applied fields of *images* along with 2D images as a method of diagnostic imaging, and because humans have been observed as a series of cross sections, in other words, a collection of 2D images, etc. Their 3D-ness is likely not particularly considered, and so the term "image" is used naturally, without any particular sense of incongruity

Remark 1.2. Generally speaking, there are two ways to handle images in which the spacing between cross sections is larger. One is to just treat it as a 3D image, taking voxels not as cubes but as rectangular solids. The other is to use some appropriate method to interpolate new cross sections between the existing ones in a manner such that the sampling spacing becomes as similar as possible in all three directions. In reality, the sampling distance in each direction will not be at an integral ratio; thus, creating precisely cubical elements (in other words, voxels that are exact cubes) will not be possible. Some image processing algorithms can be directly applied to non-cubic elements; however, the majority of processes cannot, and those will be limited to approximating values within a given range of precision. When measuring certain features on digital images, it therefore will be necessary to verify the image acquisition process and then make any necessary corrections.

This is also related to the equipment and methods used for imaging and digitalization. For example, when the imaging is performed on digital processing equipment, the sampling distance will be determined by the capabilities of the imaging device, and so the quality of the resulting image will depend on the device used. For example, for cross-sectional images generated by the medical imaging devices such as X-ray CT or magnetic resonance imaging (MRI), factors such as the capabilities of the imaging devices and the meaning of the data obtained, as well as the burden placed upon the patient, must be taken into consideration. Recent X-ray CT devices allow for the reconstruction of cross sections at an arbitrary cross-sectional spacing (reconstruction pitch) after acquisition of the sensing data.

On the other hand, in the case of microscopic imaging of pathological samples, digitalization is sometimes performed by creating a continuous image (a micrograph) from scans of cross sections after exposure by sequential shaving of the specimen. In such a case, the spacing of cross sections is determined at the point where the photograph is taken or the specimen is shaved, but selection of the sampling distances within the cross section is limited only by the capabilities of the scanner, leaving a wide degree of freedom.

1.2 What does "3D image" mean?

The terms "3D image" and "3D image processing" are generally used with a wide variety of meanings. This section and the one following it give a simple overview of those meanings.

1.2.1 Dimensionality of the media and of the subject

It is first necessary to make a clear distinction between the *dimensionality of the media* (or, the *dimensionality of the data structure*) and that of the *subject* (or *content*).

The former refers to the dimensionality of the space (media) that contains the record of the image. When density values for each point in an n-dimensional space are recorded, the result is referred to as an n-dimensional image. For example, an image drawn on a 2D plane such as paper is a 2D image, and an image recorded in a 3D space is a 3D image. For an n-dimensional digital image, density values are recorded in an n-dimensional array.

Dimensionality of the subject refers to the dimensionality of that *thing* (*scene*) that is recorded in the image, or to that object that is the main *subject of processing*. For example, an image that records a 3D scene or a 3D object might be called a 3D image, even if it is recorded on paper. Similarly, a 3-dimensional scene drawn using computer graphics is referred to as 3D graphics, even when displayed on a 2D screen.

1.2.2 Types of 3D images

The meaning of the word "dimension" discussed above is used with a variety of meanings. The following are differing types of what each are called 3D images:

(1) *Image data that are recorded (stored) in a 3D array:* This is a 3D image (a continuous image, or a digital image) of the type described in Section 1.1, and the main type discussed in this book. Specific examples are given in the following section and subsequently throughout the book, starting in Chapter 2. More specifically, however, this book is most concerned with 3D images in which recorded data are related not only to visible surfaces, but also to structures internal to the subject.

(2) *Images depicting 3D scenes and 3D objects:* In this case, the term 3D image is used despite the fact that it is a picture, photograph, or graph drawn on a 2D space (paper, etc.). In actuality, however, we will limit this to those images in which steps have been taken so that the image will be recognized by the viewer as that of a 3D scene or object.

(3) *Images intentionally created so as to create a stereoscopic effect (a sense of 3-dimensionality) in the viewer:* This would refer to, for example, a pair of 2D images intended to be viewed with one eye each (a stereogram). The image described in Remark 1.3 falls into this category.

(4) *Images in which the density value itself contains information related to a 3D space:* For example, range images and certain types of relief contour maps (see Remark 1.4).

(5) *Special images in which the form of a 3D object is recreated optically:* This would include various types of holograms.

(6) *2D dynamic images:* This refers to a time series of 2D images that record changes over time (movement of an object, etc.) in the subject scene. These images are also recorded in a 3D array, but the coordinate axes are spatiotemporal, measuring 2D positioning in space along with time, and so in that sense are not truly isotropic. An extension of this type would be a 4D image that records the changes over time of a 3D image as described in (1) (in other words, a 3D movie).

Of the above, only images of the type described in (1) contain information related to the overall structure of a 3D object, including its interior. In this book, when it is necessary to make a distinction with other types, such images will sometimes be called *true 3D images* or *voxel construction images*.

Remark 1.3. There exist a variety of different ways to create images that cause a feeling of reality or immersion in the viewer of a 3D space. Projection of images onto extremely large, curved screens or domed screens is one example. Such methods cause the viewer to visually interpret themselves as being inside of a surrounding 3D environment. Of course, actual objects are not recreated, and so only those faces shown in the picture can be seen. The viewer could not move so as to see the opposite side of an object, for example.

Aside from this, there are methods by which an image is created so that the same light rays or wave fronts as when viewing the actual object are visualized by the observer. Examples are holograms and volumegraphs [Dohi00, Nakajima00]. These examples allow viewers to change, to some extent, the visible face of an object by changing their point of view.

1.2.3 Cues for 3D information

Given a 2D image, or two to three 2D images (2D in the sense that they are drawn on a plane or that the dimensionality of the media is 2), the following types of cues contain information related to the third dimension and create a 3D effect, or a sense of depth (Fig. 1.1):

(1) In a single image
  - Shading (object surface brightness or changes therein)
  - Shadows (changes in brightness of an object brought about by blockage of light upon it by another object)
  - Occlusion (the hiding of a background object by a foreground object)
  - Deformation of known patterns by the surface of the subject (deformations of slit light due to surface irregularities, etc.)
  - Drawings using perspective transformations (shapes drawn using methods of perspective)
  - Blurring and contrast (for example, drawing objects far away as blurred)
  - Hues (for example, drawing objects far away with a bluish tinge)
  - Reflections (reflection of another object on the surface of the subject)
(2) In two or more images
  - A combination of multiple images of the same object, depicting a different angle (a multi angle image). Examples of this are pairs of images corresponding to the information brought in by each of the right and left eye (stereocorrespondence), or tri directional design drawings.
(3) In images that include motion
  - Objects that move quickly on the screen appear to be closer, while those moving more slowly appear to be farther away.

Using a 2D image to understand the state of a 3D scene (the positioning of objects, etc.) based on these limited cues is a topic of primary importance in the field of computer vision. Depending on the cues used, these problems have names of the form "shape from X," for example, "shape from shading," "shape from texture," etc. [Horn86] see also Section 1.4. Because these cues contain at least some information related to the 3D object, they are sometimes called 2.5D images.

1.2.4 Specific examples of 3D images

This section discusses several specific examples, focusing on true and near-true 3D images (see Fig. 1.2).

(a) Computed tomography (CT)

CT, an X ray-based method first made practical in the early 1970s, uses the Radon transform to measure the strength of X-rays penetrating a human

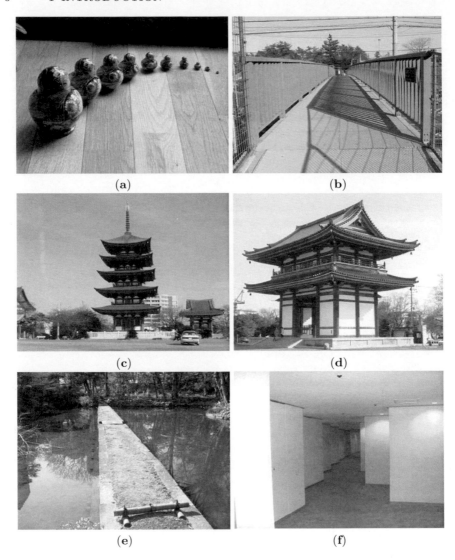

Fig. 1.1. Cues to depth perception in a monocular image: (**a**) Arrangement of the same shape of figures with shading; (**b**) perspective - a pedestrian overpass; (**c**) perspective - a five-storied pagoda; (**d**) perspective - a gate of a Buddhist temple; (**e**) perspective - a passage across a pond in Japanese garden; (**f**) perspective - a passage of a hotel.

body from multiple directions (a 1D projection) to recreate a 2D cross section. This is referred to as X-ray CT [Bankman00, Ritman03]. Later, the method was further developed by moving the subject (a human body) parallel to the device and continuously rotating the X-ray tubes and sensor system. By doing

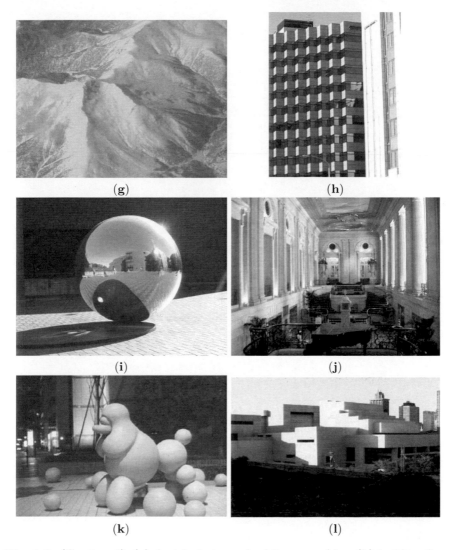

Fig. 1.1. (Continued): (**g**) Aerial photograph of Japanese Alps; (**h**) building faces of changing brightness; (**i**) spherical monument with metallic surface in a museum; (**j**) perspective of a hall in a hotel; (**k**) sculptures with smooth surfaces lit by street light; (**l**) building faces of different brightness.

so multiple parallel cross sections are created, allowing for continuous scanning of the subject. Methods also developed for extremely high-speed imaging of slices, allowing a specific portion of the patient to be recreated in 3D through the use of tens up to hundreds of parallel images (helical or spiral CT, or multi slice CT). At present, this method allows for the creation of images that are

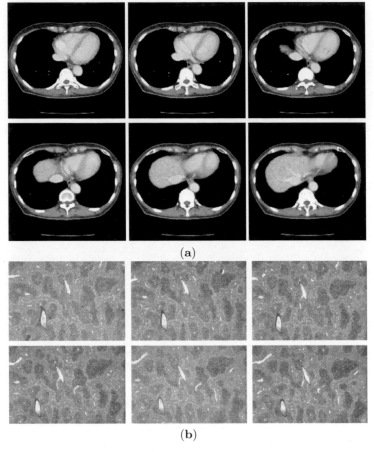

Fig. 1.2. Examples of 3D images: (**a**) Slices of CT images of the human body; (**b**) microscope images of tissue sections.

the closest to true 3D. Recent devices are approaching true 3D images with an approximately isotropic resolution of 1 mm [Bankman00, Ritman03]. These images require large amounts of data, and in a medical setting there is a good chance that many images, for example, $512 \times 512 \times 512$ 3D gray-scale images, might be created.

The principles behind CT also are being applied to other fields. One well-known example is emission CT, where radioactive isotopes (RIs) are injected into patients, and then gamma ray emissions are acquired to recreate cross sections (see Remark 1.4). X-ray CT has also started to be used for the internal inspection and measurement of industrial products. New applications are also attracting attention, including, for example, applications to computer-aided design (CAD), precise measurement of products, and internal inspection of machine parts while the device is in operation [Hardin00]. In each case, the

X-ray attenuation coefficient at specific points within the object is measured, and this along with spatial changes show the internal structure of the subject, allowing use of the data as 3D shape information. Currently, recording similar resolutions both between and within slices is somewhat difficult, with spacing between slices tending to be to some extent larger. Developments in the technology are extremely rapid, however, and so such problems will likely be improved soon.

Remark 1.4. More specifically, this is referred to by names such as positron emission tomography (PET) and single photon emission CT (SPECT). These technologies are attracting attention as ways to measure brain functioning. As with X-ray CT, the measurement of the integral of attenuation along the path of an X-ray is required. Recent devices allow for imaging while simultaneously performing X-ray CT.

(b) Magnetic resonance imaging

Magnetic resonance imaging (MRI) is a technique in which the subject is placed within a magnetic field that is altered at a specific frequency, causing the subject to emit signals at the spin resonance frequencies of the nuclei of its component atoms, and the strength of those emissions are measured. By placing the subject in a precisely controlled magnetic field and controlling information from signal detection positions, the strength of the resonance signal at any arbitrary point and surrounding micro scale area can be measured, even from within the subject [Bankman00]. The strength of the resonance signal gives the number (ratio) of atoms corresponding to the signal in that area. At present the technique is used mainly on human subjects as a way to view hydrogen ratios, making it an effective tool in cancer and tumor diagnosis, as well as acquiring information about brain, heart, muscle, and other soft tissue form and composition. Isotropic data are more easily obtained than with the X-ray CT method described above, though some distortion is caused by empty cavities. Types of information that can be obtained using this method are still increasing rapidly.

(c) Tissue sample microscopy

In medicine, examination of pathological samples is performed by hardening an actual sample, shaving off slices in thicknesses measured in microns, and then observing those slices under an optical microscope. By taking and digitalizing sequential photographs of the image in the microscope (or by connecting a CCD camera to directly acquire images from the microscope), a 3D image can be obtained. When using this technique, however, it is difficult to keep the distancing within the slice and between slices the same, and aligning the position of adjacent slices is problematic. In theory large-scale 3D images of up to $1000 \times 1000 \times 500$ elements can be obtained, but digitalization requires extreme effort, and building up a 3D structure can be difficult. Nonetheless the technique is an extremely important one, as it allows judgments to be made based on direct observation of the actual sample (see Fig. 1.2).

(d) Artificial imaging

This refers to computer-based creation of the image data in their entirety, with an array of 3D data created as a time series and used as the subject of visualization. Some examples include the behavior of physical phenomena based on numerical solutions to differential equations (the behavior of fluids, deformation of materials, electromagnetic field strengths, etc.), saving image data as voxel data for use in computer graphics, creating a virtual space and storing it as voxel data, etc. As computer performance continues to improve, computer simulations have rapidly become increasingly more important as a fundamental method of scientific research. Computational physics is one example. In such cases, it is typical for data resulting from computer experiments to be created and stored as large-scale voxel structure data and visualization tools used to make viewing of the data possible. Along with the increasing importance of such methods, a variety of techniques has been developed for visualization and is currently an important topic in 3D image processing [IEEE95c, Johnson06].

(e) Range imaging

A range image is one in which a reference point (or reference plane, generally the location of the point of view or that of the measuring device) is chosen, and the distance from that point to the surface of all objects forward from the point is measured and recorded. Systems measuring propagation times from reflected lasers or ultrasound (called "range finders") are used to find the distance to reflective surfaces. Similar devices include fish detectors, ultrasound equipment used in medical imaging, and display screens on radar receivers. These devices do not allow internal structures to be recorded, but can handle applications related to external surface forms. Though these cannot be called true 3D images, they can be thought of as 3D in the sense that they can measure the distance to complex curved surfaces from multiple directions, the representation of which requires the use of a 3D space. The devices have been used in a variety of methods and areas, including the use of lasers to record the shape of human faces and bodies, the input of simple 3D shapes, examination of the image of human organs using ultrasound, observation of micron-order surface features on VLSI components using confocal microscopy, etc.

A somewhat analogous scenario is to take a 2D gray-scale image $f(x, y)$ as a surface in 3D space described by x, y, f. Taking this perspective one can analyze the features of the 3D curve, which is taken as a part of 2D image processing. Extending this to a true 3D image as discussed above makes it a 4D image (see Chapter 6).

Standard X-ray images of the human body (meaning not CT, but rather the previous standard imaging) is not quite so precise, yet it too has its own depth of information. In fact, by examining several X-ray images taken at different angles, one can to some extent recreate a 3D image showing the internal structure of organs and blood vessels.

(f) Animated images

A true 3D image is stored in a 3D array and moreover has three axes (i, j, k), indicating position in space. In other cases, a time series of 2D images (in other words, an animation) may be stored in a 3D array and treated as a single 3D image. In such cases these objects are treated as true 3D images having rectangular image elements (in most cases, the direction of the time axis and that of the other axes will represent different physical meanings and resolutions), but generally they are not referred to as 3D images. Instead they are often called spatiotemporal images. (In other cases, images may show foreground and background relationships between objects due to occlusion, or as discussed above an otherwise 2D image may carry some 3D information. Such images are often called 2.5D images.) Video and television images are trivial examples. Some processing, for example, tracking and measuring the movement of specific objects in an image or editing support, is effectively performed when the image is treated as a 3D one. There has been interesting research in recent years related to creating a virtual environment (including temporal changes) within a computer in real time, based on a 3D space created using images from multiple TV cameras, and furthermore adding 3D image data for objects that do not actually exist. This is referred to as mixed reality [Ohta99].

(g) Variable focus microscopy images

By using a device that can view a single object from a fixed angle, making fine adjustments to the position of the focus surface (that object surface on which the focus is aimed), and taking a series of photographs after moving the focus surface by tiny amounts, one can create a composite image that records surface irregularities in the direction of the optic axis. This allows for distance measurements between points on the visible surface of the object along the primary axis of the photographic lens. A 3D image of those surface irregularities then can be created. If the object of study is transparent, then observation of its internal structure is also possible. A well-known example of such a device is the confocal laser microscope. Examples of applications include microscopy of tissue samples from living specimens and examination of surface features on VLSI devices [Ichikawa94, Ichikawa95, Ichikawa96, Vitria96]. See also [Geissler99].

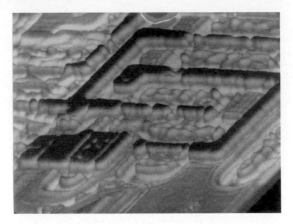

Fig. 1.3. Example of a 3D image. Surface of a sample of a VLSI observed by a confocal microscope [Ichikawa96].

1.3 Types and characteristics of 3D image processing

1.3.1 Examples of 3D image processing

Taking "3D image" in its meaning as described above, then "3D image processing" will mean the process of creation, display, transmission, identification, etc., of such a 3D image. The following are a few examples.

(a) Processing of true 3D images

This is literal 3D image processing and refers to all processing performed on true 3D images, especially to their display, measurement, identification, and understanding. This type of processing is the main focus of this book.

(b) Comprehension of 3D objects and 3D scenes

This refers to making computers identify and comprehend the state of 3D objects and scenes on the basis of a single or relatively small number of 2D images. When doing so, cues such as those described in Section 1.2.3 are utilized. As described previously, this is a core theme in the field of computer vision. Unless otherwise specified, this is often what the phrase "3D processing" refers to [Watt98, Kanatani90, Horn86].

(c) Creation and display of semi-3D images in 2D

This refers to the display (rendering) of an image that appears to the human eye to be in 3D (i.e., types (2) and (3) in Section 1.2.2 above) on a 2D screen such as a computer display. Such processing lies within the realm of computer graphics and is also called 3D graphics. Important features include determination of shapes using the laws of perspective (perspective projections) and creation of shading and shadows using a variety of supplied methods (reflectivity models of the object surface, correspondence relationships between distance and density values, characteristics related to the shape of the object and the shape of light sources, characteristics of component materials, etc.).

(d) Creation and display of 3D images using optical and visual effects

A variety of 3D images of types (3) and (4) as described in Section 1.2.2, such as stereovision and holograms, can be created and displayed.

(e) Stereology

When only a small number of cross sections of the 3D object can be observed, mainly geometric and statistical methods can be applied to whatever information can be ascertained from them to obtain information about the 3D space. Active research into such attempts has been ongoing over the past two or three decades in a wide variety of applied fields, including biology, pathology, crystallography, and mineralogy. The methodology also has been to some extent theoretically systematized and is now called stereology. Academically, stereology is included in a field called the science of form, and active research continues. In recent years, advances in imaging and computer technology have made possible the measurement of entire spaces in other areas, and so interest has waned. The underlying logic remains valid, however, and there remain cases where for some subjects information can be obtained only from only a very limited number of cross sections, and so this remains an important basic method. See, for example, the original articles by [Toth72, Weibel79], etc.

1.3.2 Virtual spaces as 3D digital images

True 3D images are recordings of some characteristic value for an entire 3D space, including both the interiors and exteriors of any objects. When those values are read into a computer, the subjects, or an overall 3D structure, are recorded therein. Viewing such as a virtual reality (VR), one can say that the objects (or the space) have been *virtualized* and now reside within the computer. Of course, such objects are no longer restrained by the laws of reality and can be manipulated as desired. This is an important perspective, and presents great possibilities for VR technology applications. For example, taking CT imaging of a human subject as a representative example of a true 3D image, that image represents a *virtualized human body* within the computer. This makes it possible to perform a number of actions that are difficult to perform on an actual human body, such as observations, examinations (for example, virtual endoscopy [Toriwaki00, Toriwaki04]), and simulated surgeries [Taylor96]).

1.3.3 Characteristics of 3D image processing

The following is a simple summary of some of the characteristics of 3D image processing, as compared to 2D image processing (in particular, transformations, recognition, and understanding).

(a) As compared to human recognition and understanding of images

Not everything is understood about human pattern recognition capabilities, but they are extremely powerful, at least in the case of 2D images. Furthermore, humans have a high level of intellectual ability with regard to understanding 3D conditions (the form and relative location of objects) based on visual input from a 2D source. Reproducing such capabilities in a computer is a central problem in the field of computer vision, yet as of today in most cases the abilities of computers lag far behind that of humans. The 3D images treated in this book, on the other hand, while perhaps limited by the capabilities of imaging technology, retain information about all points in the 3D space, including the interiors of subjects. Humans, it would seem, go through a process of combining 2D images, cross sections, to mentally build a 3D structure. Strictly speaking, we cannot yet guarantee that such a process is actually occurring, but when viewed from the outside it seems as if that is indeed the case.

For computers, on the other hand, moving from two dimensions to three is simply a routine extension to the processing of data held in an array, and is not fundamentally different. Computers can easily access any given image element in either two or three dimensions, but humans are not able to directly view the internals of a 3D image. Furthermore, because true 3D images also include all information about the internal structure of the subject, complex processing related to the recovery of a 3D image from a 2D source, such as occlusion or stereopsis, is unnecessary. In that regard, computer processing is even preferable to human vision.

Moreover, while most true 3D images are of completely new things that until very recently humans have had no contact with, most 2D images are of things that humans have been in constant contact with since the days of the wall paintings of Altamira and Lascaux. As such, it probably would be extremely difficult for a human viewer to have a direct comprehension of a 3D image in the same manner as with a 2D image.

(b) Amounts of data

As compared with 2D images, 3D images represent massive amounts of data. A single X-ray CT image, for example, may be $512 \times 512 \times 512$ bytes, while images from tissue sample microscopy may be as large as $3000 \times 2000 \times 500$ bytes. This has huge effects on all aspects of the image processing system. Already, data transfer between sensors and processors poses a significant problem in CT devices.

(c) The importance of display technology

As described in (1) above, it is difficult for humans to have a direct comprehension of 3D images. The use of appropriate display rules (visibility rules) is therefore extremely important, not only when displaying the results of processing input image files, but also in researchers' evaluation of intermediate results. Processing information contained within a 3D image for display onto a 2D screen is in a sense the opposite of the problem posed by computer vision. This technology is currently within the realm of computer graphics or of information visualization. Three-dimensional image processing is therefore a new field, requiring an integration of image pattern recognition and computer graphics. This also has a deep connection to virtual reality, and therefore has an even greater significance in this age of multimedia processing.

(d) Properties of image geometry

Several properties arise in 3D images that did not exist in 2D images. Typical examples include the existence of knots, links, and holes. In general, the topological characteristics of figures are extremely complex. As a result, the design and evaluation of related algorithms, for example, axis (surface) thinning, edge tracing, etc., becomes more difficult. A large portion of this book is devoted to analysis of such topics.

(e) Diversity of density values

The physical meaning of density values is not limited to image subjects and their recordings, but will vary greatly according to the space they are contained in and the measurement (imaging) technologies used, even when the same subject is being treated. An example is given in Table 1.1. According to these factors, the characteristics and content of detected edges, outlines, high density areas, etc., will be very different.

1.3.4 Objectives in 3D image processing

When processing true 3D images, one must consider whether the 3D image will be directly manipulated during processing. The following are some objectives to keep in mind when making that decision:

Table 1.1. Examples of meanings of density values in 3D images.

X-ray CT images	attenuation coefficient of X-ray at a small volume of an object
magnetic resonance images	strength of resonance signals at a small volume element of an object
ultrasound images	absorption, reflection, or transmission coefficient of ultrasound wave at a small volume element
confocal laser microscopi images	strength of reflected light or distance to the surface of an object
positron emission CT (PET)	absorption rate of γ-ray at a small volume of an object

(1) Applying some processing methodology to a set of independent 2D images and using the result to build or reconstruct the 3D image (*2D image processing with 3D image reconstruction*)

(2) Processing each cross section, but during processing taking into consideration the status and consistency of neighboring slices (for example, vertical relationships), and using such processing methods as necessary. (Here, this will be referred to as *2.5D processing*)

(3) Performing 3D processing on 3D image data (*3D processing*).

The decision also will be dependent upon the characteristics of the input image. When the sampling distance between cross sections is large as compared to the resolution (size of pixels) within cross sections, if additional cross sections will not be inserted, then 2.5D processing may be effective. On the other hand, if a true 3D image with approximately similar resolutions is obtained, the 3D processing should be used whenever possible. Conversely, as humans excel at intuitive judgments related to 2D images, starting out with the 2D image processing with 3D image reconstruction discussed in (1) above may not be without merit.

The focus of this book is 3D image processing. If a true 3D image of the subject is available, then the 3D processing of (3) above should be performed whenever possible. However, in actual practice the other two methods also should be put to use as circumstances demand. One must also keep in mind that the condition of the input image or the computing environment may force such decisions.

Let's look at an example. Figure. 1.4 shows a schematic image containing an arboroid structure like that of a bronchial tube. Here, ellipsoids might be extracted from 2D cross-sectional images of the tube using 2D image processing, and the extracted ellipsoid structures smoothly connected to extract

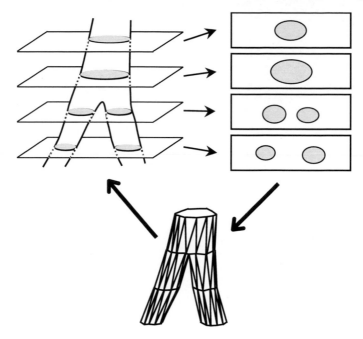

Fig. 1.4. A 3D image constructed from a sequence of cross sections.

the arboroid structure. Such a procedure (2D processing with 3D image reconstruction) would be worthwhile if the distance between cross sections is large as compared to the resolution within cross sections. In order to make such a method work, however, the structure must extend in a direction near perpendicular to the plane group of cross sections. If the direction that the figure predominantly extends in is not known beforehand, then features that run parallel to the cross sections may be lost.

When extracting the ellipsoids from the cross sections (the 2D images), implementing a method by which processing of the nth cross section will only extract those ellipsoidal forms that form a vertical overlay with those in the immediately preceding $(n-1)$th cross section also might be an appropriate technique by which to make smooth vertical connections in the perpendicular direction of the subject. Such a technique would be a natural method when there is some degree of spacing between cross sections.

As an alternative method, standard 3D processing technique might, for example, use a 3D difference filter and threshold processing to extract a 3D edge surface and then perform 3D axis thinning to find diagram cores. If the distance between cross sections is sufficiently small (for example, within about twice the size of the picture elements used in the cross sections), then processing might consist of the use of appropriate methods (linear interpolation, etc.) to fill in additional cross sections, or conversely elements from within the cross section may be pruned so as to form a sufficiently isotropic true 3D image. Some 3D processing algorithms can be applied even to images with differing resolutions in each directional axis (images created from rectangular solid picture elements), taking such anisotropy into consideration without modification of the source images (one example is the distance transform of Section 5.5).

On the other hand, the construction of a 3D image by appropriately connecting a group of given shapes that depict cross-sectional forms is also important and has been studied extensively in the field of computer graphics [Watt98]. Figure. 1.4 shows a schematic diagram. As can be predicted from the figure, the inclusion of branchings or features running parallel to the cross sections will make processing more difficult.

1.4 The contents of this book

Of the types described above, this book is a systematic explanation of the fundamentals of processing true 3D digital images. Its content is divided into two parts, the geometric characteristics of 3D digital forms (in other words, the digital geometry of 3D forms), and fundamental algorithms for 3D image processing. The latter is written assuming knowledge of the former. Methods of visualization of 3D gray-scale images are also described, because, as discussed in Section 1.3.3, visualization is an indispensable tool not only with regard to the development of processing methodologies for individual images, but also for all aspects of the study and learning of digital geometry, as well as the development and evaluation of algorithms.

Chapter 2 begins with a formal and precise definition of *3D digital image*. Next, image processing is defined algebraically as *calculations on images*, or as a *mapping defined within an image space*, and then *compositions* of image calculations (both serial and parallel compositions) are defined. Additionally, the executable form of a representative case of application to a digital image is presented. From this, understanding and development of image processing algorithms can be performed effectively.

Chapter 3 introduces localized processing of 3D gray-scale images, with the focus on density value manipulations such as smoothing filters, difference filters, Laplacians, and region expansion. Most of these methods can be directly expanded from 2D graphic processing equivalents, and so are relatively easy to understand.

Chapters 4 and 5 are concerned with the geometric properties of 3D digital images and the basic processing algorithms that are associated with them. These chapters are the most important in the book, from the standpoint that they deal with those characteristics specific to 3D, and are what make the book a unique work.

First, in Chapter 4 we will discuss the fundamentals of what is referred to as digital geometry, defining such terms as neighborhood, connectivity, simplex, deletability, path, and distance metric, and we will discuss their properties. We will also consider Euler numbers, connectivity indexes, and distance functions as features of the topology of 3D digital shapes. Some specific algorithms that compute these values also will be given.

Chapter 5 explains some processing algorithms that will probably be necessary for 3D image analysis, such as labeling, axis thinning, surface thinning, border tracing, distance transformation, skeleton extraction, and figure restoration. Here our goal will be understanding not only the content of the processing performed, but also the structure and design methodology of the algorithm. We will make as clear as possible the required capabilities of such processing, along with requirements that must be fulfilled (for example, topology preservation, deletability testing, Euclid distance calculations, and figure restorability), and give specific examples.

Whereas Chapter 5 is solely concerned with shape forms (and geometric properties), Chapter 6 discusses thinning, ridge line tracing, and gray weighted distance transformations used on gray-scale images as examples of transformations required to incorporate density value information.

As described before, Chapter 7 describes display (rendering) algorithms used as visualization tools for 3D gray-scale images. The discussion is not one of computer graphics in general, but rather focuses on observation tools for gray-scale data. Specifically, the use of ray casting for the generation of images is discussed, for example, particular surface rendering and shading models, ray tracing, volume rendering, and gradient shading.

2

MODELS OF IMAGES AND IMAGE OPERATIONS

2.1 Introduction

In order to study methods of image processing, theoretically we need to first make clear what the *image* to be processed is and what is meant by *processing an image*. In this chapter we present a theoretical model of digitized images and the processing of these images. For the convenience of explanation, let us start our discussion with a two-dimensional image.

In Section 2.2, we define both a (two-dimensional or 2D) continuous image and a (2D) digitized image as a function of two variables and a 2D array, respectively. Relationships between images, such as *equality* and *greater than*, are introduced later in Subsection 2.2.6.

In Section 2.3, we give the formal description of image processing using the definitions of images above. Application of an image process algorithm is defined as *mapping* from one image space onto another. In other words, a process that generates a new image from an input image is formulated as a kind of operator on an image space. Relationships between image operators are defined based on the relationships between images. Operations between two or more image operations are then introduced in the similar way to those among images. Two different types of compositions of image operations, called *parallel composition* and *serial composition*, are explained in detail.

In the last section, Section 2.4, image operations are classified based on their features. We will discuss several important families of operations (or types of algorithms) such as sequential type, parallel type, local operations, iterative operations, and shift invariant operations. Concepts and methods to treat images and image process algorithms discussed here will be used very effectively in the following chapters to study characteristics of each algorithm theoretically and to extend their applications to wider area of practical image processing problems.

2.2 Continuous and digitized images

2.2.1 Continuous images

We will begin with the modeling of a 2D image with a 2D continuous image as a digitized image is obtained by *digitizing* a continuous one.

An image, specifically a 2D image, is defined as a scalar function of two variables $f(x, y)$, where f denotes a gray value at a point (x, y) on an image plane. We call this a *continuous image*. The physical meaning of the value of f varies according to the individual imaging process. A few examples are as follows:

(1) drawings on a sheet of paper: reflectivity.
(2) photographic negative recording of an outdoor scene: the transmission co-efficient is proportional to the amount of light energy exposed to the film. This usually represents the intensity of the light reflected by the object in the scene.
(3) medical X-ray image: attenuation coefficient to X-ray of an object.
(4) ultrasound image: the intensity of the sound wave reflected by an object.
(5) thermogram: the temperature on the surface of an object.

We simply call the value of f *image density* or *gray value*.

Remark 2.1 (Density). In some cases the terms *intensity* and *density* are clearly distinguished from each other. The intensity refers to the amount of light energy exposed to a sensor, and the density represents the logarithm of the intensity. It is said that the response to a light stimulus for the human visual system is approximately proportional to the logarithm of the light energy exposed to the eye [Hall79].

2.2.2 Digitized images

A continuous image is digitized via a two-step procedure: *sampling* and *quantization*.

(a) **Sampling**: There are two ways to understand sampling. The first is that a function $f(x, y)$ representing a continuous image is sampled at points (*sampling points*) of an ordered array (such as a rectangular array or square lattice) or a triangular array (or triangular lattice). The second approach is to consider an image plane as being divided into a set of small cells of the same shape and size, called *image cells*, *image elements*, or *pixels*. The average of values of f over each cell is considered as the density value of the image at the center point of the cell. Usually a square cell or a hexagonal cell is adopted in practical applications. Two interpretations are eventually possible if we consider the sampling point as the center point of an image cell. Note that the square lattice corresponds to the square pixel system and the triangular lattice to the hexagonal pixel system (Fig. 2.1).

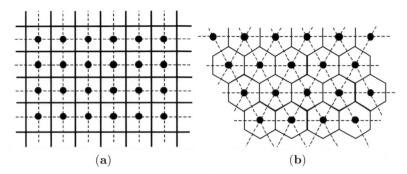

(a)   (b)

Fig. 2.1. Sampling of a 2D image (•: Sample point; solid and broken lines: pixel):
(**a**) Sampling with a square pixel (or a square lattice); (**b**) sampling with a hexagonal
pixel (or a triangular lattice).

(b) **Quantization**: The density value at each pixel (or sampling point) is assigned to one of the finite set of integers selected as suitable. This process is
called *quantization*. Quantization is in principle the same as that of a uni-
variate function, such as a time-varying signal transmitted in the communication system. Typically, a set of integers $0, 1, 2, \ldots, 2^m$, $m = 5 \sim 12$
is employed to represent the density values of a digitized image. A digitized image defined in this way takes only integer density values. This is
almost always true in applications in which only the finite number of bits
are available. It is not so convenient, however, for the theoretical analysis
of image processing, because in many image operations such as smoothing, differentiation and spatial frequency enhancement, density values of
an output image may in principle take on an arbitrary real value. Therefore, we assume that a digitized image can take arbitrary real values as
its density values unless stated otherwise.

The size of an image is always finite in practical cases. In the theoretical
considerations in this book, we treat both an image of the finite size and that
of the infinite size. From now on we will consider that a digitized image is
sampled at the square lattice or is divided into square pixels unless stated
otherwise. An image is called *binary image* if the density at any pixel assumes
only two values. We assign *0* and *1* to the densities of a digitized binary
image unless defined otherwise. Pixels of a binary image with values *0* and *1*
are called 0-*pixels* and 1-*pixels*, respectively. An image that may take various
different density values is called *gray-tone image*.

Let (i, j) denote a pixel location in the i-th row and the j-th column, and
$\mathbf{F} = \{f_{ij}\}$ denote a digitized image in which the value of the density at a
pixel (i, j) is given by f_{ij}. We represent an arbitrary pixel in the way such as
a pixel P, a point P, a pixel P $= (i, j)$, and a pixel $\boldsymbol{x}$.

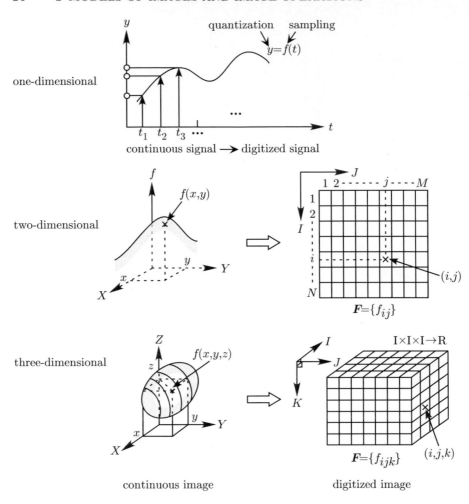

Fig. 2.2. Digitization of signals and images.

2.2.3 Three-dimensional images

In this section, we will address 3D images.

A *3D continuous image* is defined by a scalar (real) function of three variables $f(x, y, z)$, where f represents a characteristic value at a point (x, y, z) in 3D space.

A 3D continuous image is digitized in the same way as the 2D case; that is, a function f is sampled at points of a cubic ordered array (3D grid or 3D lattice of sample points). Otherwise, the 3D space is divided into a set of small cubic cells, and the value of the function f averaged over each cube is assigned it . Hence, the cube is called *volume cell* or *voxel* instead of a pixel in

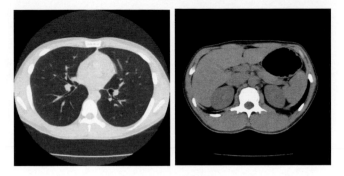

Fig. 2.3. Examples of CT slice images.

the 2D case. Quantization of density values is identical to that of a 2D image (Fig. 2.2).

A voxel at the i-th row and the j-th column on the k-th plane is denoted by a voxel (i, j, k). The notation $\boldsymbol{F} = \{f_{ijk}\}$ is employed to represent a 3D digitized image (or simply a 3D image) in which the density value at a voxel (i, j, k) is given by f_{ijk}. We usually understand the contents of a 3D image by observing the array of 2D successive slices $\boldsymbol{F}_k = \{f_{ij(k)}\}$ for different ks, whereas a computer accesses the 3D array directly. An example of a 3D digital image is a set of cross sections of the human body obtained by CT or computed (computerized) tomography system and MRI (magnetic resonance imaging) system used in medicine (Fig. 2.3).

The physical meaning of the value of the function f is quite different from those of 2D images. In 3D images values of f_{xyz} represent values of characteristic features of an object at a point (x, y, z) and at the small volume element including it. The contents vary according to the measurement technology employed in the imaging device. A few examples are shown below.

(1) X-ray CT image: Attenuation or absorption factor to the X-ray of an object.
(2) PET (positron emission CT) image: Intensity of γ-ray emitted from the volume element of an object.
(3) MRI (magnetic resonance imaging): Strength of magnetic resonance at the volume element of an object.
(4) 3D ultrasound image: The intensity of the ultrasound wave reflected by an object.

Remark 2.2 (3D lattice). An advantage of using a sampling point lattice is that results known in physics, crystallography, and other fields can be used effectively. A few well-known examples of lattices in 3D space are shown in Fig. 2.4. In 3D image processing, use of voxels corresponding to those lattices is also required. From the viewpoint of ease of treating voxels, the cubic lattice is used in most practical applications.

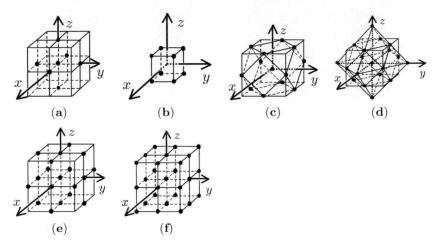

Fig. 2.4. Lattice in 3D space and a neighborhood: (**a**) Cubic lattice 7 (6-neighborhood); (**b**) cubic lattice 8; (**c**) face-centered cubic lattice 13 (12-neighborhood); (**d**) face-centered cubic lattice 19 (18-neighborhood); (**e**) cubic lattice 19 (18-neighborhood); (**f**) cubic lattice 27 (26-neighborhood).

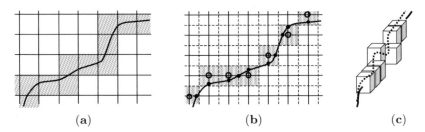

Fig. 2.5. Digitization of a 2D and a 3D line figure: (**a**) Digitization by pixel (2D); (**b**) digitization by grid (2D); (**c**) digitization by voxel (3D).

2.2.4 3D line figures and digitization

Digitization of a line figure in the 3D space must be discussed in full, because a line figure has no width. Let us consider first the case of a 2D line figure. The following two methods are used in the digitization of a 2D line figure (Fig. 2.5).

(1) **Digitization by pixel**: Divide the continuous plane into pixels. A pixel which a line figure passes is assigned the value *1*, and otherwise the value *0*. Since the probability that a line figure exactly passes through the border of a pixel is regarded as zero, a resulting digital line figure always becomes 4-connected.

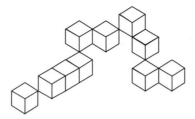

Fig. 2.6. Simple arc.

(2) **Digitization by grid**: Superimpose a grid on an image plane. Each grid point is regarded as a center point of a pixel. At an every cross point of a line figure and the grid, the nearest grid point is given a 1-pixel. The resulting digital line figure is then 8-connected.

Both methods are utilized with a 3D image. In the first case, a voxel (a cube) that a line figure passes through becomes a 1-voxel and the other a 0-voxel (voxel digitization). A 6-connected figure[†] is always obtained, if we disregard the probability that a line figure passes exactly through a vertex or a face shared by two voxels.

In the second method, a 3D grid plane is put on the 3D space, and cross points between a line figure and the 3D grid are calculated. Each 3D grid point is regarded as the center point of a cubic voxel. Then at each cross point between the 3D grid and the line figure, the nearest grid point is selected and a 1-voxel is put there. A resultant line figure obtained by this digitization method is always 26-connected[†]. More detailed discussion is found in [Jonas97].

Remark 2.3 (Simple arc). In the simplest form of a line figure, only two voxels have one 1-voxel in their k-neighborhoods and all other voxels have exactly two 1-voxels in their k-neighborhoods. We call such a figure *simple* (*k-connected*[†]) *digital curve*, or briefly *simple arc*. Two voxels that have only one neighboring 1-voxel are called *edge voxel* (edge point) and others are called *connecting voxels* (connecting point) (Fig. 2.6).

The direction from an arbitrary 1-voxel on a digital line figure toward the other 1-voxel in the k-neighborhood can be represented by using a code specific to each direction (such as integers $1, 2, \ldots, 26$) (Fig. 2.7). This code is called the *direction code* or *chain code*. A simple digital arc is exactly defined by the start point and a sequence of the chain code.

Desirable properties of the digitization of a 3D line figure were explained in [Jonas97] as introduced below.

[†] The term "k-connected" will be explained in detail in Section 4.1.2.

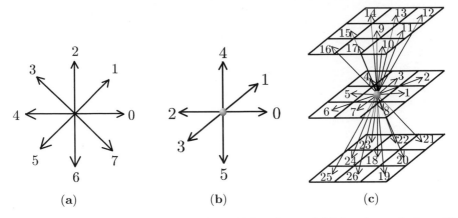

Fig. 2.7. Chain code representation for a 3D line figure: (**a**) Direction code for a 2D line figure (8-connectivity); (**b**) direction code for a 3D line figure (6-connectivity); (**c**) direction code for a 3D line figure (26-connectivity).

(1) *Axis symmetry*: Digital expression is symmetrical with respect to the coordinate transformation or the exchange of coordinate axes. According to the expression adopted in the text, the expression of a 3D line figure is invariant with respect to exchange among i, j, and k and the inversion of the order of numbering.

(2) *Direction symmetry*: By exchanging a starting point and an end point, the order of the direction codes and each direction itself are both inverted.

(3) *Shift invariance*: A digital expression does not vary by a shift of an original line figure by integer times of the sampling interval.

(4) *Finite memory*: Digital expression of a line figure does not depend on an arbitrarily distant part of a curve. That is, local change in a line figure causes only local change in its digital expression.

(5) *Line segment property*: A digital expression of a line segment in the continuous space is a digital arc.

(6) *Projection property*: A digital expression of a projection of a 3D curve to $x - y$ plane is coincident to the projection of a 3D digital expression of the same curve to the same $x - y$ plane.

(7) *Minimal property*: Digitization of a curve in the 3D continuous space is a result of the minimization of the distance (bias, discrepancy) in some sense between an original continuous curve and its digital expression.

(8) *Compactness*: The number of codes (the number of chain codes, for example) required for the digital expression of a given curve is minimal under the condition that all of the above are satisfied.

These are only a guideline, as a method of digitization to satisfy all of them does not seem to exist.

Relationships between properties of a line figure in the continuous space and its digitized version should be discussed under the assumption that digitization satisfies at least several of the above conditions. For example, what condition should be satisfied in order that a given 26-connected digitized curve is a digitized version of a line segment in 3D continuous space? Although a relatively clear solution has been obtained for a 2D line figure [Rosenfeld74, Kim82a, Kim82b], it cannot be extended easily to a 3D figure [Kim83, Kim84]. Another example is the estimation of the length of an original line figure from a chain code expression [Kiryati95, Chattopadhyay92, Klette85, Kim83, Amarunnishad90]. These problems can be studied theoretically by first assuming a method to map a curve in continuous space onto digitized space.

2.2.5 Cross section and projection

A cross section of a 3D continuous image $f(x, y, z)$ along an arbitrary plane H (= a distribution of density values on the plane H) is considered as a 2D image. We call this *cross section* (*profile*) of an image f (by a plane H).

The integration of density values of a 3D continuous image $f(x, y, z)$ along the perpendicular line to the plane H is called *projection* of f to the plane H. The projection to the plane H is also a 2D image on the plane H.

For example, the cross section by the horizontal plane $z = z_0$ is given by

$$f_{\text{cross}}(x, y; z_0) = f(x, y, z)|_{z=z_0}. \tag{2.1}$$

The projection of a 3D image $f(x, y, z)$ to the plane H is represented as

$$f_{\text{proj}}(x, y) = \int_{-\infty}^{\infty} f(x, y, z)dz. \tag{2.2}$$

A cross section and a projection of a 3D digitized image are defined in the same way (Fig. 2.8). For example, the cross section at $k = k_0$:

$$f_{\text{cross}}(k_0) = \{f_{ijk_0}\}, \tag{2.3}$$

the projection to the $i - j$ plane:

$$f_{\text{proj}}(k) = \{\sum_{k=1}^{K} f_{ijk}\}. \tag{2.4}$$

Calculation of a cross section by a plane of an arbitrary direction and a projection to an arbitrary plane are not always easy for 3D images. Various algorithms to calculate them have been studied in computer graphics and visualization. Both a cross section by the plane of an arbitrary direction and a projection to an arbitrary plane as well as the cross section along a curved surface are often used in medical applications.

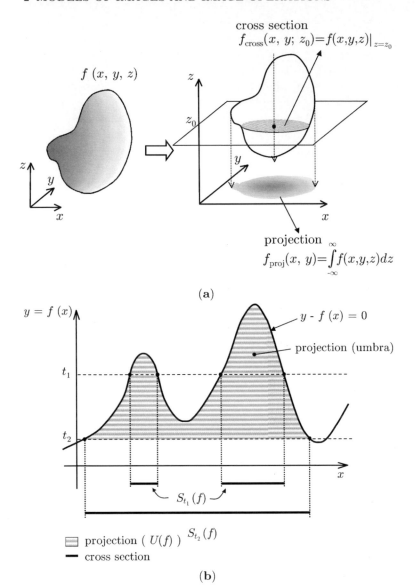

Fig. 2.8. Cross section and projection: **(a)** Cross section and projection (1); **(b)** cross section and projection (2).

Remark 2.4 (Cross section and projection). Two terms, *cross section* and *projection*, are used also in different ways as follows (Fig. 2.8).

Definition 2.1. Consider a continuous one-valued real function $f(x, y, z)$ and a real value t (called *level* or *threshold value*). Then, *cross section* of f at a level t is defined as follows.

$$S_t(f) \equiv \{(x, y, z) \in D;\ f(x, y, z) \geq t\}, \qquad (2.5)$$

where D is the domain of the function f = the region of all points (x, y, z) such that their density values are larger than or equal to t .

Then, a 3D continuous function $f(x, y, z)$ is represented in the form

$$f(x, y, z) = \sup\{t \in \mathrm{R};\ (x, y, z) \in S_t(f)\}, \qquad (2.6)$$

where R = set of all real numbers = supremum of the level t such that a cross section includes a point (x, y, z). If all cross sections are given, then the function f is fixed uniquely.

In a 3D image in which density values are quantized into M levels, there exist M cross sections. The cross section at a level k is the set of all voxels such that density values are larger than or equal to k. Inversely, the density value of a voxel (x, y, z) is equal to the maximum level such that a cross section includes the voxel (x, y, z).

Definition 2.2. Consider a 4D space (i, j, k, f). Then, the set of points (i, j, k, f) such that $f(i, j, k) \geq t$ is called *umbra* (or *projection*) of the image $f(i, j, k)$ and denoted by $U(f)$. That is,

$$U(f) \equiv \{(i, j, k, f);\ f(i, j, k) \geq t\} \qquad (2.7)$$

Inversely, given the umbra $U(f)$, then $f(i, j, k)$ is determined by

$$f(i, j, k) = \sup\{t;\ (i, j, k, f) \in U(f)\} \qquad (2.8)$$
$$(= \text{the maximum of } t \text{ in the umbra, when } (x, y, z) \text{ is fixed.})$$

Intuitively, the umbra is the subspace of the 4D space (i, j, k, f) below the curved surface $t = f(i, j, k)$ including the surface itself.

Thus both the cross section and the umbra (projection) are sets of points, although the cross section is in the 3D space and the umbra in the 4D space, respectively. We can consider a binary image that takes the value *1* on the set (cross section or umbra) and takes *0* otherwise. According to the terminology of the set theory, they are characteristic functions of sets called cross section and umbra, respectively. All of cross sections or umbras are equivalent to the original 3D image itself. In other words, a 3D gray-tone image can be described equivalently by a 4D binary image or by a set of 3D binary images.

2.2.6 Relationships among images

For formal treatment of an image and an image operation we will give a formal definition of a digitized image as follows.

Table 2.1. Binary relations among images.

Relation	Definition	Notation
Equality ($\boldsymbol{F}$ is equal to $\boldsymbol{G}$)	$f_{ijk} = g_{ijk}, \forall(i,j,k) \in \mathrm{I} \times \mathrm{I} \times \mathrm{I}$	$\boldsymbol{F} = \boldsymbol{G}$
Comparison ($\boldsymbol{F}$ is smaller than $\boldsymbol{G}$) ($\boldsymbol{G}$ is larger than $\boldsymbol{F}$)	$f_{ijk} < g_{ijk}, \forall(i,j,k) \in \mathrm{I} \times \mathrm{I} \times \mathrm{I}$	$\boldsymbol{F} < \boldsymbol{G}$
($\boldsymbol{F}$ is smaller than or equal to $\boldsymbol{G}$) ($\boldsymbol{G}$ is larger than or equal to $\boldsymbol{F}$)	$f_{ijk} \leq g_{ijk}, \forall(i,j,k) \in \mathrm{I} \times \mathrm{I} \times \mathrm{I}$	$\boldsymbol{F} \leq \boldsymbol{G}$

Definition 2.3 (Digitized image). (A *3D digitized image* is defined as a mapping

$$\mathrm{I} \times \mathrm{I} \times \mathrm{I} \to \mathrm{R} \tag{2.9}$$

where I is the set of whole integers, and R is the set of all real numbers. An element (i,j,k) of the direct product $\mathrm{I} \times \mathrm{I} \times \mathrm{I}$ is called *voxel* (or simply *point*), and the image of the voxel (i,j,k) by this mapping is called *density*.

An image in which the density value at a voxel (i,j,k) is given by f_{ijk} is denoted as $\boldsymbol{F} = \{f_{ijk}\}$.

The set of all images is called an image space and is denoted by $\mathcal{P}$. If a density value f_{ijk} is equal to *0* or *1* for all voxels (i,j,k), then $\boldsymbol{F} = \{f_{ijk}\}$ is called *binary image*. The set of all binary images is denoted by $\mathcal{P}_\mathcal{B}$. The term *gray-tone image* is used when we need to show explicitly that a density f_{ijk} takes an arbitrary value. A gray-tone image $\boldsymbol{F} = \{f_{ijk}\}$ is called a *semipositive image* if $f_{ijk} \geq 0$ for all i, j, and k and a *constant image* of the value C if $f_{ijk} = C$ (a constant) for all i, j, and k. If an image $\boldsymbol{F}$ is a semi-positive image, the set of all positive voxels and all 0-voxels in $\boldsymbol{F}$ is denoted by $R(\boldsymbol{F})$ and $\overline{R}(\boldsymbol{F})$, respectively. They also may be referred to as the *figure* and the *background*. A digitized image is simply called an *image* unless the possibility of a misconception exists.

Relationships among these digitized images are defined below and can be effectively utilized for analysis of image operators.

Definition 2.4 (Binary relation). Binary relations between two images $\boldsymbol{F} = \{f_{ijk}\}$ and $\boldsymbol{G} = \{g_{ijk}\}$ are given as shown in Table 2.1, which are based upon relations between density values f_{ijk} and g_{ijk}.

2.3 Model of image operations

We will now present a theoretical model of image operations and examine basic properties of image operations. An image operation is defined as a mapping from a set of images to another set of images. By using this model and relationships between images we introduce binary relationships between two operators such as *equal to* and *greater (less) than* (in Section 2.3.2).

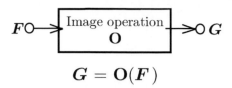

$$G = \mathbf{O}(F)$$

Fig. 2.9. Unary operation of an image.

In 2.3.4 we discuss *an operation among image operations* which is a process to generate a new image operation by combining two or more operations. Two operations introduced here - *a parallel composition* and *a serial composition* - are widely used in the following chapters. We will also present basic properties of image operations such as inverse, iterative operation, and commutative and distributive laws.

Finally in Subsection 2.3.5 we introduce several important operators including a shift operator and position (shift) invariant operators.

2.3.1 Formulation of image operations

We will give a formal definition of image processing as a basis of theoretical study in subsequent chapters. A process that generates a new image from an input image is theoretically formulated as a unary operator on an image space as follows.

Definition 2.5 (Unary operator). A process to derive a new image from a given image is defined as a *unary operator* on an image space or as a mapping from an image space $\mathcal{P}_1$ onto $\mathcal{P}_2$, that is,

$$\text{mapping } \mathbf{O} : \mathcal{P}_1 \to \mathcal{P}_2 \tag{2.10}$$

where $\mathcal{P}_1$, and $\mathcal{P}_2$ are subsets of $\mathcal{P}(= $ the set of all images $)$ which are called *domain* and *range* of the mapping $\mathbf{O}$, respectively. The set of all operators is called an *operator space* and is denoted by $\mathbf{O}$. The image that is obtained by applying an operator $\mathbf{O}$ to an image F is expressed by $\mathbf{O}(F)$ (Fig. 2.9).

An operator in which the domain is a set of binary images is called a *binary image operator*.

An operator $\mathbf{I}$ such that

$$\mathbf{I}(F) = F, \ \forall F \in \mathcal{P}_1, \tag{2.11}$$

is called an *identity operator* with the domain $\mathcal{P}_1$. The identity operator does not cause any effect on an image in its domain.

2.3.2 Relations between image operators

We can define the relationships between two image operators based upon those between images presented in 2.2.6.

Definition 2.6 (Relation between image operators). For two operators $\mathbf{O}_1$ and $\mathbf{O}_2$ with the common domain $\mathcal{P}_1$,

$$\mathbf{O}_1(\mathbf{F}) = \mathbf{O}_2(\mathbf{F}), \ \forall \mathbf{F} \in \mathcal{P}_1 \leftrightarrow \mathbf{O}_1 = \mathbf{O}_2, \qquad (2.12)$$

$$\mathbf{O}_1(\mathbf{F}) > \mathbf{O}_2(\mathbf{F}), \ \forall \mathbf{F} \in \mathcal{P}_1 \leftrightarrow \mathbf{O}_1 > \mathbf{O}_2. \qquad (2.13)$$

Other relations such as $<$, $\leq$, and $\geq$ between image operators are defined in the same way.

2.3.3 Binary operators between images

An operator generating a new image from two input images also plays an important role in the analysis of image processing algorithms.

Definition 2.7 (Binary operator). A mapping:

$$\mathcal{P}_1 \times \mathcal{P}_2 \to \mathcal{P}_3, \qquad (2.14)$$

where $\mathcal{P}_1$, $\mathcal{P}_2$, and $\mathcal{P}_3$ are arbitrary subsets of the image space is called a *binary operator between images* (or simply *binary operator*). Here, $\mathcal{P}_1 \times \mathcal{P}_2$ and $\mathcal{P}_3$ are *domain* and *range* of the mapping.

The notation, $\mathbf{H} = \phi(\mathbf{F}, \mathbf{G})$, or $\mathbf{H} = \mathbf{F} * \mathbf{G}$, is employed to state that an image $\mathbf{H} = \{h_{ijk}\}$ is derived from images $\mathbf{F} = \{f_{ijk}\}$ and $\mathbf{G} = \{g_{ijk}\}$ by the above mapping. If the following equation holds among $\mathbf{F}$, $\mathbf{G}$, and $\mathbf{H}$,

$$h_{ijk} = \phi(f_{ijk}, g_{ijk}), \forall (i, j, k) \in \mathrm{I} \times \mathrm{I} \times \mathrm{I}, \qquad (2.15)$$

where $\phi(x, y)$ is an arbitrary real function of two variables independent of i, j, and k, then the operation is called a *pointwise operation* on $\mathbf{F}$ and $\mathbf{G}$.

The density value at a voxel (i, j, k) in an output of a pointwise operation is calculated by using density values at the voxel of the same location (i, j, k) in two input images and the function ϕ defining the operation. The form of the function should be common to all voxels (Fig. 2.10).

Many pointwise operations can be defined by using different functions $\phi(x, y)$ in Eq. 2.15. In each of these specific cases we use an appropriate symbol instead of $*$ to represent the particular pointwise operation. Most commonly used examples are given in Table 2.2.

A pointwise operation on two images is regarded as a set of arithmetic operations performed on all voxels independently of each other. Thus they satisfy several general rules similar to those of real numbers as follows:

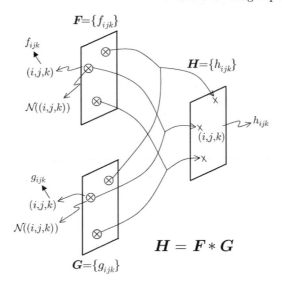

Fig. 2.10. Binary operation among images.

Table 2.2. Examples of pointwise operations among images.

	Definition	Notation
(1) Addition	$\phi(x, y) = x + y$	$\boldsymbol{H} = \boldsymbol{F} + \boldsymbol{G}$
(2) Subtraction	$\phi(x, y) = x - y$	$\boldsymbol{H} = \boldsymbol{F} - \boldsymbol{G}$
(3) Multiplication	$\phi(x, y) = x \times y$	$\boldsymbol{H} = \boldsymbol{F} \times \boldsymbol{G}$
(4) Division	$\phi(x, y) = x \div y$	$\boldsymbol{H} = \boldsymbol{F} \div \boldsymbol{G}$
(5) Max	$\phi(x, y) = \max(x, y)$	$\boldsymbol{H} = \boldsymbol{F} \wedge \boldsymbol{G}$
(6) Min	$\phi(x, y) = \min(x, y)$	$\boldsymbol{H} = \boldsymbol{F} \vee \boldsymbol{G}$
(7) Logical sum	$\phi(x, y) = x \oplus y$	$\boldsymbol{H} = \boldsymbol{F} \oplus \boldsymbol{G}$
(8) Logical product	$\phi(x, y) = x \otimes y$	$\boldsymbol{H} = \boldsymbol{F} \otimes \boldsymbol{G}$
(9) Logical difference	$\phi(x, y) = x \ominus y$	$\boldsymbol{H} = \boldsymbol{F} \ominus \boldsymbol{G}$

* (7)(8) and (9) in the table are binary image operators applied to binary images $\boldsymbol{F}$ and $\boldsymbol{G}$, and x and y are binary variables

$$\text{commutative law:} \quad \boldsymbol{F} + \boldsymbol{G} = \boldsymbol{G} + \boldsymbol{F}, \ \boldsymbol{F} \times \boldsymbol{G} = \boldsymbol{G} \times \boldsymbol{F} \quad (2.16)$$

$$\text{right distributive law:} \ (\boldsymbol{F} + \boldsymbol{G}) \times \boldsymbol{H} = (\boldsymbol{F} \times \boldsymbol{H}) + (\boldsymbol{G} \times \boldsymbol{H}) \quad (2.17)$$

$$\text{associative law:} \quad (\boldsymbol{F} + \boldsymbol{G}) + \boldsymbol{H} = \boldsymbol{F} + (\boldsymbol{G} + \boldsymbol{H}),$$
$$(\boldsymbol{F} \times \boldsymbol{G}) \times \boldsymbol{H} = \boldsymbol{F} \times (\boldsymbol{G} \times \boldsymbol{H}) \quad (2.18)$$

2.3.4 Composition of image operations

Let us consider generating a new image operation by composing or combining two or more procedures. This process is formulated as *operations among image operations.* Two types of compositions - *parallel composition* and *serial composition* - are important for our objectives.

Definition 2.8 (Parallel composition). A parallel composition (by a pointwise operation "$*$") of arbitrary two operators $\mathbf{O}_1$ and $\mathbf{O}_2$ that share a common domain $\mathcal{P}_0$ is defined as follows:

$$(\mathbf{O}_1 * \mathbf{O}_2)(\boldsymbol{F}) \equiv \mathbf{O}_1(\boldsymbol{F}) * \mathbf{O}_2(\boldsymbol{F}), \ \forall \boldsymbol{F} \in \mathcal{P}_0. \tag{2.19}$$

The parallel composition is denoted by $\mathbf{O}_1 * \mathbf{O}_2$ in general, and a more appropriate symbol may be used instead of the asterisk to designate a particular type of composition (e.g., $(\mathbf{O}_1 + \mathbf{O}_2)(\boldsymbol{F}) \equiv \mathbf{O}_1(\boldsymbol{F}) + \mathbf{O}_2(\boldsymbol{F})$).

The parallel composition $\mathbf{O}_1 * \mathbf{O}_2$ represents the processing that generates an image $\boldsymbol{H}$ by applying the pointwise operation $*$ to the result of the operator $\mathbf{O}_1$ applied to an image $\boldsymbol{F}$ and that of the operator $\mathbf{O}_2$ applied to an image $\boldsymbol{G}$ (Fig. 2.11 (a)).

Definition 2.9 (Serial composition). *Serial composition* of two arbitrary operators $\mathbf{O}_1$ and $\mathbf{O}_2$, denoted by $\mathbf{O}_1 \cdot \mathbf{O}_2$, is defined as follows:

$$(\mathbf{O}_1 \cdot \mathbf{O}_2)(\boldsymbol{F}) \equiv \mathbf{O}_1(\mathbf{O}_2(\boldsymbol{F})), \tag{2.20}$$

where the domain of $\mathbf{O}_1$ is assumed to be coincident with the range of $\mathbf{O}_2$. The domain of $\mathbf{O}_1 \cdot \mathbf{O}_2$ is equal to the domain of $\mathbf{O}_2$; the serial composition $\mathbf{O}_1 \cdot \mathbf{O}_2$ means the processing that is equivalent to applying the operator $\mathbf{O}_1$ to the output of the operator $\mathbf{O}_2$ (Fig. 2.11 (b)).

Remark 2.5. More specifically, a serial composition $\mathbf{O}_1 \cdot \mathbf{O}_2$ can be defined well if the range of the operator $\mathbf{O}_2$ is contained in the domain of the operator $\mathbf{O}_1$. The requirement that the domain of $\mathbf{O}_1$ should be coincident with the range of $\mathbf{O}_2$ is added only for the sake of simplicity in theoretical analysis.

Two basic operators, the *inverse* and the *power* of an operator, are defined using these compositions as follows.

Definition 2.10 (Inverse, the power of an operator). The result of n times of serial compositions of the same operator $\mathbf{O}$ is called n-th *power* of the operator $\mathbf{O}$ and is denoted by $\mathbf{O}^n$. That is,

$$\mathbf{O}^n \equiv \mathbf{O} \cdot \mathbf{O}^{n-1}, \ n \geq 2, \tag{2.21}$$

where we assume that $\mathbf{O}^{n-1}$ always exists and its range is included in the domain of $\mathbf{O}$ for all $n \geq 2$.

For a given operator $\mathbf{O}$, if there exists an operator $\mathbf{O}'$ such that

$$\mathbf{O}' \cdot \mathbf{O} = \mathbf{O} \cdot \mathbf{O}' = \mathbf{I} \ (= \text{identity operator}) , \tag{2.22}$$

then $\mathbf{O}'$ is called the *inverse operator* of $\mathbf{O}$ and is denoted by $\mathbf{O}^{-1}$.

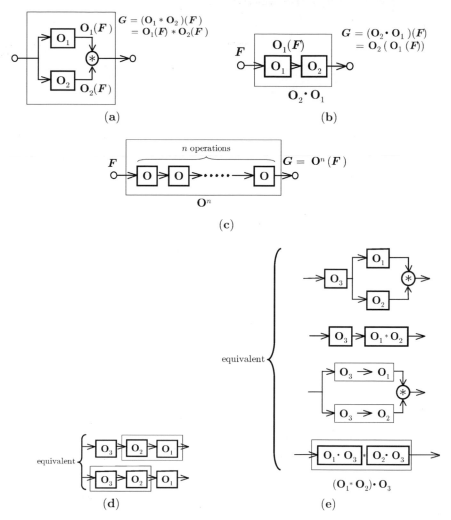

Fig. 2.11. Composition of image operations: (**a**) Parallel composition; (**b**) serial composition; (**c**) iterative composition (n-th power); (**d**) associative law of serial compositions; (**e**) distributive law.

Furthermore, $\mathbf{O}^{-n}$ is defined as follows:

$$\mathbf{O}^{-n} \equiv \mathbf{O}^{-1} \cdot \mathbf{O}^{-(n-1)}, n \geq 2, \tag{2.23}$$

where we assume that $\mathbf{O}^{-(n-1)}$ exists and its range is included in the domain of $\mathbf{O}^{-1}$ for all $n \geq 2$ (Fig. 2.11 (c)).

To represent iterative application of more than one operator, we use notations similar to those of real numbers. For example,

$$\sum_{i=1}^{n} \mathbf{O}_i = \mathbf{O}_1 + \mathbf{O}_2 + \ldots + \mathbf{O}_n = (\ldots((\mathbf{O}_1 + \mathbf{O}_2) + \ldots) + \mathbf{O}_n, \qquad (2.24)$$

$$\prod_{i=1}^{n} \mathbf{O}_i = \mathbf{O}_n \cdot \mathbf{O}_{n-1} \cdot \ldots \cdot \mathbf{O}_2 \cdot \mathbf{O}_1 = (\ldots(\mathbf{O}_3 \cdot (\mathbf{O}_2 \cdot \mathbf{O}_1))\ldots). \qquad (2.25)$$

These algebraic operations among image operators have the following property.

Property 2.1. For arbitrary image operators $\mathbf{O}_1$, $\mathbf{O}_2$, and $\mathbf{O}_3$, the following relations hold:

$$(\mathbf{O}_1 \cdot \mathbf{O}_2) \cdot \mathbf{O}_3 = \mathbf{O}_1 \cdot (\mathbf{O}_2 \cdot \mathbf{O}_3) \qquad \text{(associative law)}, \qquad (2.26)$$

$$(\mathbf{O}_1 * \mathbf{O}_2) \cdot \mathbf{O}_3 = (\mathbf{O}_1 \cdot \mathbf{O}_3) * (\mathbf{O}_2 \cdot \mathbf{O}_3) \text{ (right distributive law)}, \quad (2.27)$$

where we assume that domains and ranges of relating operators satisfy appropriate conditions such that compositions " $\cdot$ " and "$*$" in these equations are meaningful (Fig. 2.11 (d), (e)).

Remark 2.6. The left distributive law

$$\mathbf{O}_3 \cdot (\mathbf{O}_1 * \mathbf{O}_3) = (\mathbf{O}_3 \cdot \mathbf{O}_1) * (\mathbf{O}_3 \cdot \mathbf{O}_1) \qquad (2.28)$$

does not hold true in general, and requires proof of correctness for individual cases. In serial composition, $\mathbf{O}_1 \cdot \mathbf{O}_2$ is not always equal to $\mathbf{O}_2 \cdot \mathbf{O}_1$.

2.3.5 Basic operators

Let us introduce here a few basic image operators that are relatively simple but important in the subsequent parts of the text.

(a) Monotonic operator

Definition 2.11 (Monotonicity). An operator $\mathbf{O}$ with the domain $\mathcal{P}$ is said to be *monotonic* if the following relation holds:

$$\mathbf{O}(\boldsymbol{F}) \geq \mathbf{O}(\boldsymbol{G}), \ \forall \boldsymbol{F} \in \mathcal{P}, \ \forall \boldsymbol{G} \in \mathcal{P} \text{ such that } \boldsymbol{F} \geq \boldsymbol{G}. \qquad (2.29)$$

For example, an operator $\mathbf{O}_1$ which maps a set of binary images onto a set of binary images may replace some of 1-voxels by 0-voxels, but never changes 0-voxels. Then the operator $\mathbf{O}_1$ is monotonic if that figures (a set of all 1-pixels) in a binary image $\boldsymbol{F}$ cover figures in $\boldsymbol{G}$ implies that figures in the output of the operator $\mathbf{O}_1$ for $\boldsymbol{F}$ cover figures in the output of $\mathbf{O}_1$ for $\boldsymbol{G}$ for arbitrary binary images $\boldsymbol{F}$ and $\boldsymbol{G}$. The local minimum filter and the local maximum filter are examples of the monotonic operator. Thinning discussed in Chapter 4 and 5 is not monotonic, although it never changes 0-voxels. In fact, a circle is reduced to an isolated single pixel by thinning, but a long stick-like figure that is smaller than the circle may be converted to a long thin line segment by thinning.

(b) Shift operator

Definition 2.12 (Shift operator). An operator $\mathbf{O}$ which derives an image $\boldsymbol{G} = \{g_{ijk}\}$ from an image $\boldsymbol{F} = \{f_{ijk}\}$ by the equation

$$g_{ijk} = f_{i-p,j-q,k-r}, \ (p,q,r) \in \mathrm{I} \times \mathrm{I} \times \mathrm{I} \qquad (2.30)$$

is called a *shift operator* and denoted by $\mathbf{T}[p,q,r]$ where p, q, and r are integer parameters.

The shift operator $\mathbf{T}[p,q,r]$ translates an input image by p voxels in the i-direction, q voxels in the j-direction, and r voxels in the k-direction.

Property 2.2. The following holds concerning a shift operator:

(1) Defining operators $\mathbf{D} \equiv \mathbf{T}[1,0,0]$, $\mathbf{R} \equiv \mathbf{T}[0,1,0]$, and $\mathbf{B} \equiv \mathbf{T}[0,0,1]$, the inverses $\mathbf{D}^{-1}$, $\mathbf{R}^{-1}$ and $\mathbf{B}^{-1}$ exist, and

$$\mathbf{T}[p,q,r] = \mathbf{D}^p \cdot \mathbf{R}^q \cdot \mathbf{B}^r, \ (p,q,r) \in \mathrm{I} \times \mathrm{I} \times \mathrm{I} \qquad (2.31)$$

(2) For two shift operators $\mathbf{T}[p,q,r]$ and $\mathbf{T}[u,v,w]$,

$$\mathbf{T}[p,q,r] \cdot \mathbf{T}[u,v,w] = \mathbf{T}[u,v,w] \cdot \mathbf{T}[p,q,r] = \mathbf{T}[u+p,v+q,w+r]. \quad (2.32)$$

(3) The following left distributive laws hold:

$$\mathbf{T}(\boldsymbol{F} * \boldsymbol{G}) = \mathbf{T}(\boldsymbol{F}) * \mathbf{T}(\boldsymbol{G}), \ \forall \mathbf{T} \in \mathcal{T}, \ \forall \boldsymbol{F}, \forall \boldsymbol{G} \in \mathcal{P}, \qquad (2.33)$$

$$\mathbf{T} \cdot (\mathbf{O}_1 * \mathbf{O}_2) = (\mathbf{T} \cdot \mathbf{O}_1) * (\mathbf{T} \cdot \mathbf{O}_2), \ \forall \mathbf{T} \in \mathcal{T}, \ \forall \mathbf{O}_1, \forall \mathbf{O}_2 \in \mathcal{O} \ (2.34)$$

where $\mathcal{T}$ is the set of all shift operators, $\mathcal{P}$ is the set of all images, $\mathcal{O}$ is the set of all image operators, and $*$ is an arbitrary pointwise operation of two images (or parallel composition of image operators).

(c) Point operator

Definition 2.13 (Point operator). *Point operator* is defined as the operator that calculates the output $\boldsymbol{G} = \{g_{ijk}\}$ by the equation

$$g_{ijk} = \psi(f_{ijk}), \ \forall(i,j,k) \in \mathrm{I} \times \mathrm{I} \times \mathrm{I} \qquad (2.35)$$

where $\boldsymbol{F} = \{f_{ijk}\}$ is an input image and ψ is an arbitrary real function.

Thus, in a point operator the output gray value at a voxel (i,j,k) is determined only by the input gray value at the voxel of the same location. Various point operators are defined by selecting different functions for ψ. Some point operators are denoted by symbols specific to them. Examples are shown in Table 2.3.

Property 2.3. The parallel and serial compositions of arbitrary two point operators are point operators.

Table 2.3. Examples of point operations.

	Definition $\psi(x)$	Notation
(1) Multiplication by constant	$\psi(x) = cx$	**M**[c]
(2) Substitution of constant	$\psi(x) = c$	**S**[c]
(3) Addition and subtraction by constant	$\psi(x) = x + c$	**A**[c]
(4) Power by constant	$\psi(x) = x^c$	**P**[c]
(5) Exponential	$\psi(x) = e^x$	**EXP**
(6) Logarithmic	$\psi(x) = \log(x)$	**LOG**
(7) Absolute value	$\psi(x) = |x|$	**ABS**
(8) Thresholding (1)	$\psi(x) = \begin{cases} x, & \text{if } x \geq t \\ 0, & \text{if } x < t \end{cases}$	**U1**[t]
(9) Thresholding (2)	$\psi(x) = \begin{cases} x, & \text{if } x > t \\ 0, & \text{if } x \leq t \end{cases}$	**U2**[t]
(10) Thresholding (3)	$\psi(x) = \begin{cases} 1, & \text{if } x \geq t \\ 0, & \text{if } x < t \end{cases}$	**U3**[t]
(11) Thresholding (4)	$\psi(x) = \begin{cases} 1, & \text{if } x > t \\ 0, & \text{if } x \leq t \end{cases}$	**U4**[t]
(12) Idempotent	$\psi(x) = x$	**I**
(13) Negation	$\psi(x) = 1 - x$	**N**

(d) Shift-invariant operator

Definition 2.14 (Shift invariance). An operator **O** is said to be *shift invariant* (or *position invariant*) if it is commutative with a shift operator **T**, that is, if the following equation holds:

$$\mathbf{O} \cdot \mathbf{T} = \mathbf{T} \cdot \mathbf{O}, \ \forall \mathbf{T} \in \mathcal{O}_T \tag{2.36}$$

where $\mathcal{O}_T$ is the set of all shift operators.

Both the serial and the parallel compositions of shift invariant operators are again shift invariant. A point operator and a shift operator itself are always shift invariant.

2.4 Algorithm of image operations

In the last section, an image operator was defined as a mapping on an image set or an algebraic operation applied to a set of images. It is another problem, however, to perform such an operation with a general purpose computer or a special purpose image processor. In this section, we will examine in more detail concrete algorithms to perform unary operators of images. After giving a formal expression as a general image operation, we will introduce several important types of algorithms including a sequential type, a parallel type, and local parallel operations.

2.4.1 General form of image operations

In order to obtain an output image $G = \{g_{ijk}\}$ of an image operation $\mathbf{O}$, we need to clearly determine the procedure to calculate the density value g_{ijk} of the output image $G = \{g_{ijk}\}$ for all (i, j, k)s. Thus a very general form of an image operation is represented by

$$g_{ijk} = \phi_{ijk}(\mathbf{F}), \ \forall (i, j, k) \in \mathcal{S} = I \times I \times I, \tag{2.37}$$

where ϕ_{ijk} is an appropriate multivariable function, $\mathcal{S}$ is a set of all integer triads (i, j, k) corresponding to the numbers of rows, columns, and planes, and $\mathbf{F} = \{f_{ijk}\}$ is an input image. For example, an image generation process in a kind of imaging system is modeled by the equation

$$g_{ijk} = \sum_{(p,q,r)\in\mathcal{S}} h(p, q, r; i, j, k) f_{pqr}, \ \forall (i, j, k) \in \mathcal{S}. \tag{2.38}$$

Note here that the form of the function ϕ_{ijk} in Eq. 2.37 may depend on (i, j, k), the position on the relating image space, and the calculation of one density value g_{ijk} at a voxel (i, j, k) of an output image requires all of density values in an input image $\mathbf{F}$.

2.4.2 Important types of algorithms

An image operator may be implemented or executed by different types of algorithms. From the viewpoint of algorithms, we describe here several important aspects of an image operation characterizing how to implement an operation defined as a mapping on an image set.

(a) Local and global operations

In some classes of image operations, density values of an input image $\mathbf{F} = \{f_{ijk}\}$ in a small finite area around a voxel (i, j, k) are used to calculate an output density value g_{ijk} at the voxel (i, j, k). That is, the output density g_{ijk} is obtained by the equation,

$$g_{ijk} = \phi_{ijk}(\{f_{pqr}; (p, q, r) \in \mathcal{N}_{ijk}((i, j, k))\}) \tag{2.39}$$

where

$$\mathcal{N}_{ijk}((i, j, k)) \equiv \{(i + p, j + q, k + r); (p, q, r) \in \mathcal{S}_{ijk}\} \tag{2.40}$$

and $\mathcal{S}_{ijk}$ is an appropriate subset of the set of all integer triads $I \times I \times I$.

The subarea of the image space $\mathcal{N}_{ijk}((i, j, k))$ is called the *neighborhood* of (i, j, k). Note that $\mathcal{N}_{ijk}((i, j, k))$ may or may not include the voxel (i, j, k) in it. The operation defined by Eq. 2.39 is called a *local operation* if the size of the neighborhood $\mathcal{N}_{ijk}((i, j, k))$ (= the number of voxels contained in

Table 2.4. Examples of neighborhood.

	Notation	Definition
6-neighborhood	$\mathcal{N}^{[6]}\{(i,j,k)\}$	$\{(i+p,j+q,k+r); |p|+|q|+|r|=1\}$
18-neighborhood	$\mathcal{N}^{[18]}\{(i,j,k)\}$	$\{(i+p,j+q,k+r); 1 \le |p|+|q|+|r| \le 2\}$
26-neighborhood	$\mathcal{N}^{[26]}\{(i,j,k)\}$	$\{(i+p,j+q,k+r); p,q,r=0,\pm 1\}$
$3 \times 3 \times 3$ neighborhood	$\mathcal{N}_{333}\{(i,j,k)\}$	$\{(i+p,j+q,k+r); \max(|p|,|q|,|r|)=1\}$
		$\{(i+p,j+q,k+r); \max(|p|,|q|,|r|) \le 1\}$
		$= \mathcal{N}^{[26]}\{(i,j,k)\} \cup (i,j,k)$
$K \times L \times M$ neighborhood	$\mathcal{N}_{KLM}\{(i,j,k)\}$	$\{(i+p,i+q,k+r);$
		$-[(K-1)/2] \le p \le [K/2]$
		$-[(L-1)/2] \le q \le [L/2]$
		$-[(M-1)/2] \le r \le [M/2]\}$
k-th order $K \times L \times M$ neighborhood	$\mathcal{N}^{[m]}\{(i,j,k)\}$	$\{i+k'p,j+k'q,k+k'r \ (k'=1,2,3,\ldots)\}$

$\mathcal{N}_{ijk}((i,j,k)))$ is sufficiently small compared with the size of an input image. If it is comparable to the image size, the process is called a *global operation* (Fig. 2.12). Obviously, only local information about an input image is used to determine an output gray value of each voxel in a local operation. For example, the discrete Fourier transform (DFT) is a typical global operation, and most of procedures discussed in Chapters 3, 4, 5, and 6 of the text are local ones.

Remark 2.7. By the word *local*, we mean that only voxels close to the current voxel (i,j,k) are referred to, as well as that the number of referred voxels are small. Hence we do not regard the shift operator as a local one despite its use of only one density value of an input image for calculating one output density value.

Examples of the neighborhood frequently used are shown in Table 2.4. In particular, $3 \times 3 \times 3$ voxels centered at a voxel (i,j,k), that is,

$$\mathcal{N}_{ijk}((i,j,k)) = \{(i+p,j+q,k+r); \ p,q,r=0,1,-1\} \tag{2.41}$$

are employed most frequently.

(b) Parallel type and sequential type

If the Eq. 2.39 has the form

$$g_{ijk} = \phi_{ijk}(f_{i_1 j_1 k_1}, f_{i_2 j_2 k_2}, \ldots, f_{i_n j_n k_n}), \ \forall (i,j,k) \in I \times I \times I,$$
$$(i_n, j_n, k_n) \in \mathcal{N}_{ijk}((i,j,k)), \ \forall n(N \ge n \ge 1) \tag{2.42}$$

where ϕ_{ijk} is an arbitrary N-variable function, N is an arbitrary integer, and $\mathcal{N}_{ijk}((i,j,k))$ is the neighborhood of the voxel (i,j,k), an image operation is called *parallel (type) operation*.

The operation is called *sequential (type) operation* if it is presented by the equation

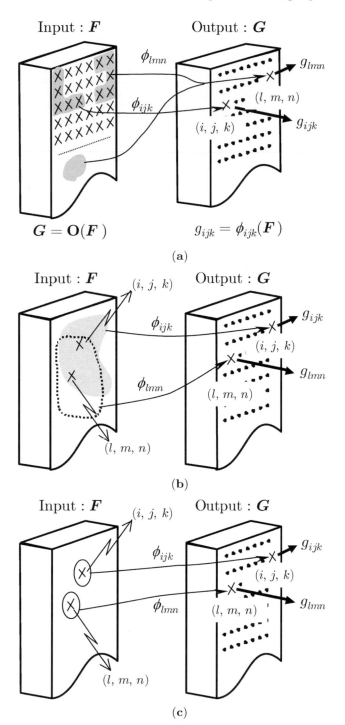

Fig. 2.12. Types of execution of image operations: (**a**) Image processing - general form; (**b**) global operation; (**c**) local operation.

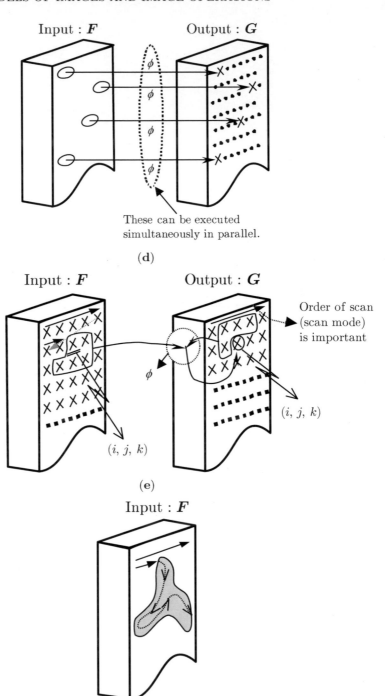

Fig. 2.12. (Continued) Types of execution of image operations (continued): (**d**) Parallel type operation; (**e**) sequential type operation; (**f**) tracing type operation.

$$g_{ijk} = \phi_{ijk}(g_{i_1 j_1 k_1}, g_{i_2 j_2 k_2}, \ldots, g_{i_m j_m k_m},$$
$$f_{i_{m+1} j_{m+1} k_{m+1}}, \ldots, f_{i_{n-1} j_{n-1} k_{n-1}}, f_{i_n j_n k_n}),$$
$$(i_n, j_n, k_n) \in \mathcal{N}_{ijk}((i, j, k)), \ \forall n (N \geq n \geq 1) \tag{2.43}$$

where ϕ_{ijk} is an arbitrary n-variable function, and m and n are arbitrary integers such that $n \geq m \geq 1$. The right-hand side of the Eq. 2.43 must not contain g_{ijk} itself (Fig. 2.12 (d),(e)).

The parallel and the sequential type of operations are characterized as follows:

[Parallel type]

(1) An output value g_{ijk} is determined using the gray values of an input image $\boldsymbol{F} = \{f_{ijk}\}$ only.
(2) Values of g_{ijk} for different (i, j, k)s can be calculated independently (and concurrently if suitable hardware is available).

[Sequential type]

(1) An output value g_{ijk} at a voxel (i, j, k) is determined by using both an input image $\boldsymbol{F} = \{f_{ijk}\}$ and part of an output image $\boldsymbol{G} = \{g_{ijk}\}$ at voxels for which values already have been obtained.
(2) Output values must be computed one by one, sequentially, in a predetermined order.

Many image operations can be performed by either type of algorithm. In such cases, we distinguish the operation (the function) in general and the method of execution by using the term *algorithm* to refer to the latter case. In some classes of sequential operations the order of calculation among voxels depends upon an input image. In the case of operations called *tracing type* we start at a suitably selected initial voxel and proceed to the adjacent voxel sequentially according to the set of predetermined rules based upon densities of an input and/or an output image (Fig. 2.12 (f)).

A *shift invariant local operation*, sometimes called *local parallel operation*, or simply *filtering operation*, is most important for practical applications. Specific types of them utilizing the *3 × 3 × 3* neighborhood have been called *mask operation* or simply *neighborhood logic* in the literature.

The order of processing among all voxels, that is, the order in which voxels are processed, is of critical importance in a sequential operation (or a sequential algorithm). A frequently used order in the sequential operation is called *raster scan*, examples of which are shown in Fig. 2.13. One of them (mode I, for example) is called *forward raster* and the other (mode II) *backward raster*.

Remark 2.8 (Existence of sequential operation). Whether a sequential operation exists or not which is equivalent to an arbitrarily given parallel operation is a theoretically interesting problem which has not been solved completely. The idea of the sequential type operation was shown by Rosenfeld first

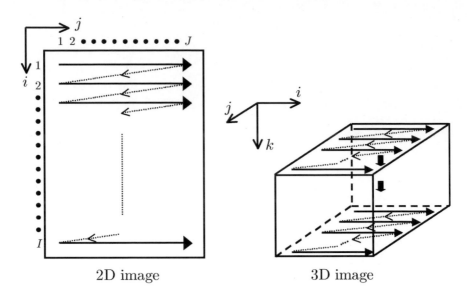

Fig. 2.13. Raster scan.

for 2D image processing concerning the distance transformation and the skeleton (see Chapter 5) [Rosenfeld67]. The above issue was also referred to very briefly there. This problem was discussed by Yamashita et al. [Yamashita83] from a more general viewpoint, being related to the geometrical shape of the neighborhood and the type of the raster scan employed.

(c) Iterative operation

An operation defined or represented by a sequence of one or more operations applied repeatedly a number of times is called an *iterative operation*. Iterations are terminated either after the resultant output image satisfies predetermined requirements (*data dependent*) or after a given number of repetitions (*data independent*).

An iterative operation is regarded as the serial composition of one or more identical (or very similar) operations. That is, an iterative operation **O** is represented in the following form:

$$\mathbf{O} = \mathbf{O}_n \cdot \mathbf{O}_{n-1} \cdot \ldots \cdot \mathbf{O}_2 \cdot \mathbf{O}_1 \qquad (2.44)$$

where $\mathbf{O}_i$s are identical operations or the same class of operations with different values of parameters. In most practically important iterative operations, $\mathbf{O}_i$ is a parallel local operation with the *3 × 3 × 3* neighborhood.

The significance of the iterative operation is summarized as follows.

(1) A very complicated parallel local operation can be implemented by the iteration (or serial composition) of relatively simple parallel local operations.

(2) A global operation may be realized by iterative use of operations $\mathbf{O}_i$, even if $\mathbf{O}_i$ is a local operation with a very small neighborhood.

(3) A certain type of the recursive expression is derived to specify an image operation which is difficult to represent by a closed form. This often simplifies theoretical analysis of the behavior of image operations. In fact, a data-dependent operation cannot be expressed by an explicit form beforehand. By using the iterative form, on the other hand, we may give a smart explicit representation of such operation with some parameters including the number of iterations. Examples of iterative local parallel operations which are of practical importance include distance transformation, fusion (morphological operation), and thinning.

3

LOCAL PROCESSING OF 3D IMAGES

In this chapter we discuss the basics of 3D local operations using density values in small subareas of an input image. A smoothing filter, a difference filter, and features of the curvature of a surface are explained in detail.

3.1 Classification of local operations

3.1.1 General form

The general form of a local process was given in Section 2.4.2 as shown below.

Definition 3.1 (Local processing, local operation). The output density g_{ijk} is obtained by the equation,

$$g_{ijk} = \phi_{ijk}(\{f_{pqr}; (p, q, r) \in \mathcal{N}_{pqr}((i, j, k))\}) \tag{3.1}$$

where

$$\mathcal{N}_{pqr}((i, j, k)) \equiv \{(i + p, j + q, k + r); (p, q, r) \in \mathcal{S}_{ijk}\}, \tag{3.2}$$

$\mathcal{S}_{ijk}$ is an appropriate subset of the set of all integer triads $I \times I \times I$.

The subarea of the image space $\mathcal{N}_{pqr}((i, j, k))$ is called the *neighborhood* of (i, j, k). This means that a density value at a voxel (i, j, k) of an output image is calculated by a function ϕ_{ijk} using the density values of an input image $\boldsymbol{F} = \{f_{ijk}\}$ in the neighborhood $\mathcal{N}_{pqr}((i, j, k))$. We call the function ϕ_{ijk} a *local function*. In the most general case, both the neighborhood and the local function may be changeable according to their location on an image. In the explanation in this book, however, it is assumed that they are the same over the whole of an image to be processed, unless claimed otherwise (*position-invariant processing*).

Remark 3.1. Local processes are sometimes called *filtering* and *mask processing*. More specific names such as $* * *$ *filter* and $* * *$ *operator* are also used for these processes. For example, terms such as edge detection filter, difference filter, Gaussian filter, and smoothing filter are often used.

3.1.2 Classification by functions of filters

(a) Smoothing filter

This is a filter designed to suppress random variations of density values in the neighborhood of an image called a *smoothing filter*. The basic policy of its design is:

(i) To calculate a simple (or a weighted) average of density values in the neighborhood.
(ii) To detect an outlier (a voxel of a density value extraordinarily different from other voxel's density values) and suppress its value.

(b) Difference filter, edge extraction (detection) filter

This is a filter that calculates local differences in density values called a (*spatial*) *difference filter*. These filters are used to detect parts of input images in which the differences in local density values are relatively large and can be used to define these differences.

(c) Local pattern matching (local template matching)

A typical pattern (or a density value distribution) in the subarea of a shape and the size of the image neighborhood is used as a template, and the similarity measure (or the degree of matching) between the subarea of an input image and the template is calculated for each voxel of the input image.

(d) Local statistics filter

Various statistics of density values in the neighborhood area are calculated for each voxel of an input image. An example of these statistics is as follows: average, variance, median, maximum, minimum, k-th order statistics, range, etc. Sometimes, a filter is denoted by the name of the calculated statistics, such as a *median filter* and a *range filter*.

(e) Morphological filter

Morphological operations are performed on each voxel between subarea patterns (template) defined beforehand and on subarea patterns of an input image in the neighborhood.

3.1.3 Classification by the form of a local function

The concrete form of a local operation (or a filter) discussed here is determined by the local function ϕ in Eq. 3.1. Filters also are classified by the local function ϕ.

(a) Linear filter

A linear filter is a filter defined by a local linear function. In other words, the output value for each voxel is calculated by a linear combination (the weighted sum) of density values on an input image in the neighborhood of each voxel. Formally it is represented by Eq. 3.3.

$$\textbf{Linear filter LF } [\textbf{W}] : \textbf{F} = \{f_{ijk}\} \rightarrow \textbf{G} = \{g_{ijk}\}$$

$$g_{ijk} = \sum_{p=1}^{P} \sum_{q=1}^{Q} \sum_{r=1}^{R} w_{pqr} \cdot f_{i-[P/2]+p, j-[Q/2]+q, k-[R/2]+r} \tag{3.3}$$

Here a neighborhood of $P \times Q \times R$ voxels is employed. A set of filter parameters w_{pqr} is called a *weight matrix* or *mask*, and these are often illustrated by a 3D array of the size $P \times Q \times R$. Since a weight can take 0, the generality is not lost by considering only this parallelepiped neighborhood.

(b) Difference filter

The local function of this type of filter contains the calculation of the difference between density values of an input image. The simplest form is the calculation of the difference of two voxels adjacent to each other. Most edge detection filters such as Laplacian are operated by the difference filter as shown in Section 3.3.

(c) Local statistics filter

The local statistics filter introduced in the previous section is also considered to define a local function.

3.2 Smoothing filter

Most smoothing filters in 2D image processing can easily be applied to a 3D image. We present a few examples.

3.2.1 Linear smoothing filter

If a negative value is not contained in a weight matrix in Eq. 3.3, the filter has a smoothing effect when used on a local function. The weight values are selected according to individual applications. If all weights are 1, the filter is called a *uniform weight smoothing filter* and represented by UF. This is equivalent to the filter of which the output at each voxel is the sum (or average) of density values in the neighborhood of an input image. A uniform weight smoothing filter with the $3 \times 3 \times 3$ neighborhood is most frequently used due to the simplicity of its calculation. The decomposition to a serial composition of three 1D UFs is also possible as in a 2D case.

Uniform weight linear filter UF $[C]: \boldsymbol{F} = \{f_{ijk}\} \rightarrow \boldsymbol{G} = \{g_{ijk}\}$

$$g_{ijk} = \sum c \cdot f_{ijk}. \tag{3.4}$$

$\sum$ represents the sum over all voxels in the neighborhood $\mathcal{N}((i,j,k))$

We assume $c = 1$ in the sequel, if not described otherwise.

In order to describe explicitly that a weight $\boldsymbol{W}$ of the size of the neighborhood $P \times Q \times R$ voxels is employed, we use the notation

Linear filter LF $[\boldsymbol{W} \, P \times Q \times R]: \boldsymbol{F} = \{f_{ijk}\} \rightarrow \boldsymbol{G} = \{g_{ijk}\}.$ $\qquad$ (3.5)

The fast algorithm of the recursive type is available in the same way as the 2D **UF** [Preston79].

A weight matrix derived based on the probability density of Gaussian distribution is frequently employed to smooth an input image in practical applications. This type of filter is called a *Gaussian filter*.

Remark 3.2 (Gaussian distribution). The probability density function of the 3D Gaussian distribution (normal distribution) $p(x_1, x_2, x_3)$ is given as follows

$$p(x_1, x_2, x_3) = (2\pi)^{-3/2} |\boldsymbol{\Sigma}|^{-1/2} \exp\{-(\boldsymbol{x} - \boldsymbol{\mu})^t \boldsymbol{\Sigma}^{-1} (\boldsymbol{x} - \boldsymbol{\mu})/2\}$$

$$\boldsymbol{x} = (x_1, x_2, x_3)^t$$

$$\boldsymbol{\mu} = (\mu_1, \mu_2, \mu_3)^t = \text{mean vector}$$

$$\boldsymbol{\Sigma} = \begin{pmatrix} \sigma_{11} & \sigma_{12} & \sigma_{13} \\ \sigma_{21} & \sigma_{22} & \sigma_{23} \\ \sigma_{31} & \sigma_{32} & \sigma_{33} \end{pmatrix} = \text{covariance matrix} \tag{3.6}$$

To derive a weight matrix, we assume that the origin is located at the center voxel of the neighborhood. Therefore, we assume the mean vector as $(0, 0, 0)$. An arbitrarily selected positive definite matrix can be given as a covariance matrix $\boldsymbol{\Sigma}$. A scale factor may be neglected. Thus we determine each element of the weight matrix by the equation.

$$\exp\{-(\boldsymbol{x} - \boldsymbol{\mu})^t \boldsymbol{\Sigma}^{-1}(\boldsymbol{x} - \boldsymbol{\mu})\} \tag{3.7}$$

3.2.2 Median filter and order statistics filter

The median filter is a filter that outputs at each voxel (i, j, k) the median of density values of an input image in the neighborhood of (i, j, k). Formally it is defined as follows.

Median filter MED $: \boldsymbol{F} = \{f_{ijk}\} \rightarrow \boldsymbol{G} = \{g_{ijk}\}$

$$g_{ijk} = \text{ the median of } \{f_{pqr}; (p, q, r) \in \mathcal{N}((i, j, k))\} \qquad (3.8)$$

$$\mathcal{N}((i, j, k)) = \text{ the neighborhood}$$

This filter changes the density distribution of an input image into a smoother one by replacing the density value f_{ijk} of a voxel (i, j, k) by the median of density values in its neighborhood. Extraordinary density values can be eliminated without being affected by its absolute value, and the filter can preserve edges to some extent. Computing cost is relatively high because sorting of density values in the neighborhood is performed at every voxel in an input image.

Remark 3.3 (Order statistics filter). The concept of the median filter is easily extended to the one that outputs the k-th order statistics (or the k-th largest density value in the neighborhood). This we call *order statistics filter* **OS**[k]. Formal description is given as follows.

Order statistics filter OS $[m] : \boldsymbol{F} = \{f_{ijk}\} \rightarrow \boldsymbol{G} = \{g_{ijk}\}$

$$g_{ijk} = \text{ the } m\text{-th largest of } \{f_{pqr}; (p, q, r) \in \mathcal{N}((i, j, k))\} \qquad (3.9)$$

$$\mathcal{N}((i, j, k)) = \text{ the neighborhood}$$

Assuming the neighborhood $\mathcal{N}((i, j, k))$ contains n $(= \text{odd})$ voxels, **OS** $[m]$ reduces to the median filter, if $m = [(n + 1)/2]$. If $m = 1$ and $m = n$, we call those filters *maximum filter* and *minimum filter*, and denote by **MAX** and **MIN**, respectively. Both **MAX** and **MIN** filter and their repetitive application are very important in the distance transformation and the fusion presented in Chapter 5 in detail. The basic structure and computation of an algorithm essentially do not depend on the dimensionality of an input image. The 1D order statistics filter has been studied in detail in the field of signal processing [Nodes82, Bovik83, Arce87, McLoughlin87]. However, some of the features such as edge preservation characteristics and the existence of kernels (an invariant component to the iterative application) may not always be extended to 3D image processing.

3.2.3 Edge-preserving smoothing

The smoothing operation changes the spatial distribution of the density values in an input image and makes it smoother. It also eliminates or weakens a significant variation in density values such as in the edges and borders of a 3D figure. Because of this, there is always a trade-off between noise reduction by smoothing and the edge detection (detection of abrupt change) in density values.

A method to deal with this difficulty is by smoothing while preserving the edge. The basic idea is to roughly estimate the possible existence of edges before executing the smoothing procedure. One idea is to divide the neighborhood area into several smaller subareas and to consider the possibility that each subarea contains a border. A suitable measuring of density variations in each subarea must be applied to do this. A smoothing operator is executed only in the subarea, regarded as such as "no border exists in it."

The concept of edge-preserving smoothing was firstly developed for a 2D image. The extension of the idea to be applied to a 3D image is not complicated. However, the devision of the neighborhood and the estimation of the existence of a border requires careful consideration, as the result may be a serious increase in computation time. Different ideas were presented in [Tomasi98, Wong04] with applications to 3D CT and MRI images of the brain.

3.2.4 Morphology filter

Let us consider an input image $F = \{f_{ijk}\}$ and a gray-tone image $B = \{b_{ijk}; (i, j, k) \in \mathcal{N}((0, 0, 0))\}$ defined at the origin $(0, 0, 0)$ and on its neighborhood. Then we define the following two operations, dilation and erosion.

Definition 3.2 (Dilation and erosion). *Dilation* of an input image F by the structure element B is defined as

$$\text{Dilation DIL } [B] : F = \{f_{ijk}\} \to G = \{g_{ijk}\}$$

$$g_{ijk} = \max_{(p,q,r)} \{f_{pqr} + bs_{p-i,q-j,r-k}; (p, q, r) \in \mathcal{N}((i, j, k))\}. \tag{3.10}$$

Erosion of an input image F by the *structure element* B is defined as

$$\text{Erosion ERO } [B] : F = \{f_{ijk}\} \to G = \{g_{ijk}\}$$

$$g_{ijk} = \min_{(p,q,r)} \{f_{pqr} - bs_{p-i,q-j,r-k}; (p, q, r) \in \mathcal{N}((i, j, k))\}. \tag{3.11}$$

where $Bs = \{bs_{ijk}\}$ is a gray-tone image symmetric to B with respect to the origin.

The following notations are also used frequently.

$$\text{Dilation of } F \text{ by } B = F \oplus B. \tag{3.12}$$

$$\text{Erosion of } F \text{ by } B = F \ominus B. \tag{3.13}$$

Both are also called *morphological filters* with the structure element B (and with the neighborhood $\mathcal{N}((i, j, k))$. If $b_{ijk} = 0$, (i, j, k), then the dilation and erosion reduce to the maximum filter and the minimum filter, respectively.

Serial compositions shown below are called morphological operations, too. They are sometimes called the *closing* and *opening*, respectively.

$$(F \ominus B) \oplus B \quad (\text{operator expression } \mathbf{DIL}[B] \cdot \mathbf{ERO}[B]) \ (opening) \tag{3.14}$$

$$(F \oplus B) \ominus B \quad (\text{operator expression } \mathbf{ERO}[B] \cdot \mathbf{DIL}[B]) \ (closing) \tag{3.15}$$

They both can eliminate (or suppress) isolated random variations in an input image; they change a curved surface $w = f(i, j, k)$ transferring to an input image into a smoother one.

Remark 3.4. The following holds concerning the morphological operations. Putting an input image by $\boldsymbol{F} = \{f_{ijk}\}$ and an output image by $\boldsymbol{G} = \{g_{ijk}\}$,

(i) Erosion: $\boldsymbol{G} \le \boldsymbol{F}$. It eliminates an isolated protrusion smaller than a given width.
(ii) Dilation: $\boldsymbol{G} \ge \boldsymbol{F}$. It eliminates an isolated cavity or a depression smaller than the given size by filling them.
(iii) Opening: $\boldsymbol{G} \le \boldsymbol{F}$. It makes an image smoother by whittling isolated points, protrusions, and ridges smaller than the given size.
(iv) Closing: $\boldsymbol{G} \ge \boldsymbol{F}$. It makes an image smoother by filling holes, depressions, cavities, and valleys smaller than a given size.

By representing a 3D gray-tone image by a set of cross sections or a set of umbras, we treat a 3D gray-tone image only by morphological operations on a binary image or the operation on a set.

Remark 3.5. We will introduce another expression of the dilation and the erosion. Note that an input 3D image $\boldsymbol{F} = \{f_{ijk}\}$ can be regarded as a curved surface $w - f_{ijk} = 0, \forall(i, j, k)$ in the 4D space. Let us consider the subspace R_1 of this 4D space defined by

$$R_1 = \{(i, j, k); z - f_{ijk} \le 0\} = \text{umbra of } \boldsymbol{F}. \tag{3.16}$$

Next let us consider a weight function $\{w_{ijk} \in \mathcal{N}((0, 0, 0))\}$ defined on the neighborhood $\mathcal{N}((0, 0, 0))$ of the origin $((0, 0, 0))$. We denote by $R_w((0, 0, 0))$ the region $z - w_{ijk} \le 0$ ($=$ umbra of $\{w_{ijk}\}$). Then let us denote by $R_w(i, j, k)$ the result of the translation of $R_w((0, 0, 0))$ to (i, j, k). Then, the following point set $\boldsymbol{S}$

$$\boldsymbol{S} = \{(i, j, k); R_w(i, j, k) \subset R_1\} \tag{3.17}$$

is called *figure erosion* of the region R_1 by the *weight function* (the *mask function, structural element*) R_w. Furthermore, putting the region $\{(i, j, k); z - f_{ijk} \ge 0\}$ by R_2, the point set $\bar{\boldsymbol{S}}$ ($=$ the complement of $\boldsymbol{S}'$), where

$$\boldsymbol{S}' = \{(i, j, k); R_w(i, j, k) \subset R_2\} \tag{3.18}$$

is called *figure dilation* of the region R_2 by the weight function (structure element) R_w. The operations to derive the figure dilation and the figure erosion are also examples of morphological operations (Fig. 3.1).

Remark 3.6. Generally speaking, if an input image and a mask (a weight function) are both binary, a morphological operation of the image is treated as a morphological operation on the set, regardless of the dimension of an image to be processed [Haralick87, Maragos87a, Maragos87b, Matheron75, Serra82].

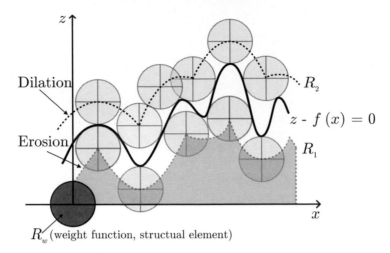

Fig. 3.1. An example of morphological operations for a 1D curve.

Applications of the morphological operation to practical image process have increased during the last ten years. In the computer aided diagnosis of medical 3D images, for example, this procedure is applied to the segmentation of organs from chest and abdominal CT images and to the nodule detection in lungs. Design of an appropriate weight or a structural element is the most important factor in such practical applications.

Remark 3.7. Let us show an example of the morphological operation. An input is a 1D image (waveform), and a mask is a circle of the radius r (Fig. 3.1). In this example, R_w = the region below the curve.

Figure erosion = the trace of the center of circles (weight) such that all the circles stay below the curve.

Figure dilation = the trace of the center of circles (weight) such that the entire circle stays above the curve or the circle touches the curve at least at one point.

3.3 Difference filter

3.3.1 Significance

When we see an unknown image (a 2D image) for the first time, we focus on the following areas:

(i) an area with subtle variation in density,
(ii) abrupt change in density values,

(iii) connections of common features.

Human vision is sufficient when working with a 2D image, making the above statements valid for this type of image. For a 3D image, however, we tend to develop methods for computer processing. At first we tend to imagine that an area of nearly uniform density suggests the existence of a 3D object. Secondly we expect that borders or edges of 3D objects may exist. A sudden change in density values will be detected by calculating the spatial difference of a 3D image.

3.3.2 Differentials in continuous space

Before proceeding to the explanation of a difference filter, we will summarize the basics of differentials of a continuous function. Let us consider a function of three variables $f(x, y, z)$. We presently assume $f(x, y, z)$ at least twice differentiable.

(a) Gradient

$$\nabla f(x, y, z) = (\partial f/\partial x) \cdot \boldsymbol{i} + (\partial f/\partial y) \cdot \boldsymbol{j} + (\partial f/\partial z) \cdot \boldsymbol{k}, \qquad (3.19)$$

where $\boldsymbol{i}$, $\boldsymbol{j}$, and $\boldsymbol{k}$ are unit vectors in x, y, and z directions, respectively.

(b) Maximum gradient

$$\|\nabla f\| = \left[(\partial f/\partial x)^2 + (\partial f/\partial y)^2 + (\partial f/\partial z)^2\right]^{1/2}. \qquad (3.20)$$

(c) Direction of the maximum gradient

$$\theta^* = \tan^{-1}\left[(\partial f/\partial y)/(\partial f/\partial x)\right]. \qquad (3.21)$$

$$\varphi^* = \tan^{-1}\{(\partial f/\partial z)/\left[(\partial f/\partial y)^2 + (\partial f/\partial x)^2\right]^{1/2}\}. \qquad (3.22)$$

(d) Coordinate transform (Fig. 3.2)

(r, θ, ϕ)(polar coordinate system) $\rightarrow (x, y, z)$(Cartesian coordinate system)
$$x = r\cos\theta\cos\phi, \ y = r\sin\theta\cos\phi, \ z = r\sin\phi. \qquad (3.23)$$

(x, y, z)(Cartesian coordinate system) $\rightarrow (r, \theta, \phi)$(polar coordinate system)
$$r = (x^2 + y^2 + z^2)^{1/2}, \ \theta = \tan^{-1}(y/x), \ \phi = \tan^{-1}(z/(x^2 + y^2)^{1/2}). \ (3.24)$$

(e) Derivative in angular direction (θ', φ')

$$(\partial f/\partial x)\cos\theta'\cos\phi' + (\partial f/\partial y)\sin\theta'\cos\phi' + (\partial f/\partial z)\sin\phi'. \qquad (3.25)$$

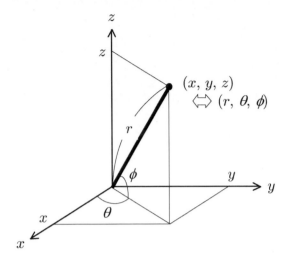

Fig. 3.2. The Cartesian coordinate system and polar coordinate system. Cartesian coordinates $(x, y, z) \leftrightarrow$ polar coordinates (r, θ, ϕ).

(f) Laplacian

$$\nabla f = (\partial^2 f/\partial x^2) + (\partial^2 f/\partial y^2) + (\partial^2 f/\partial z^2). \tag{3.26}$$

(g) Derivatives in the direction of coordinate axis

(first-order derivatives)

$$f_x = (\partial f/\partial x), \; f_y = (\partial f/\partial y), \; f_z = (\partial f/\partial z) \tag{3.27}$$

(second-order derivatives)

$$f_{xx} = (\partial^2 f/\partial x^2), \; f_{yy} = (\partial^2 f/\partial y^2), \; f_{zz} = (\partial^2 f/\partial z^2)$$
$$f_{xy} = (\partial^2 f/\partial x \partial y), \; f_{yz} = (\partial^2 f/\partial y \partial z), \; f_{zx} = (\partial^2 f/\partial z \partial x) \tag{3.28}$$

The set of these partial derivatives are often denoted in the form of matrix called *Hessian*, that is,

$$\text{Hessian} \begin{pmatrix} f_{xx} & f_{xy} & f_{xz} \\ f_{yx} & f_{yy} & f_{yz} \\ f_{zx} & f_{zy} & f_{zz} \end{pmatrix} \tag{3.29}$$

3.3.3 Derivatives in digitized space

Derivatives are approximated by differences on a digitized image. Several examples are shown below.

$$f_x = (f_{i+1,j,k} - f_{i-1,j,k})/2\Delta i \tag{3.30}$$

$$f_{xx} = (f_{i+1,j,k} - 2f_{ijk} + f_{i-1,j,k})/4\Delta i \tag{3.31}$$

$$f_{xy} = (f_{i+1,j+1,k} - f_{i-1,j+1,k} - f_{i+1,j-1,k} + f_{i-1,j-1,k})/4\Delta i\Delta j, \tag{3.32}$$

where Δi and Δj are sampling intervals (= the length of voxel edges) in the i and the j directions, respectively. They are unit length usually. The value of Δk may be larger when the interval between slices is larger than the voxel size within a slice as is often seen in CT images of the human body. Various other methods and equations to numerically evaluate differentials are found in books about numerical analysis.

Remark 3.8. Values of derivatives can be estimated by executing a curve fitting in the neighborhood of each voxel. The outline of the procedure is as follows in the case of 3D image processing:

Given an input image $\boldsymbol{F} = \{f_{ijk}\}$, we consider to fit a suitable function $\phi(x, y, z; \boldsymbol{a})$ at a voxel (i, j, k) and its neighborhood, where x, y, and z represent variables in the coordinate axes i, j, and k, and $\boldsymbol{a}$ is a parameter vector specific to the function ϕ. Then we obtain values $\underline{\boldsymbol{a}} = (\underline{a}_1, \underline{a}_2, \ldots, \underline{a}_M)$ which minimizes the following estimation error e_{ijk}

$$e_{ijk} = \sum_{(p,q,r)} [f_{pqr} - \phi(p, q, r; \underline{\boldsymbol{a}})], \tag{3.33}$$

where $\sum$ means the sum over the neighborhood $\mathcal{N}(i, j, k)$ of a voxel (i, j, k).

Next, we estimate the density f_{ijk} at a voxel (i, j, k) by $\phi(i, j, k; \underline{\boldsymbol{a}})$. Values of derivatives at the same voxel are also approximated by $\partial\phi/\partial x, \partial^2\phi/\partial x^2$, etc.

Process of calculation is obvious. The value of $\underline{\boldsymbol{a}}$ is obtained by solving the equation.

$$\partial e_{ijk}/\partial a_k = -2\sum (p, q, r)[f_{pqr} - \phi(p, q, r; \underline{\boldsymbol{a}})](\partial\phi/\partial a_k) = 0, \ k = 1, 2, \ldots, M \tag{3.34}$$

The solution is obtained from values of (i, j, k) and density values of an input image in the neighborhood $\mathcal{N}((i, j, k))$. The calculation process is simplified by putting the origin at the center of the neighborhood $\mathcal{N}((i, j, k))$, because it is enough to calculate values of $\phi_x(0, 0, 0; \underline{\boldsymbol{a}})$, $\phi_{xx}(0, 0, 0; \underline{\boldsymbol{a}})$, etc., without using values of $\phi_x(0, 0, 0; \underline{\boldsymbol{a}})$ etc. at a general position of (i, j, k). The underlying idea here is the same as the processing of a 2D image as is seen in [Haralick81, Haralick83]. Examples of applications to 3D images are found in [Brejl00, Hirano03].

3.3.4 Basic characteristics of difference filter

Derivatives are approximated by differences in digital image process. A local processing to perform this is called a *difference operation* (*difference operator*, *difference filter*). Basic characteristics of difference filters are almost the same as those of 2D images. We neglect the details here and will discuss the most important features.

(i) The simplest form of the difference filter is one in which the difference between densities of two voxels (denoted by P and Q for explanation) is calculated. In this case, the output for an edge running in the direction near the line connecting two voxels P and Q is small. On the other hand, for an edge perpendicular to the direction connecting P and Q, the output will be a larger difference value. Therefore, the response of a difference filter strongly depends on both the direction of the difference and that of an edge. This type of difference filter is called a *directional-type* filter. A filter giving a significant output to any direction of edges is called an *omnidirectional-type* filter.The directional type is effective if we have precise knowledge of the edge direction or if we want to detect only edges of restricted directions. However, the omnidirectional-type filter is preferred if we do not have enough knowledge about the edge direction or if detecting the edges of all directions is necessary.

(ii) We can derive an omnidirectional filter from directional filters. This is called *omnidirectionalization*. Details of this procedure are explained in Subsection 3.3.5.

(iii) The difference in density between two voxels separated in a definite distance from each other may be used instead of the difference between adjacent voxels. By adjusting the distance k between two voxels for which the density difference is calculated, we can design a filter that may respond to edges and borders (*line detection type*) and to a massive figure (*mass detection type*). This feature is basically common to 2D image processing [Preston79].

(iv) A disadvantage of the difference filter is that it is too sensitive to random noise. This sensitivity is prevented by applying a smoothing filter before applying a difference filter or by developing a filter that has both smoothing and difference calculation functions. This type of filter we call a *smoothed difference filter*. Formally this is regarded as the serial composition of a smoothing operator and a difference operator. If both operators are linear, their serial composition is also linear.

3.3.5 Omnidirectionalization

Let us first apply a few relatively simple difference filters (*element filters*) to obtain the final output by calculating a suitable function of those outputs. We call this process the *integration* of element filters. An omnidirectional filter may be created by integrating directional filters. This is called *omnidirectionalization*. Denoting n operations with those n element filters by $\mathbf{O}_1, \mathbf{O}_2, \ldots, \mathbf{O}_n$, the final output is the parallel composition of element operators $\mathbf{O}_1, \mathbf{O}_2, \ldots, \mathbf{O}_n$.

Let us denote by f_p an output value of an element filter $\mathbf{O}_p$ at a voxel (i, j, k) $(p = 1, 2, \ldots, n)$. Then, the following examples show the output of an omnidirectionalized filter f_g.

$$(1) \ f_q = \sum_{p=1}^{n} f_p, \ \left(\text{or } f_q = \sum_{p=1}^{n} f_p/n\right). \tag{3.35}$$

$$(2) \ f_q = \sum_{p=1}^{n} \|f_p\|, \ f_q = \sum_{p=1}^{n} f_p^2. \tag{3.36}$$

$$(3) \ f_q = \text{order statistics of } \{|f_p|\}. \tag{3.37}$$
$$(\max\{|f_p|\}, \min\{|f_p|\}, \text{median of}\{|f_p|\}, \text{etc.})$$

3.3.6 1D difference filters and their combinations

The simplest form of a difference filter is one in which voxels used for calculation are arranged along a line segment. This we call a *simple difference filter*. Examples are shown below:

1st order difference
$$\mathbf{LDF}_1[p, q, r] : \mathbf{F} = \{f_{ijk}\} \rightarrow \mathbf{G} = \{g_{ijk}\},$$
$$g_{ijk} = f_{i-p,j-q,k-r} - f_{i+p,j+q,k+r} \tag{3.38}$$

2nd order difference
$$\mathbf{LDF}_2[p, q, r] : \mathbf{F} = \{f_{ijk}\} \rightarrow \mathbf{G} = \{g_{ijk}\},$$
$$g_{ijk} = f_{i-p,j-q,k-r} + f_{i+p,j+q,k+r} - 2f_{ijk} \tag{3.39}$$

1st order difference - rotationary type
$$\mathbf{LDF}_{\text{rot1}}[r, \theta, \phi] : \mathbf{F} = \{f_{ijk}\} \rightarrow \mathbf{G} = \{g_{ijk}\},$$
$$g_{ijk} = f_1(r, \theta, \phi) - f_2(r, \theta, \phi) \tag{3.40}$$

2nd order difference - rotationary type
$$\mathbf{LDF}_{\text{rot2}}[r, \theta, \phi] : \mathbf{F} = \{f_{ijk}\} \rightarrow \mathbf{G} = \{g_{ijk}\}.$$
$$g_{ijk} = f_1(r, \theta, \phi) + f_2(r, \theta, \phi) - 2f_{ijk} \tag{3.41}$$

In the rotationary type above, two voxels $(i \pm r \cos\theta \sin\phi, j \pm r \sin\phi \sin\theta, k \pm r \cos\theta)$ are selected at each voxel (i, j, k), so that they are located separately by r from the voxel (i, j, k) and symmetrically with respect to (i, j, k) in the directional angles ϕ (Fig. 3.3). Then, $f_1(r, \theta, \phi)$ and $f_2(r, \theta, \phi)$ in the above rotationary type represent input density values at these voxels.

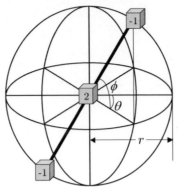

θ, ϕ : Rotation angle
r : Radius of a filter

Fig. 3.3. A 3D simple difference filter. This figure shows a second-order difference filter. A first-order difference filter is obtained by making a center weight to be zero.

Remark 3.9. Omnidirectionalization results of the rotational-type filters mentioned above are called *rotational difference filter*. Results were applied to 3D chest CT images to detect lung cancer [Shimizu93, Shimizu95a, Shimizu95b]. Several examples are:

$$g_{ijk}^{(p)}(r) = \max_{(\theta,\phi)}\{g_{ijk}^{(p)}(r,\theta,\phi); 0 < \theta, \phi \leq \pi\}. \tag{3.42}$$

$$g_{ijk}^{(p)}(r) = \min_{(\theta,\phi)}\{g_{ijk}^{(p)}(r,\theta,\phi); 0 < \theta, \phi \leq \pi\}. \tag{3.43}$$

$$g_{ijk}^{(p)}(r) = \sum_{\theta}\sum_{\phi} g_{ijk}^{(p)}(r,\theta,\phi) \; (p = 1, 2). \tag{3.44}$$

3.3.7 3D Laplacian

A 3D Laplacian is derived naturally from the sum of the output of three second-order difference filters as is shown below, or of the sum of all outputs of the first-order difference filters for all directions.

$$g_{ijk} = f_{i+r,j,k} + f_{i,j+r,k} + f_{i,j,k+r} + f_{i-r,j,k} + f_{i,j-r,k} + f_{i,j,k-r} - 6f_{ijk}. \tag{3.45}$$

Representations by masks are shown in Fig. 3.4 for $r = 1$, and other variations are given in Table 3.1 and 3.2.

3.3.8 2D difference filters and their combination

New types of 3D filters are derived by calculating a suitable function of outputs of 2D filters on two parallel planes placed on the opposite side of a voxel

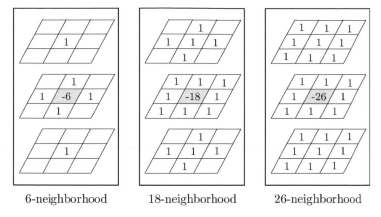

6-neighborhood   18-neighborhood   26-neighborhood

Fig. 3.4. Examples of a weight function of 3D Laplacian.

Table 3.1. A Laplacian on the 3D 26-neighborhood.

Element filter (assuming $r = 1$)
(1) The form of $g_{ijk} = f_{i-1,j,k} + f_{i+1,j,k} - 2f_{ijk}$ (three directions)
(2) The form of $g_{ijk} = f_{i-1,j-1,k} + f_{i+1,j+1,k} - 2f_{ijk}$ (six directions)
(3) The form of $g_{ijk} = f_{i-1,j-1,k-1} + f_{i+1,j+1,k+1} - 2f_{ijk}$ (four directions)

Sum of 3 element filters $\rightarrow$ 6-neighbor Laplacian
Sum of 9 element filters of (1) and (2) $\rightarrow$ 18-neighbor Laplacian
Sum of 13 element filters of (1), (2) and (3) $\rightarrow$ 27-neighbor Laplacian

(i, j, k). For instance, 2D filters on planes $(i = i - 1)$ and $(i = i + 1)$ are applied first, and then the sum of their outputs may be considered as the output at the voxel (i, j, k). Even if 2D filters are omnidirectional, a resulting 3D filter may become directional, if we employ only one pair of planes. On the contrary, a resulting 3D filter may become omnidirectional even if we use directional ones in 2D planes.

Figure 3.5 shows an example of a 3D difference filter derived from a pair of two 2D 4-neighbor Laplacians. The obtained 3D filter is directional, because only one pair of filters arranged in the k-direction is employed there. Note here that both 2D filters are omnidirectional in 2D planes.

Other examples are illustrated in Figs. 3.6 and 3.7. Those in Fig. 3.6 were derived from 2D Sobel filters. The Sobel filter in Fig. 3.7 was derived directly from a 3D image. Examples of operators for edge detection in a 3D image are given in Table 3.2.

Remark 3.10. The directional characteristics of 2D and 3D filters in synthesizing 3D ones from 2D ones are as follows:

(i) (2D, directional) $\rightarrow$ (3D, directional) $\rightarrow$ (3D, omnidirectional)

Table 3.2. The weight matrix (mask) of edge detection filters for a 3D image.

C_{ijk} (i,j,k)	111	112	113	121	122	123	131	132	133	211	212	213	221	222	223	231	232	233	311	312	313	321	322	323	331	332	333	A	B	C	D
Simple 1st order difference					-1																		1					○	6	1	○
Hyperplane fitting type		-1		-1	-1	-1		-1												1		1	1	1		1		○	18	1	○
Hyperplane fitting type	-1	-1	-1	-1	-1	-1	-1	-1	-1										1	1	1	1	1	1	1	1	1	○	26	1	○
Optimization type		α		α	-1	α		α												γ		γ	1	γ		γ		○	18	1	○
Optimization type	β	α	β	α	-1	α	β	α	β										δ	γ	δ	γ	1	γ	δ	γ	δ	○	26	1	○
Sobel type		-2		-2	-3	-2		-2												2		2	3	2		2		○	18	1	○
Sobel type	-1	-2	-1	-2	-3	-2	-1	-2	-1										1	2	1	2	3	2	1	2	1	○	26	1	○
Minimum difference		☆		☆	☆	☆		☆		☆	☆	☆	☆	@	☆	☆	☆	☆		☆		☆	☆	☆		☆		✕	18	1	✕
Minimum difference	☆	☆	☆	☆	☆	☆	☆	☆	☆	☆	☆	☆	☆	@	☆	☆	☆	☆	☆	☆	☆	☆	☆	☆	☆	☆	☆	✕	26	1	✕
Range difference type					☆						☆		☆	☆	☆		☆						☆					✕	6	1	✕
Range difference type		☆		☆	☆	☆		☆		☆	☆	☆	☆	☆	☆	☆	☆	☆		☆		☆	☆	☆		☆		✕	18	1	✕
Range difference type	☆	☆	☆	☆	☆	☆	☆	☆	☆	☆	☆	☆	☆	☆	☆	☆	☆	☆	☆	☆	☆	☆	☆	☆	☆	☆	☆	✕	26	1	✕
Simple 2nd order difference					1									-2									1					○	6	2	○
Laplacian		1		1	1	1		1		1	1	1	1	-18	1	1	1	1		1		1	1	1		1		✕	18	2	○
Laplacian	1	1	1	1	1	1	1	1	1	1	1	1	1	-26	1	1	1	1	1	1	1	1	1	1	1	1	1	✕	26	2	○

(a) Empty cells in the table mean the value 0.
(b) In the optimization type, $\alpha = -1/\sqrt{2}$, $\beta = -1/\sqrt{3}$, $\gamma = 1/\sqrt{2}$, $\delta = 1/\sqrt{3}$.
(c) In the minimum difference type, the value of @ - the minimum of ☆ is calculated as an output.
(d) In the range difference type, the maximum of ☆ - the minimum of ☆ is output.

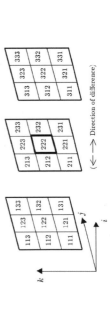

$(\longleftrightarrow$ Direction of difference)

113	123	133
112	122	132
111	121	131

213	223	233
212	222	232
211	221	231

313	323	333
312	322	332
311	321	331

Notation

A: Directionality
  ○ : directional
  ✕ : omnidirectional
B: Connectivity (see Chapter 4)
C: Order of the difference
D: Linearity ○:linear, ✕:nonlinear

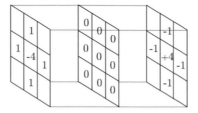

Fig. 3.5. An example of a 3D difference filter derived by arranging two 2D Laplacians. A 3D directional filter is obtained from 2D omnidirectional ones.

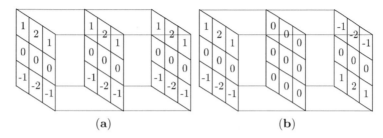

(a) (b)

Fig. 3.6. The combination of 2D Sobel filters for deriving 3D filters: (a) Juxtaposition of three 2D filters; (b) difference of two 2D directional filters. Both are obtained from 2D directional filters and are directional as 3D filters.

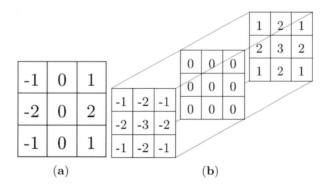

(a) (b)

Fig. 3.7. The extension of a 2D Sobel filter to a 3D Sobel filter: (a) 2D Sobel filter; (b) 3D Sobel filter.

(ii) (2D, directional) → (3D, omnidirectional)
(iii) (2D, omnidirectional) → (3D, directional) → (3D, omnidirectional)
(iv) (2D, omnidirectional) → (3D, omnidirectional)

Remark 3.11. Large numbers of 2D filters have been developed for various applications and have been studied theoretically and experimentally. Most of their structures and properties are extended straightforward to 3D image

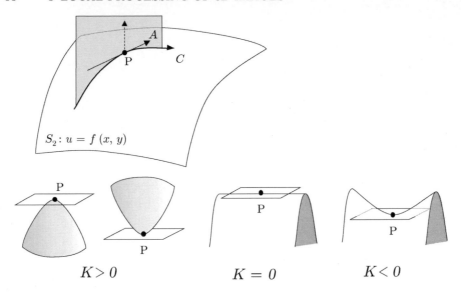

Fig. 3.8. An illustration of a curved surface according to values of curvature (K means Gaussian curvature).

processing. The procedure of extension is obvious, hence they are not discussed in this book. Examples contain curve fitting in local areas such as in the Heuckel operator, Laplacian-Gaussian, and the use of zero crossings, recursive and nonrecursive filters that are frequently discussed in digital signal processing, linear filters designed in the spatial frequency domain, separability of filters and fast algorithms, etc. The 3D difference filters were perhaps first reported in [Liu77, Herman78], and the optimization type was found in [Zucker79, Zucker81]. In some 3D cases the computation cost may become too much. The physical meaning of some of these filters may not be applicable to 3D image such as the similarity between the response of the human vision and the DOG (difference of Gaussian) filter.

3.4 Differential features of a curved surface

Consider a 3D continuous image $f(x, y, z)$ and a 4D hypersurface $S : u = f(x, y, z)$. At an arbitrary point P on this surface, there exist three principal curvatures. We denote them by k_1, k_2, and k_3. They are calculated as follows (see Fig. 3.8 also).

Let us denote the first and the second derivatives of a 3D gray-tone continuous image $u = f(x, y, z)$ by f_x, f_y, and f_{xx}, and f_{xy}, etc. Then we consider the following two matrices, $\mathbf{F}_1$ and $\mathbf{F}_2$.

(the first fundamental form)

$$\mathbf{F}_1 = \begin{pmatrix} 1 + f_x^2 & f_x f_y & f_x f_z \\ f_y f_x & 1 + f_y^2 & f_y f_z \\ f_z f_x & f_z f_y & 1 + f_z^2 \end{pmatrix} \tag{3.46}$$

(the second fundamental form)

$$\mathbf{F}_2 = -1/D \begin{pmatrix} f_{xx} & f_{xy} & f_{xz} \\ f_{yx} & f_{yy} & f_{yz} \\ f_{zx} & f_{zy} & f_{zz} \end{pmatrix} \tag{3.47}$$

where

$$D = (1 + f_x^2 + f_y^2 + f_z^2)^{1/2}. \tag{3.48}$$

Then, principal curvatures k_1, k_2, and k_3 of a hypersurface S are obtained as eigen values of a matrix

$$\mathbf{W} = \mathbf{F}_1^{-1}\mathbf{F}_2. \tag{3.49}$$

Relations among them are classified as summarized below.

(i) Signs and orders in their sizes (*20* cases).
(ii) Orders in sizes of their absolute values and zero and nonzero (*26* cases).
(iii) The sign of the sum $k_1 + k_2 + k_3$ (*3* cases).

There exist *1560* cases of all these combinations. Noting that we can assume $|k_1| \geq |k_2| \geq |k_3|$ without loss of generality, consideration of only *20* cases is enough. They are given in Table 3.4.

These curvatures represent local shape futures of the surface S at a point P and its vicinity. We could imagine shapes of a hypersurface from the analogy on a 2D image (= shape of a 3D surface).

Sets of points satisfying various conditions may be utilized as shape features of surfaces in the 3D space and a hypersurface in the 4D space such as equidensity surface, a surface of a 3D object and border surface, for example, [Enomoto75, Enomoto76, Nackman82] for a 2D image, and [Watanabe86, Thirion95, Monga95, Brechbuhler95, Hirano00].

However, differential features are defined only at a differentiable point for a continuous image. For a digitized image, the method to calculate difference, the method of digitization, and the effect of random noise must be taken into account.

Remark 3.12. For a 2D continuous image $f(x, y)$, consider a curved surface $S_2 : u = f(x, y)$, a point P on it, and a tangent A of the curved surface (Fig. 3.8). Consider next a plane that includes a tangent A and the normal of S_2 at P. Then let us obtain an intersecting line C between this plane and the surface S_2. Since C is a curve on a 2D plane, the curvature at a point P can be treated in the frame of 2D geometry. Because the curvature depends on a tangential line A, we call this curvature the normal curvature of the surface S_2 at a point P in the direction A (Fig. 3.8).

Table 3.3. A possible set of principal curvatures in a 4D curved surface.

Number	Simple principal curvature criterion	Absolute value criterion	Mean curvature criterion
1	$k_1 > k_2 > k_3 > 0$	$|k_1| > |k_2| > |k_3| > 0$	$k_1 + k_2 + k_3 > 0$
2	$k_1 > k_2 > k_3 = 0$	$|k_1| > |k_2| > |k_3| = 0$	//
3	$k_1 > k_2 = k_3 > 0$	$|k_1| > |k_2| = |k_3| > 0$	//
4	$k_1 > k_2 = k_3 = 0$	$|k_1| > |k_2| = |k_3| = 0$	//
5	$k_1 = k_2 > k_3 > 0$	$|k_1| = |k_2| > |k_3| > 0$	//
6	$k_1 = k_2 > k_3 = 0$	$|k_1| = |k_2| > |k_3| = 0$	//
7	$k_1 = k_2 = k_3 > 0$	$|k_1| = |k_2| = |k_3| > 0$	//
8	$k_1 = k_2 = k_3 = 0$	$|k_1| = |k_2| = |k_3| = 0$	$k_1 + k_2 + k_3 = 0$
9	$k_1 > k_2 > 0 > k_3$	$|k_1| > |k_2| > |k_3| > 0$	$k_1 + k_2 + k_3 > 0$
10	//	$|k_1| > |k_2| = |k_3| > 0$	//
11	//	$|k_1| > |k_3| > |k_2| > 0$	//
12	//	$|k_1| = |k_3| > |k_2| > 0$	//
13	//	$|k_3| > |k_1| > |k_2| > 0$	//
14	//	//	$k_1 + k_2 + k_3 = 0$
15	//	//	$k_1 + k_2 + k_3 < 0$
16	$k_1 > k_2 = 0 > k_3$	$|k_1| > |k_3| > |k_2| = 0$	$k_1 + k_2 + k_3 > 0$
17	//	$|k_1| = |k_3| > |k_2| = 0$	$k_1 + k_2 + k_3 = 0$
18	//	$|k_3| > |k_1| > |k_2| = 0$	$k_1 + k_2 + k_3 < 0$
19	$k_1 = k_2 > 0 > k_3$	$|k_1| = |k_2| > |k_3| > 0$	$k_1 + k_2 + k_3 > 0$
20	//	$|k_1| = |k_2| = |k_3| > 0$	//
21	//	$|k_3| > |k_1| = |k_2| > 0$	//
22	//	//	$k_1 + k_2 + k_3 = 0$
23	//	//	$k_1 + k_2 + k_3 < 0$
24	$k_1 = k_2 = 0 > k_3$	$|k_3| > |k_1| = |k_2| = 0$	//
25	$k_1 > 0 > k_2 > k_3$	$|k_1| > |k_3| > |k_2| > 0$	$k_1 + k_2 + k_3 > 0$
26	//	//	$k_1 + k_2 + k_3 = 0$
27	//	//	$k_1 + k_2 + k_3 < 0$
28	//	$|k_1| = |k_3| > |k_2| > 0$	//
29	//	$|k_3| > |k_2| > |k_1| > 0$	//
30	//	$|k_3| > |k_1| = |k_2| > 0$	//
31	//	$|k_3| > |k_1| > |k_2| > 0$	//
32	$k_1 > 0 > k_2 = k_3$	$|k_1| > |k_2| = |k_3| > 0$	$k_1 + k_2 + k_3 > 0$
33	//	//	$k_1 + k_2 + k_3 = 0$
34	//	//	$k_1 + k_2 + k_3 < 0$
35	//	$|k_1| = |k_2| = |k_3| > 0$	//
36	//	$|k_2| = |k_3| > |k_1| > 0$	//
37	$k_1 = 0 > k_2 > k_3$	$|k_3| > |k_2| > |k_1| = 0$	//
38	$k_1 = 0 > k_2 = k_3$	$|k_2| = |k_3| > |k_1| = 0$	//
39	$0 > k_1 > k_2 > k_3$	$|k_3| > |k_2| > |k_1| > 0$	//
40	$0 > k_1 > k_2 = k_3$	$|k_2| = |k_3| > |k_1| > 0$	//
41	$0 > k_1 = k_2 > k_3$	$|k_3| > |k_2| = |k_1| > 0$	//
42	$0 > k_1 = k_2 = k_3$	$|k_1| = |k_2| = |k_3| > 0$	//

The normal curvature $k(A)$ varies as a function of the direction A when we rotate the tangential line A around the normal of the surface S_2 at a point P. Then the maximum k_1 and the minimum k_2 of $k(A)$ and other values calculated from them are called as follows. They are regarded as features of local shape of the surface.

k_1, k_2 ; principal curvature $\hspace{6cm}$ (3.50)

$H = (k_1 + k_2)/2$; mean curvature $\hspace{4.5cm}$ (3.51)

$K = k_1 \cdot k_2$; total curvature or Gauss curvature $\hspace{2.8cm}$ (3.52)

Directions of tangents corresponding to k_1 and k_2 ; principal directions (3.53)

The outline of local shapes on a surface of a 2D image (or a 3D surface) is illustrated in Fig. 3.8 and Table 3.4.

3.5 Region growing (region merging)

3.5.1 Outline

A procedure called *region growing* (*region merging*) or more generally most region-based segmentation procedures can be applied to a 3D image directly. We will only explain them briefly.

   Region growing is a procedure starting from suitably selected set of voxels (initial regions, initial voxels) and expands them sequentially by adding adjacent voxels or regions while incorporating predetermined conditions. The core of the region-growing algorithm consists of the following three parts:

(i) Selection of starting voxels (or regions).
(ii) Expansion (growing, merging) of regions .
(iii) Testing of terminating condition.

There are two typical procedures for the third step: a fixed rule (a *procedure-independent rule*) and a *procedure-dependent rule*. For example, a maximum voxel number for a region may be given beforehand (procedure-independent rule). Alternatively, the procedure may be terminated unless a new voxel involved in a merging condition is found (a procedure-dependent rule).

3.5.2 Region expansion

The kernel of the algorithm is the iterative execution of the second and the third step of the above procedure summarized as follows:

Algorithm 3.1 (Region growing). Iterate the following for $k = 1, 2, \ldots$. Denote by R_k the region that has been detected when the k-th iteration of processing starts. For $k = 1, R_1$ has been assumed to be given by the other procedure.

Table 3.4. The classification of local shapes in a 3D curved surface: (**a**) Classification by principal curvatures k_1 and k_2; (**b**) classification by Gaussian curvature K and mean curvature H.

(**a**)

	$k_2 < 0$	$k_2 = 0$	$k_2 > 0$
$k_1 < 0$	peak	ridge line	saddle
$k_1 = 0$	ridge line	planar	valley line
$k_1 > 0$	saddle	valley line	hollow

(**b**)

	$K > 0$ (elliptic)	$K = 0$	$K < 0$ (saddle like)
$H < 0$	peak	ridge line	saddle (ridge-line like)
$H = 0$		planar	minimal surface
$H > 0$	hollow	valley line	saddle (valley-line like)

(1) Stop if a given terminating rule is satisfied. Otherwise, select candidate of a voxel or a set of voxels r_k (test) to be added to R_k according to the procedure given beforehand. Stop if a candidate voxel set is not found.

(2) Calculate features of r_k (test) and test whether they satisfy the criteria for expansion (or merging).

(3) Replace R_k by $R_k \cup r_k$ (test) if r_k(test) meets the criteria. $k \leftarrow k+1$, and go to (1). Otherwise stop.

(4) If there exist more than one candidate sets r_k (test) in (1), execute (1) $\sim$ (3) for all of them. If more than one R_k exists when the whole of the procedure starts, apply (1) $\sim$ (3) for all of them.

The most important steps of the algorithm are the criteria for expansion in (2) and selection of the candidate set in (1). Both of them determine the performance of the algorithm. Examples that used (2) are many of the algorithms:

(a) A set of voxels with properties similar to those in regions already extracted.

(b) A set of voxels neighboring to voxels extracted past or connected to them in the predetermined way.

Voxels of density values within a suitable range around the average voxel density previously extracted, that are 26-adjacent to regions extracted in the past, are examples of the simplest criteria.

The expansion process may be executed either sequentially or in parallel. A candidate may be tested and merged as soon as it is detected. In the other case, after all possible candidates have been detected at a suitable time point, they may be tested and merged at the same time.

Region growing is the grouping of voxels or is regarded as a kind of clustering of voxels based upon their features. Geometrical features, in particular, with properties relating to connectivity are taken into account during the execution of the algorithm. The region growing used was effective to extract the whole of a region connected to the starting regions. In order to extract more than one separate object the entire procedure must be repeated many times.

Region growing is frequently used in the processing of 3D CT images in medicine, to segmentate organs in the human body such as the bronchus and chest vessels, the stomach, liver, colon etc [Kitasaka02a, Yokoyama03]. Region growing is suitable to extract the entire objects spreading in a relatively large area in an input 3D image. However, detection of a smooth surface and deciding on exact locations of borders are difficult to accomplish by region growing only [Duda01].

4

GEOMETRICAL PROPERTIES OF 3D DIGITIZED IMAGES

A digitized binary image contains only two groups of voxels, 1-voxels and 0-voxels. We assume for now that we have interest in the set of 1-voxels and will call it a *figure*. The other set we call the *background*. Properties of a digitized figure are often very different from those of ordinary figures in the continuous space. Treating geometrical properties of digitized figures is called *digital geometry*. In this chapter, we briefly introduce the basics of digital geometry before discussing them further. The most important basic concepts of digital geometry are shown in Fig. 4.1.

In Section 4.1, after introducing the basic concepts of neighborhood and connectivity, we discuss three important topological features including genus, connectivity indexes, and the relationship between them. Then we explain the concept of deletability of 1-voxels and the condition under which an arbitrary algorithm preserves topological features of a figure in a binary image. We also show a simple proof of this condition using the above topological features.

In this chapter we will deal with binary images only. We assume that images consist of cubic voxel arrays of I rows, J columns, and K planes. It is also assumed that the first row, the I-th row, the first column, the J-th column, the first plane, and the K-th plane are all filled with 0-voxels. These rows, columns, and planes are called the *frame* of an image.

4.1 Neighborhood and connectivity

4.1.1 Neighborhood

As is shown in Fig. 4.1, we will start the discussion of geometrical properties of a binary image with the neighborhood and the connectivity and will introduce a connected component. As it was already stated in Section 2.4.2 we define the neighborhood as follows:

Definition 4.1 (Neighborhood). The *neighborhood* of a voxel (i, j, k), denoted by $\mathcal{N}_{ijk}((i, j, k))$, is defined by the equation

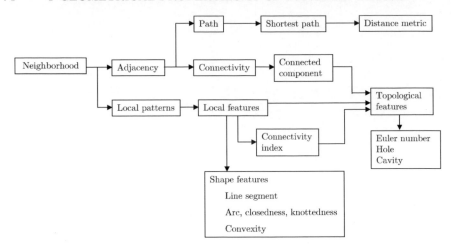

Fig. 4.1. Basic concept of digital geometry.

$$\mathcal{N}_{ijk} \equiv \{(i+p, j+q, k+r); (p,q,r) \in \mathcal{S}'_{ijk}\}\ \ \mathcal{S}' \subset \mathcal{S}(\equiv I \times I \times I), \qquad (4.1)$$

where I is the set of all integers and $\mathcal{S}'_{ijk}$ is a suitably given set of integer triads.

Here we consider only the neighborhood that does not depend on the position (i, j, k). Examples of the neighborhood were given in Table 2.4 and Fig. 4.2. Three of them – the 6-neighborhood, the 18-neighborhood, and the 26-neighborhood – are most frequently used in practical applications and often denoted in the following way (Fig. 4.2)

$$\mathcal{N}^{[6]}(\boldsymbol{x}_0) = \{\boldsymbol{x}_p, p \in S_1\}, \qquad (4.2)$$

$$\mathcal{N}^{[18]}(\boldsymbol{x}_0) = \{\boldsymbol{x}_p, p \in S_1 \cup S_2\}, \qquad (4.3)$$

$$\mathcal{N}^{[26]}(\boldsymbol{x}_0) = \{\boldsymbol{x}_p, p \in S_1 \cup S_2 \cup S_3\}, \qquad (4.4)$$

where S_1, S_2, and S_3 are sets of integers and show the numbers given to voxels in $3 \times 3 \times 3$ neighborhood as in Fig. 4.2. We also use two other numbering systems as shown in the system T and U in Fig. 4.2.

Remark 4.1. Considering a voxel is a cube in a digitized image, then

(i) any of voxels in the 6-neighborhood of a voxel $\boldsymbol{x}$ shares at least one face of the voxel $\boldsymbol{x}$,

(ii) any of voxels in the 18-neighborhood of a voxel $\boldsymbol{x}$ shares at least one edge of the voxel $\boldsymbol{x}$,

(iii) any of voxels in the 26-neighborhood of a voxel $\boldsymbol{x}$ shares at least one vertex of the voxel $\boldsymbol{x}$.

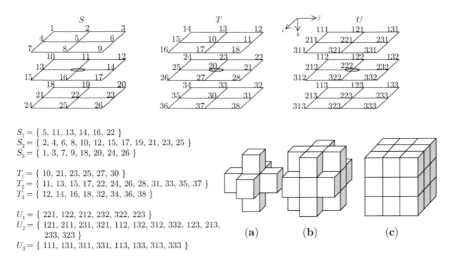

$S_1 = \{ 5, 11, 13, 14, 16, 22 \}$
$S_2 = \{ 2, 4, 6, 8, 10, 12, 15, 17, 19, 21, 23, 25 \}$
$S_3 = \{ 1, 3, 7, 9, 18, 20, 24, 26 \}$

$T_1 = \{ 10, 21, 23, 25, 27, 30 \}$
$T_2 = \{ 11, 13, 15, 17, 22, 24, 26, 28, 31, 33, 35, 37 \}$
$T_3 = \{ 12, 14, 16, 18, 32, 34, 36, 38 \}$

$U_1 = \{ 221, 122, 212, 232, 322, 223 \}$
$U_2 = \{ 121, 211, 231, 321, 112, 132, 312, 332, 123, 213,$
$\qquad 233, 323 \}$
$U_3 = \{ 111, 131, 311, 331, 113, 133, 313, 333 \}$

(a)   **(b)**   **(c)**

Fig. 4.2. Notations of voxels in the neighborhood and three basic neighborhoods: **(a)** 6-neighborhood $= S_1$; **(b)** 18-neighborhood $= S_1 \cup S_2$; **(c)** 26-neighborhood $= S_1 \cup S_2 \cup S_3$.

If two voxels $\boldsymbol{x}$ and $\boldsymbol{y}$ satisfy the relation "$\boldsymbol{x} \in \mathcal{N}^{[6]}(\boldsymbol{y})$," it is said that $\boldsymbol{x}$ and $\boldsymbol{y}$ are 6-adjacent to, each other, or that $\boldsymbol{x}$ is 6-adjacent to $\boldsymbol{y}$, etc. The 18- and 26-adjacency are also defined in the same way.

Remark 4.2. If the neighborhood of a voxel (i, j, k) is symmetrical in respect to (i, j, k), $\boldsymbol{x} \in \mathcal{N}^{[k]}(\boldsymbol{y})$ implies $\boldsymbol{y} \in \mathcal{N}^{[k]}(\boldsymbol{x})$, and vice versa. This is not always true otherwise or if the neighborhood is asymmetrical.

Remark 4.3. As was stated in Section 2.4.2, a neighborhood of a voxel $\boldsymbol{x}$ in general may or may not contain the voxel $\boldsymbol{x}$ itself. For example, the 6- and the 26- neighborhood of $\boldsymbol{x}$ does not contain the central voxel $\boldsymbol{x}$, but the $K \times L \times M$ neighborhood of $\boldsymbol{x}$ includes the voxel $\boldsymbol{x}$.

4.1.2 Connectivity and connected component

Let us define the concept of connectivity between two voxels based on the neighborhood.

Definition 4.2 (Connectivity). Two voxels $\boldsymbol{x}_1$ and $\boldsymbol{x}_2$ with a common value are said to be 6-*connected* (18-*connected*, 26-*connected*), if a sequence of voxels $\boldsymbol{y}_0(= \boldsymbol{x}_1), \boldsymbol{y}_1, \ldots, \boldsymbol{y}_n(= \boldsymbol{x}_2)$ exists, such that each $\boldsymbol{y}_i$ is in the 6-neighborhood (18-neighborhood, 26-neighborhood) of $\boldsymbol{y}_{i-1}(\forall i(1 \leq i \leq n)$ and all $\boldsymbol{y}_i$s have the same value as $\boldsymbol{x}_1$ and $\boldsymbol{x}_2$. It is clear that 6-connectedness, 18-connectedness, and 26-connectedness thus defined gives a kind of *equivalence relationship* among voxels with the value *1* (or value *0*).

Remark 4.4 (Equivalence relationship). Given a set, assuming two arbitrary elements of the set, we can decide whether a predetermined relationship "∼" holds or not. If the relationship "∼" satisfies all of the following laws, we call it an *equivalence relationship*.

(i) $x \sim x$ (reflective law)
(ii) If $x \sim y$, then $y \sim x$ (symmetric law)
(iii) If $x \sim y$ and $y \sim z$, then $x \sim z$ (transitive law)

If $x \sim y$, it is said that x *is equivalent to* y. The set of all voxels equivalent to a voxel x is called an *equivalence class* of x.

Definition 4.3 (Connected component). All voxels in an image can be classified into different classes by making voxels connected to each other belong to the same class. Each class derived from this procedure is called a *connected component*. More precisely, each equivalence class of voxels defined by 6-connectedness is called a 6-connected component. An 18-connected component and a 26-connected component are defined in a similar way. A connected component of 0-voxels is called a 0-*component*, and that of 1-voxels is called a 1-*component*.

Definition 4.4 (Cavity). Any connected component of 0-voxels that is not connected to the frame of an image is called a *cavity*.

Definition 4.5 (Hole, handle). Let us consider a connected component of 1-voxels C. Then consider a figure F_C in the continuous space obtained by combining all 1-voxels in C. Each 1-voxel is treated as a cube here. The figure F_C is called a *continuous figure corresponding to* C. The surface of this continuous figure F_C is a closed curved surface in the continuous 3D space. Then if this closed surface has a hole (handle), we call this hole (handle) a *hole* (*handle*) of the connected component C (Fig. 4.3).

Definition 4.6 (Simply connected, multiply connected). A connected component of 1-voxels with none of hole and cavity is said to be *simply connected*, and otherwise, *multiply connected*.

Remark 4.5 (18′-Connectivity). Although any of 6-, 18-, or 26-connectivity may be adopted for the analysis of any particular problem, care must be taken to avoid a contradiction concerning the connectivity of 1-voxels and that of 0-voxels. It is required that only the pairs of connectivity listed in Table 4.1 are used. Here the 18′-connectivity is introduced for preserving theoretical consistency. Definitions of the 18′-connectivity and the 18′ neighborhood are the same as those of the 6-connectivity except the configuration given in Fig. 4.4. This local configuration of six voxels is regarded as a plane of six voxels in the 18′-connectivity case and as a loop of six voxels in the 6-connectivity case.

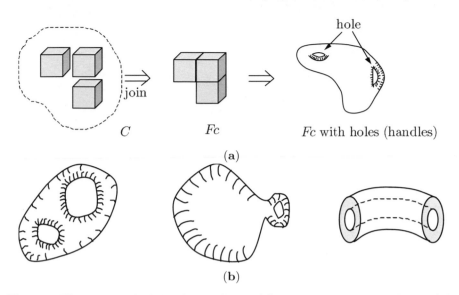

Fig. 4.3. Illustration of a hole of a 3D figure: (**a**), and a few examples of holes (**b**). A figure in the left of (**b**) has two holes and the other two have one hole for each.

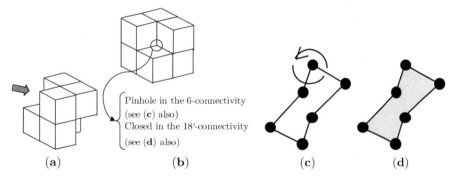

Fig. 4.4. Illustration of 18′-connectivity: All voxels drawn here are 1-voxels and 0-voxels are not presented here. This configuration is regarded as a loop in the 6-connectivity (**c**), and as a surface in the 18′-connectivity (**d**).

There may be more than one (occasionally large numbers of) connected components in a 3D input image. On the computer, we distinguish each component from each other giving it a label. One method to assign a label to a component is to store an integer to each 1-voxel in such a way that all 1-voxels belonging to the same component have the same integer value, and 1-voxels of different components have different integers. This integer is called a *label* of a component, and the procedure to give labels to all 1-voxels is called *labeling*. A labeling algorithm will be shown in the next chapter.

Table 4.1. Acceptable pairs of connectivity for 1-voxels and 0-voxels.

1-voxel m	0-voxel $\underline{m}$
6-connectivity	26-connectivity
18-connectivity	18$'$-connectivity
18$'$-connectivity	18-connectivity
26-connectivity	6-connectivity

Remark 4.6. Labels usually will be positive integers because the value *0* is used as the label of the background.

There may exist more than one holes and cavities in one component. A continuous figure corresponding to a 1-component in Definition 4.5 has the same number of closed surfaces of cavities as that of cavities, in addition to the outside surface of the component. A hole may exist on either of an outside surface and a surface of a cavity. Examples of a handle are a center hole of a doughnut, a floater, a coffee cup with a handle (one hole), a pot with two handles, an eyeglass frame, pants (two holes), and the sponge (many holes). Conceptually, a hole in a 2D figure corresponds to a cavity of a 3D figure. A hole (handle) is the concept specific to a 3D figure.

Remark 4.7. It seems that an explicit definition of a handle (or a hole) in a 3D figure has not been given in literature. In [Lee93], for example, the number of handles was explained from the viewpoint of the "nonseparating cut." Also *linkage* and the *knot* of a 3D figure were discussed also, although algorithms to treat them were not been shown.

For a continuous 3D figure, on the other hand, the following is known as one possible definition. Consider a division of a 1-component C into a set of simplexes. Then the number of handles (holes) of the 1-component C is defined as the number of independent 1D homology classes.

4.2 Simplex and simplicial decomposition

Simplex is one of most basic concepts in the study of topological properties for a continuous figure. This is a typical example of a figure representing all figures of each dimension as a concrete form realizing the concept of dimensionality. For example, a point (zero dimension), a closed segment (one-dimension), a triangle (two-dimension) and a tetrahedron (three-dimension) are simplexes of lower dimensions.

We need to extend these simplexes to a digitized image. One way to perform this is given in Fig. 4.5.

Definitions of them are given as follows.

Definition 4.7 (Simplex). *Simplexes* used for decomposition of a 3D digitized image should be defined as follows:

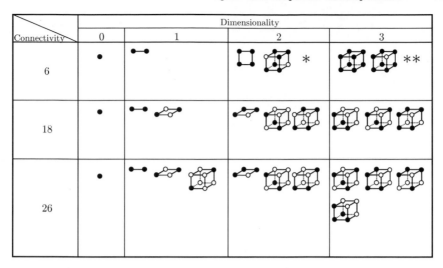

Fig. 4.5. Simplexes in a 3D figure: Black circles show 1-voxels and white ones 0-voxels. In the 18′-connectivity case a pattern with ∗ is added to the 6-connectivity case, and only the pattern with ∗∗ is considered as a 3D simplex.

(1) 0-simplex = each of 1-voxels.
(2) 1-simplex = pair of two 1-voxels neighboring each other.
(3) 2-simplex = a set of three 1-voxels, any one of which is adjacent to the remaining two voxels, or a set of four voxels that exist on the same plane and any one of which is adjacent to two of the remaining three voxels.
(4) 3-simplex = a set of four 1-voxels, any one of which is adjacent to all of the remaining three voxels, or a set of five or more 1-voxels that do not exist on the same plane and make a closed polyhedron with the minimum number of faces.

The 1-, 2-, and 3-simplexes are called *edge element*, *face element*, and *volume element*, respectively. Concrete forms of simplexes vary according to the type of the connectivity. We show in Fig. 4.5 all of the different possible simplexes for four types of connectivity.

Let us assume that a figure is given in the 3D space and let us express this figure as the set sum of simplexes. This expression in the form of the set sum is called *simplicial decomposition* if it satisfies the following requirements (Fig. 4.6).

(1) Neighboring two face elements share only one common 1-voxel or share only one common edge element.
(2) Connections between a face element and an edge element happen either in the form that one of vertexes of the edge element coincides with one of vertexes of the face element or that the edge element coincides with one of edges of the face element.

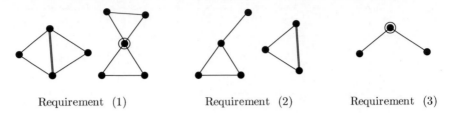

Requirement (1)   Requirement (2)   Requirement (3)

Fig. 4.6. Illustration of requirements to the simplicial decomposition.

(3) Two edge elements are connected by one common vertex only.

The simplicious decomposition for a given 3D image is not always uniquely determined for a given figure.

4.3 Euler number

We will now introduce a widely used topological property of a figure called the Euler number or the genus.

Definition 4.8 (Euler number, genus). Consider a 3D digitized figure C and its simplicious decomposition. Then the *Euler number* (*genus*) $\mathcal{E}$ of a figure (a connected component) C is defined by

$$\mathcal{E}(C) = n_0 - n_1 + n_2 - n_3, \tag{4.5}$$

where n_ks denote the numbers of k-dimensional simplexes (k-simplexes). The value of the Euler number varies according to the type of the connectivity.

The following equation is known as *Euler-Poincare's formula* in the field of topology.

Property 4.1.
$$\mathcal{E} = b_0 - b_1 + b_2, \tag{4.6}$$

where b_0 = number of 1-components (0-dimensional Betti number), b_1 = number of holes in all of 1-components (1-dimensional Betti number), b_2 = number of cavities in all of 1-components (2-dimensional Betti number). For a given binary image $\boldsymbol{F}$, the sum of the Euler numbers of all connected components in $\boldsymbol{F}$ is called the Euler number of an image $\boldsymbol{F}$.

Remark 4.8. The Euler number $\mathcal{E}(C)$ of a 3D figure C defined above is intuitively described as follows.

$$\mathcal{E}(C) = 1 - \text{the number of handle in } C + \text{the number of cavities in } C. \tag{4.7}$$

For the whole of a binary image F that includes more than one figure in it, the following is obtained by adding the above equation over all the figures in F. The Euler number of an image F,

$$
\begin{aligned}
\mathcal{E}(F) = \ & \text{the number of connected components in } F \\
& - \text{the number of handles in } F \\
& + \text{the number of cavities in } F
\end{aligned} \tag{4.8}
$$

Remark 4.9. The Euler number of a 3D figure C is alternatively given by the Euler number of a continuous figure defined in Definition 4.5. If we need to differentiate the Euler number by Def. 4.8 and the one using the above method, the one by Def. 4.8 is called the *volume Euler number*, and the above one the *face Euler number*. A 3D figure of the minimum size occupies at least one voxel. Its boundary surface is a closed surface and has a cavity inside it. Therefore, the face Euler number is

$$
1 - 0 (= \text{number of handles}) \ + 1 (= \text{number of cavities}) \ = 2. \tag{4.9}
$$

If a figure does not have a handle, the face Euler number is twice the volume Euler number.

Remark 4.10. For a 2D image the Euler number $\mathcal{E}_{2D}$ was defined as

$$
\mathcal{E}_{2D} = \text{the number of connected component } - \text{the number of holes .} \tag{4.10}
$$

The natural extension of this to a 3D image is the volume Euler number.

4.4 Local feature of a connected component and topology of a figure

A topological property of a 3D binary image is summarized in numbers of connected components, handles, and cavities. The number of connected components is apparent in the labeling. Algorithms will be presented in the next chapter. The number of cavities also can be found in the same way after inverting 1 and 0 of a given image. The number of handles is presently difficult to count directly.

Counting numbers of simplexes (n_0, n_1, n_2, n_3, in Eq. 4.5) is an exhaustive procedure and requires much computation time. Then, by using Eq. 4.5 and by solving Eq. 4.6 or 4.7 with respect to the number of holes, the number of holes is indirectly known.

An image processing algorithm changes shapes of 3D figures in an input image by replacing parts of 1-voxels by 0-voxels and 0-voxels by 1-voxels. Then, if none of the following occur by the execution of the algorithm, this algorithm (or processing) is said to be *topology-preserving* (or *to preserve topology*):

(1) separation of a connected component, hole, and cavity
(2) vanishment of a connected component, a hole, and a cavity
(3) creation of a new hole, cavity, and connected component

We have here a local feature which is effective in knowing shape features relating to topology. Let us introduce several such features below.

Definition 4.9 (Deletability). A 1-voxel x is *deletable* (strictly, m-*deletable* where m represents the type of connectivity; $m = 6, 18, 18', 26$), if its deletion (= conversion into a 0-voxel) preserves topology of an input image.

Definition 4.10 (Connectivity number). The *connectivity number* (CN) $Nc^{(m)}(x)$ at a 1-voxel x is defined as follows:

$$Nc^m(x) = \mathcal{E}^{(m)}(\underline{x}) - \mathcal{E}^{(m)}(x) + 1, \qquad (4.11)$$

where $\mathcal{E}^{(m)}(x)$ and $\mathcal{E}^{(m)}(\underline{x})$ denote the values of the Euler number of a 3D figure before and after deletion of a 1-voxel x, respectively, and m denotes the type of connectivity ($m = 6, 18, 18'$, and 26).

Definition 4.11 (Connectivity index). In a $3 \times 3 \times 3$ neighborhood consisting of a 1-voxel x and its 26-neighborhood, we define the following three features, called *component index*, *hole index*, and *cavity index*, respectively.

Component index $R^{(m)}(x)$ = the number of m-connected components that are connected to x and exist in the 18-neighborhood for $m = 6$ and $18'$ (in the 26-neighborhood for $m = 18$ and 26). (The subpattern Q_{63} of Table 4.4 is exceptionally regarded as a single connected component for $m = 18'$).

Hole index $H^{(m)}(x)$ = the number of holes that are newly created by deletion of x, or equivalently the decrease in the number of m-connected components of 0-voxels in this subarea caused by deletion of x.

Cavity index $Y^{(m)}(x)$ = the number of cavities that are created by deleting x.

We call the triad $(R^{(m)}(x), H^{(m)}(x), Y^{(m)}(x))$ *connectivity index* at a voxel x.

Let us discuss several properties of these features. Values of these features depend on each 1-voxel x and the type of connectivity m. They represent topological properties of a local shape at x and in its $3 \times 3 \times 3$ neighborhood.

Property 4.2. The connectivity number $Nc^{(m)}(x)$ at a 1-voxel x is equal to the total amount of change Δ in the connectivity index at a voxel x caused by deletion of the 1-voxel x, that is,

$$\Delta = \text{change in the number of connected components}$$
$$- \text{change in the number of holes}$$
$$+ \text{change in the number of cavities} + 1 \qquad (4.12)$$

(Proof) The connectivity number $Nc^{(m)}(\boldsymbol{x})$ was defined as the change in the Euler number caused by the deletion of a 1-voxel $\boldsymbol{x}$ (Def. 4.10). Since the Euler number is represented as Eq. 4.5, Eq. 4.6, and Eq. 4.7, the above relation is derived immediately.

Remark 4.11. The change in the Euler number caused by the deletion of a 1-voxel $\boldsymbol{x}$ (i.e., the connectivity number) is also written as follows using the amount of change in Betti numbers.

$$Nc^{(m)}(\boldsymbol{x}) = 1 + \Delta b_0^{(m)} - \Delta b_1^{(m)} + \Delta b_2^{(m)}, \tag{4.13}$$

where $\Delta b_k^{(m)} = b_k^{(m)'} - b_k^{(m)}$, $k = 0, 1, 2$, $m = 6, 18, 18', 26$; $b_k^{(m)}$ and $b_k^{(m)'}$ are Betti numbers of the order k before and after deletion of the 1-voxel $\boldsymbol{x}$, respectively, and m denotes the type of connectivity.

Theorem 4.1. The following relation holds at an arbitrary 1-voxel $\boldsymbol{x}$ among the connectivity number $Nc^{(m)}(\boldsymbol{x})$ and the connectivity index $(R^{(m)}(\boldsymbol{x}), H^{(m)}(\boldsymbol{x}), Y^{(m)}(\boldsymbol{x}))$.

$$Nc^{(m)}(\boldsymbol{x}) = R^{(m)}(\boldsymbol{x}) - H^{(m)}(\boldsymbol{x}) + Y^{(m)}(\boldsymbol{x}) \tag{4.14}$$

where m ($m = 6, 18, 18', 26$) denotes the type of connectivity.

(Proof) See [Toriwaki02a, Toriwaki02b].

Property 4.3. Let $\boldsymbol{X} = \{\boldsymbol{x}_{10}, \boldsymbol{x}_{11}, \ldots, \boldsymbol{x}_{38}\}$ ($\boldsymbol{x}_{20}$ is excluded) denote a set of 26 voxels in the 26-neighborhood of the voxel $\boldsymbol{x}_{20}$ in Fig. 4.2. Let us regard in this notation an arbitrary 1-voxel $\boldsymbol{x}$ as $\boldsymbol{x}_{20}$ in Fig. 4.2 T. By using the notation $Nc^{(m)}(\boldsymbol{X}, \boldsymbol{x})$ instead of $Nc^{(m)}(\boldsymbol{x})$ so that we may show explicitly that the connectivity number (CN) depends on a set $\boldsymbol{X}$ as well as $\boldsymbol{x}$ itself, the following equations hold

$$Nc^{(26)}(\boldsymbol{X}, \boldsymbol{x}) = 2 - Nc^{(6)}(\underline{\boldsymbol{X}}, \underline{\boldsymbol{x}}),$$
$$Nc^{(18)}(\boldsymbol{X}, \boldsymbol{x}) = 2 - Nc^{(18')}(\underline{\boldsymbol{X}}, \underline{\boldsymbol{x}}), \tag{4.15}$$

where $\underline{\boldsymbol{X}}$ is a set of variables that are complements of elements of $\boldsymbol{X}$, that is, $\underline{\boldsymbol{X}} = \{\underline{\boldsymbol{x}}_{10}, \underline{\boldsymbol{x}}_{11}, \ldots, \underline{\boldsymbol{x}}_{38}\}$, where $\underline{\boldsymbol{x}}_{ij} = 1 - \boldsymbol{x}_{ij}$. $Nc^{(6)}(\underline{\boldsymbol{X}}, \underline{\boldsymbol{x}})$ represents the value of the CN for the configuration consisting of $\underline{\boldsymbol{x}}$ and $\underline{\boldsymbol{X}}$, instead of $\boldsymbol{x}$ and $\boldsymbol{X}$ [Toriwaki02a, Toriwaki02b].

(Proof) Note that each term relating to a voxel $\boldsymbol{x}$ in the equations to calculate the Euler number in Eq. 4.8 is also a function of the set $\boldsymbol{X}$ and the variable $\boldsymbol{x}$. Denote this term by $\Delta\mathcal{E}(\boldsymbol{X}, \boldsymbol{x})$. Then, by the definition of the CN,

$$\begin{aligned}
Nc^{(26)}(\boldsymbol{X}, \boldsymbol{x}) &= \Delta\mathcal{E}^{(26)}(\boldsymbol{X}, \underline{\boldsymbol{x}}) - \Delta\mathcal{E}^{(26)}(\boldsymbol{X}, \boldsymbol{x}) + 1 \\
&= \Delta\mathcal{E}^{(6)}(\underline{\boldsymbol{X}}, \underline{\boldsymbol{x}}) - \Delta\mathcal{E}^{(6)}(\underline{\boldsymbol{X}}, \boldsymbol{x}) + 1 \\
&= -(Nc^{(6)}(\underline{\boldsymbol{X}}, \boldsymbol{x}) - 1) + 1 \\
&= 2 - Nc^{(6)}(\underline{\boldsymbol{X}}, \boldsymbol{x}).
\end{aligned} \tag{4.16}$$

The second equation in Eq. 4.15 is also derived in the same way. Note here Eq. 4.48 and Eq. 4.49 which will be derived later.

A similar relationship holds concerning the connectivity index (R, H, Y) as is given below.

Property 4.4. Let us adopt the same notation as in Property 4.3 above, and let us express the connectivity index of the 1-voxel x_{20} by $(R^{(m)}(X, x), H^{(m)}(X, x), Y^{(m)}(X, x))$ instead of $(R^{(m)}(x), H^{(m)}(x), Y^{(m)}(x))$ so that dependency on the set X may be explicitly shown. If we define a set $\underline{X} = \{\underline{x}_{10}, \underline{x}_{11}, \ldots, \underline{x}_{38}\}$, where $\underline{x}_{ij} = 1 - x_{ij}$ as in Property 4.3, and if we denote by $(R^{(m)}(\underline{X}, x), H^{(m)}(\underline{X}, x), Y^{(m)}(\underline{X}, x))$ the connectivity index of x with the local subpattern $\underline{X}$ in its 26-neighborhood, the following relations hold.

$$R^{(6)}(X, x) - 1 = H^{(26)}(\underline{X}, x) - Y^{(26)}(\underline{X}, x)$$
$$R^{(26)}(X, x) - 1 = H^{(6)}(\underline{X}, x) - Y^{(6)}(\underline{X}, x)$$
$$R^{(18)}(X, x) - 1 = H^{(18')}(\underline{X}, x) - Y^{(18')}(\underline{X}, x)$$
$$R^{(18')}(X, x) - 1 = H^{(18)}(\underline{X}, x) - Y^{(18)}(\underline{X}, x). \tag{4.17}$$

Furthermore, $Y^{(m)}(\underline{X}, x) = 1$ if and only if $R^{(m)}(\underline{X}, x) = H^{(m)}(\underline{X}, x) = 0$, and otherwise, $Y^{(m)}(\underline{X}, x) = 0$ [Toriwaki02a, Toriwaki02b].

Theorem 4.2. Assuming that the density values of a 1-voxel x and its 26-neighborhood are given, the 1-voxel x is m-deletable if and only if the connectivity index $(R^{(m)}(x), H^{(m)}(x), Y^{(m)}(x)) = (1, 0, 0)$.

(Proof) A 1-voxel x is not deletable if it is a 3D interior voxel, that is, $Y^{(m)}(x) = 1$. Therefore, $Y^{(m)}(x)$ should be equal to zero for x to be m-deletable. Let us assume that by deleting a 1-voxel x with the connectivity index $(l, n, 0)$, α connected components and β holes are created and β' holes and γ cavities vanish. Then, $l = \alpha + \beta + 1$, and $n = \beta' + \gamma$. A voxel x is deletable if and only if

$$\alpha = \beta = \beta' = \gamma = 0. \tag{4.18}$$

Eq. 4.18 is equivalent to "$l = 1$ and $n = 0$" [Toriwaki02a, Toriwaki02b].

Corollary 4.1. 1-voxel x is m-deletable if and only if

$$Nc^{(m)}(x) = 1 \text{ and } R^{(m)} = 1. \tag{4.19}$$

For a 2D image, preservation of the values of the Euler characteristic is a necessary and sufficient condition of the topology preservation. That is, to test the deletability of a 1-pixel in a 2D figure, calculation of the Euler characteristic is enough. In a 3D image, on the contrary, preservation of the Euler characteristic does not always mean the deletability of a 1-voxel. The reason is the existence of a hole (handle). By deleting a 1-voxel, separation of a

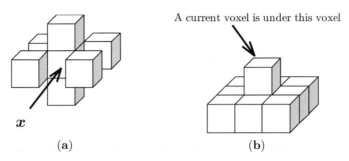

Fig. 4.7. Example of deletability: Denoting a current voxel by $\boldsymbol{x}$, (a) $Nc^{(6)}(\boldsymbol{x}) = Nc^{(18')}(\boldsymbol{x}) = 2, Nc^{(18)}(\boldsymbol{x}) = 6, Nc^{(26)}(\boldsymbol{x}) = -2$; (b) $Nc(\boldsymbol{x}) = 1$ for all types of connectivity. The left case is not always deletable. The right case is deletable for the 18- and the 26-connectivity.

connected component (increase in the Euler number by *1*) and creation of a handle (decrease in the Euler number by *1*) may occur at the same time. Such an example is illustrated in Fig. 4.7. For testing the deletability condition, we need to know values of the connectivity index $(R^{(m)}(\boldsymbol{x}), H^{(m)}(\boldsymbol{x}), Y^{(m)}(\boldsymbol{x}))$ or the connectivity number $Nc^{(m)}(\boldsymbol{x})$ and the component index $R^{(m)}(\boldsymbol{x})$. Calculation of these features is not so easy. Procedures will be presented in detail in the subsequent sections.

Remark 4.12. A deletable voxel in the sense used here is called a simple point in the literature. A method to test whether an arbitrary voxel is a simple point or not for all of four types of connectivity was first reported in [Yonekura80a, Yonekura80b, Yonekura80c, Yonekura82a, Yonekura82b, Yonekura82c, Yonekura82d]. This method is distinguished also in that explicit expressions for the deletability test were given as a set of pseudo - Boolean expressions. Several papers on the test of a simple point have been published [Bertrand94a, Bertrand94b, Bertrand96, Saha94, Bykov99, Molgouyres99, Molgouyres00]. Most of them are related to thinning algorithms of a 3D image.They presented conditions for local patterns of 0- and 1-voxels and discussed only the 6- and 26-connectivity cases. Most papers studying thinning or shrinking algorithms and their characteristics concerning topology preservation include consideration of simple point detection [Toriwaki02a, Toriwaki02b].

4.5 Local patterns and their characterization

Algorithms of local operations in binary image processing are designed by considering all possible arrangements of 1- and 0-voxels in a local area. In fact concrete contents of algorithms are fixed by giving output values correspond-

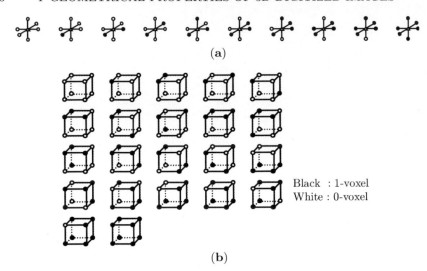

Fig. 4.8. Local patterns in the 6-neighborhood and $2 \times 2 \times 2$ local areas: (**a**) Local patterns in the 6-neighborhood. (Total is 20 cases. Figures show only the cases in which the center is a 0-voxel. Patterns symmetric to these are neglected.); (**b**) All $2 \times 2 \times 2$ local patterns.

ing to individual local pattern of an input image. The minimum size of a local area is $2 \times 2 \times 2$ voxels and the second smallest is $3 \times 3 \times 3$ voxels.

There are $2^8 = 256$ different binary patterns and $2^{27} = 134,217,728$ patterns for these local areas, respectively. This means 2^a local functions are possible, where $a = 2^8$ and 2^{27} for $2 \times 2 \times 2$ and $3 \times 3 \times 3$ neighborhoods, respectively. They will be too large to be treated by a simple exhaustive enumeration or by other intuitive methods. To understand features of each $3 \times 3 \times 3$ pattern is not easy work even for the human visual system. Thus suitable quantitative features characterizing individual patterns or a subclass of patterns are strongly desired. The connectivity index and the connectivity number introduced in the previous section are such examples.

4.5.1 $2 \times 2 \times 2$ local patterns

All $2 \times 2 \times 2$ local patterns are enumerated without much difficulty. In, fact, only 22 cases exist after excluding rotation symmetry pairs and line symmetry pairs. All of these 22 cases are shown in Fig. 4.8.

Remark 4.13. Let us present three examples of applications of $2 \times 2 \times 2$ patterns.

(a) Calculation of the Euler number: The Euler number of a 3D figure is calculated by enumerating $2 \times 2 \times 2$ patterns. Details are presented in Section 4.7.

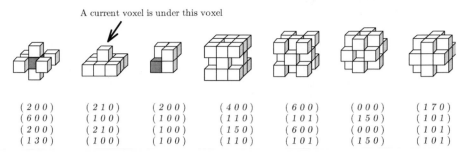

Fig. 4.9. Examples of values of connectivity index for complicated local patterns. Numbers in parenthesis show connectivity indexes (component index, hole index, cavity index). From top to bottom, 6-, 18-, 18'-, and 26-connectivity cases are given. Note that the 18-neighborhood is used in calculating the component index of the 6-connectivity case.

(b) Simplex: 3D simplexes and lower dimensional ones are found by searching $2 \times 2 \times 2$ patterns.

(c) Marching cubes algorithm: In the field of computer graphics, a polygonal surface approximating equidensity surfaces are derived by examining density values of $2 \times 2 \times 2$ voxels. The well-known algorithm to execute this is called a marching cubes algorithm [Lorensen87].

4.5.2 $3 \times 3 \times 3$ local patterns

(1) *The number of local patterns*: Let us consider a 1-voxel $\boldsymbol{x}_0$ and its $3 \times 3 \times 3$ neighborhood $\mathcal{N}_{333}(\boldsymbol{x}_0)$, centered at $\boldsymbol{x}_0$. It was shown by a simple exhaustive enumeration in [Toriwaki02b] that there are $2,852,288$ patterns excluding those derived by applying linear symmetrical transformation from other patterns. Numbers of all those patterns classified according to the number of 1-voxels and values of connectivity index are given in [Toriwaki02b].

(2) *Number of 1-voxels*: The simplest feature is the number of 1-voxels in the neighborhood. It is obvious that the number of 1-voxels may take $0 \sim 26$ in the 26-neighborhood, and that the number of patterns including k 1-voxels is $_{26}C_k$. This includes patterns that are symmetrical to each other. The number of patterns excluding those that are symmetrical to each other is not reported yet.

(3) *Connectivity index*: All possible values of the connectivity index ($R^{(m)}(\boldsymbol{x})$, $H^{(m)}(\boldsymbol{x}), Y^{(m)}(\boldsymbol{x})$) are listed in Table 4.2.

The number of possible patterns for each set of these values are enumerated and given in [Toriwaki02b]. Several examples of complicated patterns are presented in Fig. 4.9.

Table 4.2. Possible values of connectivity number and connectivity index.

6-neighborhood				26-neighborhood				18-neighborhood				18'-neighborhood			
R	H	Y	Nc	R	H	Y	Nc	R	H	Y	Nc	R	H	Y	Nc
1	7	0	-6	1	5	0	-4	1	5	0	-4	1	5	0	-4
1	6	0	-5	1	4	0	-3	1	4	0	-3	1	4	0	-3
1	5	0	-4	1	3	0	-2	1	3	0	-2	1	3	0	-2
1	4	0	-3	1	2	0	-1	1	2	0	-1	1	2	0	-1
1	3	0	-2	2	3	0	-1	0	0	0	0	0	0	0	0
2	4	0	-2	0	0	0	0	1	1	0	0	1	1	0	0
1	2	0	-1	1	1	0	0	2	2	0	0	2	2	0	0
2	3	0	-1	2	2	0	0	1	0	0	1	1	0	0	1
0	0	0	0	1	0	0	1	2	1	0	1	2	1	0	1
1	1	0	0	2	1	0	1	1	0	1	2	1	0	1	2
2	2	0	0	3	2	0	1	2	0	0	2	2	0	0	2
1	0	0	1	1	0	1	2	3	1	0	2	3	1	0	2
2	1	0	1	2	0	0	2	3	0	0	3	3	0	0	3
3	2	0	1	3	1	0	2	4	0	0	4	4	0	0	4
1	0	1	2	3	0	0	3	5	0	0	5	5	0	0	5
2	0	0	2	4	1	0	3	6	0	0	6	6	0	0	6
3	1	0	2	4	0	0	4								
3	0	0	3	5	1	0	4								
4	1	0	3	5	0	0	5								
4	0	0	4	6	0	0	6								
5	0	0	5	7	0	0	7								
6	0	0	6	8	0	0	8								

Remark 4.14. A local feature called the connectivity number (CN) was proposed in [Yokoi75] for a 2D image. The significance of this feature is summarized in four points stated below:

(i) The value of CN at a 1-pixel x represents the number of connected components existing in the 8-neighborhood of x and connected to x.

(ii) The value of CN is equal to the amount of change in the Euler number +1 caused by the deletion of a pixel x.

(iii) A 1-pixel x is deletable if and only if the value of CN $= 1$.

(iv) The value of CN is equal to the number of times for a 1-pixel x to be passed when the border of a figure is traced by the specific border following algorithm.

Extension of the CN to a 3D image inheriting all of these properties is almost impossible. In this chapter the CN of a 3D image was defined so that the second property is preserved. As a result, the first and the third properties do not hold. To compensate this limitation, a new feature, the component index, was added here; the fourth point cannot be extended to a 3D image.

4.5.3 Classification of the voxel state

The local shape of a 3D figure at a 1-voxel x_0 and its neighborhood is classified by the arrangement of 0- and 1-voxels in the $3 \times 3 \times 3$ neighborhood $\mathcal{N}_{333}(x_0)$. Let us show several examples here.

(a) Interior and border point (voxel)

We can denote the type of the connectivity of a current figure using k (k-connectivity) and that of the background by $\underline{k}$ ($\underline{k}$-connectivity), respectively. Then, a 1-voxel x_0 is called an *interior point* (*voxel*) if no 0-voxel exists in its k-neighborhood (i.e., all voxels in the k-neighborhood are 1-voxels). Otherwise the 1-voxel x_0 is called a *border point* (*voxel*). As will be described later, a cavity is created by the deletion of an interior point (voxel) (by inverting it to a 0-voxel). Therefore, the connectivity index of an interior point (voxel) is $(1, 0, 1)$.

(b) Linear connecting point and a line segment

A 1-voxel x_0 is called a *linear connecting point* if exactly two 1-voxels exist in the 26-neighborhood and are not adjacent to each other. Such a voxel x_0 is considered as the middle of an ideal line figure in 3D space. If exactly one 1-voxel exists in the 26-neighborhood of x_0, x_0 is considered as the location at the end of a line figure and is called a *linear edge point* (voxel). A line figure in general will have complicated shapes at a branching point, a crossing point, and in the vicinity of these.

   At a linear connecting point x_0, let us denote by x_1 and x_2 two 1-voxels in the 26-neighborhood of x_0. Then we define a *line element* at x by a line segment connecting a center point of voxels x_1 and x_2. Using the direction of a line segment we can define the *direction of a 3D line figure* at a point (voxel) x_0. All possible directions include *49* cases listed in Table 4.3.

   A 3D line figure with some characteristic points and line elements are illustrated in Fig. 4.10.

(c) Plane point

A figure with a unit thickness is ideally considered to be a plane or a surface. This type of figure is rarely seen in practical applications. If such a situation is realized at a 1-voxel x_0 and in its neighborhood $\mathcal{N}_{333}(x_0)$, x_0 is called a *plane point*. No decisive method has been known for detection of a plane point. Presently we only have a test to know whether any of 3D simplexes exists in the neighborhood or not.

Table 4.3. All possible 3D line elements and their lengths.

#	dx	dy	dz	$x=y=z=1$	$x=y=1,z=a$
1	2	0	0	1	1
2	0	2	0	1	1
3	0	0	2	1	a
4	2	1	0	$\frac{\sqrt5}{2}$	$\frac{\sqrt5}{2}$
5	2	-1	0	$\frac{\sqrt5}{2}$	$\frac{\sqrt5}{2}$
6	1	2	0	$\frac{\sqrt5}{2}$	$\frac{\sqrt5}{2}$
7	1	-2	0	$\frac{\sqrt5}{2}$	$\frac{\sqrt5}{2}$
8	2	0	1	$\frac{\sqrt5}{2}$	$\frac{\sqrt{a^2+4}}{2}$
9	2	0	-1	$\frac{\sqrt5}{2}$	$\frac{\sqrt{a^2+4}}{2}$
10	0	2	1	$\frac{\sqrt5}{2}$	$\frac{\sqrt{a^2+4}}{2}$
11	0	2	-1	$\frac{\sqrt5}{2}$	$\frac{\sqrt{a^2+4}}{2}$
12	1	0	2	$\frac{\sqrt5}{2}$	$\frac{\sqrt{4a^2+1}}{2}$
13	1	0	-2	$\frac{\sqrt5}{2}$	$\frac{\sqrt{4a^2+1}}{2}$
14	0	1	2	$\frac{\sqrt5}{2}$	$\frac{\sqrt{4a^2+1}}{2}$
15	0	1	-2	$\frac{\sqrt5}{2}$	$\frac{\sqrt{4a^2+1}}{2}$

#	dx	dy	dz	$x=y=z=1$	$x=y=1,z=a$
16	2	1	1	$\frac{\sqrt6}{2}$	$\frac{\sqrt{a^2+5}}{2}$
17	2	1	-1	$\frac{\sqrt6}{2}$	$\frac{\sqrt{a^2+5}}{2}$
18	2	-1	1	$\frac{\sqrt6}{2}$	$\frac{\sqrt{a^2+5}}{2}$
19	2	-1	-1	$\frac{\sqrt6}{2}$	$\frac{\sqrt{a^2+5}}{2}$
20	1	2	1	$\frac{\sqrt6}{2}$	$\frac{\sqrt{a^2+5}}{2}$
21	1	2	-1	$\frac{\sqrt6}{2}$	$\frac{\sqrt{a^2+5}}{2}$
22	1	-2	1	$\frac{\sqrt6}{2}$	$\frac{\sqrt{a^2+5}}{2}$
23	1	-2	-1	$\frac{\sqrt6}{2}$	$\frac{\sqrt{a^2+5}}{2}$
24	1	1	2	$\frac{\sqrt6}{2}$	$\frac{\sqrt{4a^2+2}}{2}$
25	1	1	-2	$\frac{\sqrt6}{2}$	$\frac{\sqrt{4a^2+2}}{2}$
26	1	-1	2	$\frac{\sqrt6}{2}$	$\frac{\sqrt{4a^2+2}}{2}$
27	1	-1	-2	$\frac{\sqrt6}{2}$	$\frac{\sqrt{4a^2+2}}{2}$
28	2	2	0	$\sqrt2$	$\sqrt2$
29	2	-2	0	$\sqrt2$	$\sqrt2$
30	2	0	2	$\sqrt2$	$\sqrt{a+1}$
31	2	0	-2	$\sqrt2$	$\sqrt{a+1}$
32	0	2	2	$\sqrt2$	$\sqrt{a+1}$
33	0	2	-2	$\sqrt2$	$\sqrt{a+1}$

#	dx	dy	dz	$x=y=z=1$	$x=y=1,z=a$
34	2	2	1	$\frac{3}{2}$	$\frac{\sqrt{a^2+8}}{2}$
35	2	2	-1	$\frac{3}{2}$	$\frac{\sqrt{a^2+8}}{2}$
36	2	-2	1	$\frac{3}{2}$	$\frac{\sqrt{a^2+8}}{2}$
37	2	-2	-1	$\frac{3}{2}$	$\frac{\sqrt{a^2+8}}{2}$
38	2	1	2	$\frac{3}{2}$	$\frac{\sqrt{4a^2+5}}{2}$
39	2	1	-2	$\frac{3}{2}$	$\frac{\sqrt{4a^2+5}}{2}$
40	2	-1	2	$\frac{3}{2}$	$\frac{\sqrt{4a^2+5}}{2}$
41	2	-1	-2	$\frac{3}{2}$	$\frac{\sqrt{4a^2+5}}{2}$
42	1	2	2	$\frac{3}{2}$	$\frac{\sqrt{4a^2+5}}{2}$
43	1	2	-2	$\frac{3}{2}$	$\frac{\sqrt{4a^2+5}}{2}$
44	1	-2	2	$\frac{3}{2}$	$\frac{\sqrt{4a^2+5}}{2}$
45	1	-2	-2	$\frac{3}{2}$	$\frac{\sqrt{4a^2+5}}{2}$
46	2	2	2	$\sqrt3$	$\sqrt{a^2+2}$
47	2	2	-2	$\sqrt3$	$\sqrt{a^2+2}$
48	2	-2	2	$\sqrt3$	$\sqrt{a^2+2}$
49	2	-2	-2	$\sqrt3$	$\sqrt{a^2+2}$

4.5.4 Voxel state and connectivity index

All possible values of the connectivity number and the connectivity index were shown in Table 4.2. The state of a 1-voxel x_0 is classified using these values also. Several examples are presented below (m denotes the type connectivity) and in Fig. 4.9.

(1) *Interior voxel*: A 1-voxel x is called an *interior voxel* if $R^{(m)}(x) = 1$, $H^{(m)}(x) = 0$, and $Y^{(m)}(x) = 1$, thus $Nc^{(m)}(x) = 2$. The cavity index $Y^{(m)}(x)$ is positive if and only if x is an interior voxel. All voxels in the m-neighborhood of an interior voxel are 1-voxels for the m-connectivity case (Fig. 4.9).

(2) *Boundary voxel*: A 1-voxel that is not a 3D interior voxel is called a 3D *boundary (border) voxel*. A boundary voxel for the m-connectivity case has at least one 0-voxel in its m-neighborhood.

(3) *Connecting voxel*: A 1-voxel x at which $Nc^{(m)}(x) = 1$ and $(R^{(m)}(x), H^{(m)}(x), Y^{(m)}(x)) = (2, 0, 0)$ is called a 3D *connecting voxel* because x has two connected components in its m-neighborhood mutually connected by x.

(4) *Isolating voxel*: A 1-voxel x at which $Nc^{(m)}(x) = 0$ and $(R^{(m)}(x), H^{(m)}(x), Y^{(m)}(x)) = (0, 0, 0)$ is called an *isolating voxel*. An isolating voxel has no 1-voxel in its m-neighborhood for the m-connectivity case.

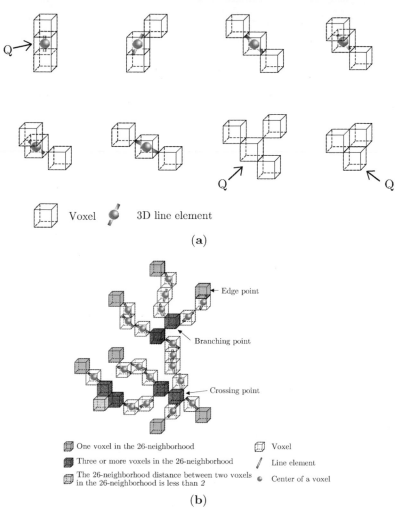

Fig. 4.10. Example of a 3D line figure and line elements: (**a**) Line element; (**b**) example of a line figure and characteristic voxels.

(5) *Two-dimensional (2D) interior voxel:* A 1-voxel $\boldsymbol{x}$ at which $Nc^{(m)}(\boldsymbol{x}) = 0$ and $(R^{(m)}(\boldsymbol{x}), H^{(m)}(\boldsymbol{x}), Y^{(m)}(\boldsymbol{x})) = (1, 1, 0)$ is called a *two-dimensional (2D) interior voxel.*

4.6 Calculation of connectivity index and connectivity number

4.6.1 Basic ideas

The following three principles are instrumental in the calculation of the Euler number, the connectivity number, and the connectivity index. We can employ any of them according to application.

(a) *Local pattern matching*: Local patterns or arrangement of 0- and 1-voxels in the neighborhood are detected by local pattern matching. Features are obtained from the types of patterns detected. Algorithms for pattern matching may vary according to input image and features required.

(b) *Use of arithmetic expression*: Values of voxels in $\mathcal{N}_{333}(\boldsymbol{x})$ are represented by binary valuables. We derive mathematical equations of those variables based upon definitions of features to be calculated. Since variables are binary, those expressions are pseudo-Boolean. The calculation of equations is performed at each voxel.

(c) *Image processing algorithm*: Regarding a local pattern in $\mathcal{N}_{333}(\boldsymbol{x})$ as a binary image, we can apply image processing algorithms to obtain results. For example, the number of connected components in $\mathcal{N}_{333}(\boldsymbol{x})$ is known by applying the labeling algorithm to $\mathcal{N}_{333}(\boldsymbol{x})$.

The second method will be most convenient for execution by computer, but suitable expressions are not always available.

4.6.2 Calculation of the connectivity index

The connectivity index $(R^{(m)}(\boldsymbol{x}), H^{(m)}(\boldsymbol{x}), Y^{(m)}(\boldsymbol{x}))$ at each 1-voxel $\boldsymbol{x}$ is calculated by the following procedure.

(1) *Component index $R^{(m)}(\boldsymbol{x})$*: $R^{(m)}(\boldsymbol{x})$ is equal to the number of connected components connected to $\boldsymbol{x}$, existing in the suitable neighborhood of $\boldsymbol{x}$ presented in Definition 4.11. Labeling is performed first in a subarea including $\boldsymbol{x}$ and its neighborhood presented above. Next, we extract all 1-voxels having the same label as that of $\boldsymbol{x}$ in the above subarea. Finally, after deleting the 1-voxel $\boldsymbol{x}$, we again perform labeling on a set of the remaining 1-voxels. The resulting number of connected components equals $R^{(m)}(\boldsymbol{x})$.

(2) *Cavity index $Y^{(m)}(\boldsymbol{x})$*: $Y^{(m)}(\boldsymbol{x}) = 0$ (voxel) for all configurations except for an interior voxel (Fig. 4.9) and $Y^{(m)}(\boldsymbol{x}) = 1$ for an interior voxel. The interior voxel is found easily by testing whether all adjacent voxels are 1-voxels or not.

(3) *Hole index $H^{(m)}(\boldsymbol{x})$*: $H^{(m)}(\boldsymbol{x})$ is obtained by substituting into Eq. 4.14 values of $R^{(m)}(\boldsymbol{x})$ and $Y^{(m)}(\boldsymbol{x})$ calculated by the above procedures and the value of $Nc^{(m)}(\boldsymbol{x})$ determined by the method presented later.

4.6.3 Calculation of the connectivity number

The connectivity number (CN) $Nc^{(m)}(\boldsymbol{x})$ is obtained by counting simplexes and using the following equation.

Property 4.5. Let $n_k^{(m)}$ and $\underline{n}_k^{(m)}$ denote the number of k-simplexes ($k = 0, 1, 2, 3$) contained in a 3D object before and after the deletion of a 1-voxel $\boldsymbol{x}$. Denoting the CN at a 1-voxel $\boldsymbol{x}$ by $Nc^{(m)}(\boldsymbol{x})$,

$$Nc^{(m)}(\boldsymbol{x}) = \Delta n_1^{(m)} - \Delta n_2^{(m)} + \Delta n_3^{(m)}, \tag{4.20}$$

where $\Delta n_k^{(m)} = n_k^{(m)} - \underline{n}_k^{(m)}$, and m represents the type of connectivity.

(Proof) Denoting the Euler number of an object before and after the deletion of a 1-voxel $\boldsymbol{x}$ by $E^{(m)}(\boldsymbol{x})$ and $E^{(m)}(\underline{\boldsymbol{x}})$, respectively,

$$E^{(m)}(\boldsymbol{x}) = n_0^{(m)} - n_1^{(m)} + n_2^{(m)} - n_3^{(m)} \tag{4.21}$$

$$E^{(m)}(\underline{\boldsymbol{x}}) = \underline{n}_0^{(m)} - \underline{n}_1^{(m)} + \underline{n}_2^{(m)} - \underline{n}_3^{(m)}, \tag{4.22}$$

and $\underline{n}_0^{(m)} - n_0^{(m)} = -1$. This and the definition of the CN imply Eq. 4.20.

Note here that changes in the number of simplexes due to the deletion of a voxel $\boldsymbol{x}$ occur in the neighborhood of $\boldsymbol{x}$ only.

Remark 4.15. For the 6-connectivity case, $\Delta n_k^{[6]}$ is given as follows.

$$\Delta n_1^{[6]} = \text{number of 1-voxels 6-adjacent to } \boldsymbol{x}. \tag{4.23}$$

$$\Delta n_2^{[6]} = \text{number of the set of } 2 \times 2 \text{ 1-voxels including } \boldsymbol{x}. \tag{4.24}$$

$$\Delta n_3^{[6]} = \text{number of the set of } 2 \times 2 \times 2 \text{ 1-voxels including } \boldsymbol{x}. \tag{4.25}$$

Property 4.6. (1) The hole index $H^{(m)}(\boldsymbol{x})$ at a 1-voxel $\boldsymbol{x}$ is equal to the amount of increase in the 1D Betti number in the 26-neighborhood of $\boldsymbol{x}$ caused by deleting $\boldsymbol{x}$. In other words, $H^{(m)}(\boldsymbol{x})$ is equal to the number of holes in the $3 \times 3 \times 3$ local area consisting of $\boldsymbol{x}$ and its 26-neighborhood created by the deletion of $\boldsymbol{x}$. It equals the number of separate connected components of 0-voxels that are connected by the deletion of $\boldsymbol{x}$.

(2) $0 \le H^{(m)}(\boldsymbol{x}) \le 7.$ $\tag{4.26}$

(3) $0 \le R^{(m)}(\boldsymbol{x}) \le 8.$ $\tag{4.27}$

(4) $-6 \le Nc^{(m)}(\boldsymbol{x}) \le 8.$ $\tag{4.28}$

[Toriwaki02a]

Theorem 4.3. The connectivity number $Nc^{(m)}(\boldsymbol{x})$ at a 1-voxel $\boldsymbol{x}$ is calculated by the following equations [Toriwaki02a, Toriwaki02b].

$$Nc^{(6)}(\boldsymbol{x}) = \sum_{h=1,3} \boldsymbol{x}_{h,0}(1 - \sum_{k \in S_1} \boldsymbol{x}_{h,k} \cdot \boldsymbol{x}_{2,k})$$

$$+ \sum_{k \in S_1} \boldsymbol{x}_{2,k}\{1 - \boldsymbol{x}_{2,k+1} \cdot \boldsymbol{x}_{2,k+2}$$

$$(1 - \sum_{h=1,3} \boldsymbol{x}_{h,0} \cdot \boldsymbol{x}_{h,k} \cdot \boldsymbol{x}_{h,k+1} \cdot \boldsymbol{x}_{h,k+2})\}. \tag{4.29}$$

$$Nc^{(18')}(\boldsymbol{x}) = \boldsymbol{x}_{1,0} + \boldsymbol{x}_{3,0} + \sum_{k \in S_1} \boldsymbol{x}_{2,k}(1 - \boldsymbol{x}_{2,k+1} \cdot \boldsymbol{x}_{2,k+2})$$

$$- \sum_{k \in S_1} \sum_{h=1,3} [\boldsymbol{x}_{h,0} \cdot \boldsymbol{x}_{h,k} \cdot \boldsymbol{x}_{2,k}(1 - \boldsymbol{x}_{h,k+2} \cdot \boldsymbol{x}_{2,k+1} \cdot \boldsymbol{x}_{2,k+2})$$

$$+ \boldsymbol{x}_{h,k+1}\{\boldsymbol{x}_{h,0} \cdot \boldsymbol{x}_{2,k+1} \cdot (\underline{\boldsymbol{x}}_{h,k} \cdot \underline{\boldsymbol{x}}_{2,k+2} \cdot \boldsymbol{x}_{2,k} \cdot \boldsymbol{x}_{h,k+2}$$

$$+ \boldsymbol{x}_{2,k} \cdot \underline{\boldsymbol{x}}_{h,k+2} \cdot \boldsymbol{x}_{h,k} \cdot \boldsymbol{x}_{2,k+2})$$

$$+ \underline{\boldsymbol{x}}_{h,0} \cdot \underline{\boldsymbol{x}}_{2,k+1} \cdot \boldsymbol{x}_{h,k} \cdot \boldsymbol{x}_{2,k} \cdot \boldsymbol{x}_{2,k+2} \cdot \boldsymbol{x}_{h,k+2}\}]. \tag{4.30}$$

$$Nc^{(18)}(\boldsymbol{x}) = 2 - \underline{\boldsymbol{x}}_{1,0} - \underline{\boldsymbol{x}}_{3,0} - \sum_{k \in S_1} \underline{\boldsymbol{x}}_{2,k}(1 - \underline{\boldsymbol{x}}_{2,k+1} \cdot \underline{\boldsymbol{x}}_{2,k+2})$$

$$+ \sum_{k \in S_1} \sum_{h=1,3} [\underline{\boldsymbol{x}}_{h,0} \cdot \underline{\boldsymbol{x}}_{h,k} \cdot \underline{\boldsymbol{x}}_{2,k}(1 - \underline{\boldsymbol{x}}_{h,k+2} \cdot \underline{\boldsymbol{x}}_{2,k+1} \cdot \underline{\boldsymbol{x}}_{2,k+2})$$

$$+ \underline{\boldsymbol{x}}_{h,k+1}\{\underline{\boldsymbol{x}}_{h,0} \cdot \underline{\boldsymbol{x}}_{2,k+1} \cdot (\boldsymbol{x}_{h,k} \cdot \boldsymbol{x}_{2,k+2} \cdot \underline{\boldsymbol{x}}_{2,k} \cdot \underline{\boldsymbol{x}}_{h,k+2}$$

$$+ \boldsymbol{x}_{2,k} \cdot \boldsymbol{x}_{h,k+2} \cdot \underline{\boldsymbol{x}}_{h,k} \cdot \underline{\boldsymbol{x}}_{2,k+2})$$

$$+ \boldsymbol{x}_{h,0} \cdot \boldsymbol{x}_{2,k+1} \cdot \underline{\boldsymbol{x}}_{h,k} \cdot \underline{\boldsymbol{x}}_{2,k} \cdot \underline{\boldsymbol{x}}_{2,k+2} \cdot \underline{\boldsymbol{x}}_{h,k+2}\}]. \tag{4.31}$$

$$Nc^{(26)}(\boldsymbol{x}) = 2 - \sum_{h=1,3} \underline{\boldsymbol{x}}_{h,0}(1 - \sum_{k \in S_1} \underline{\boldsymbol{x}}_{h,k} \cdot \underline{\boldsymbol{x}}_{2,k})$$

$$+ \sum_{k \in S_1} \underline{\boldsymbol{x}}_{2,k}\{1 - \underline{\boldsymbol{x}}_{2,k+1} \cdot \underline{\boldsymbol{x}}_{2,k+2}$$

$$(1 - \sum_{h=1,3} \underline{\boldsymbol{x}}_{h,0} \cdot \underline{\boldsymbol{x}}_{h,k} \cdot \underline{\boldsymbol{x}}_{h,k+1} \cdot \underline{\boldsymbol{x}}_{h,k+2})\}, \tag{4.32}$$

where $S_1 = \{1, 3, 5, 7\}, \boldsymbol{x}_{a,9} \equiv \boldsymbol{x}_{a,1}(a = 1, 2, 3, 4)$ and $\underline{\boldsymbol{x}}_{a,b} \equiv 1 - \boldsymbol{x}_{a,b}$.

(Proof) Eqs. 4.29 ~ 4.32 are derived from Eq. 4.11 in Def. 4.10 and values of the Euler number. Calculation of the Euler number will be discussed in detail in the next section.

4.7 Calculation of the Euler number

The Euler number is a kind of global feature characterizing the whole of a figure and a binary image. It is necessary to consider the whole of an input image or input figure for calculating the Euler number.

There are two approaches to obtaining values of the Euler number, based upon different viewpoints. Although the following procedures vary, the Euler number is accurately obtained.

(1) *Triangulation method*: We regard a voxel as a cube in the continuous space and digitization by voxels of cubes as a triangulation or a simplicial decomposition of a 3D figure. Then the Euler number $\mathcal{E}$ is obtained by Eq. 4.5 in Definition 4.8.

(2) *Simplex counting method*: The number of digital simplex (as shown in Fig. 4.5) included in an input image is counted.

We will present details of both methods in the following subsections.

4.7.1 Triangulation method

In the decomposition of a 3D object to cubes corresponding to 1-voxels, a k-dimensional simplex $(k = 0, 1, 2)$ corresponds to a vertex $(k = 0)$, an edge $(k = 1)$, and a face $(k = 2)$ of a 1-voxel, respectively, and a three-dimensional simplex reduces to a voxel itself. Thus, n_ks in Eq. 4.5 are given as follows:

$$n_0 = \text{number of vertexes of 1-voxels contained in a 3D object,} \quad (4.33)$$

$$n_1 = \text{number of edges of 1-voxels contained in a 3D object,} \quad (4.34)$$

$$n_2 = \text{number of faces of 1-voxels contained in a 3D object,} \quad (4.35)$$

and

$$n_3 = \text{number of 1-voxels contained in a 3D object.} \quad (4.36)$$

The type of connectivity should be taken into consideration here. In the case of Fig. 4.11, for example, the vertex V_1 should be counted twice for the 6-c, 18-c, and 18'-c, while only once for the 26-c, because it belongs to separating two voxels X and Y in the first three cases and not a vertex for the 26-c case. The edge e_1 should be counted twice for the 6-c, and 18-c cases, because it belongs to both of two different voxels Y and Z. Thus the result is as shown in Fig. 4.11.

To calculate the total sum of n_ks over the whole of a given 3D image, it is easiest to count them at each vertex of a 1-voxel. Let us consider, for example, a vertex V_1 and a set of $2 \times 2 \times 2$ voxels $\mathcal{S}(V)$ sharing this vertex (Fig. 4.12), and let Δn_ks $(k = 0, 1, 2, 3)$ denote the following quantities.

$$\Delta n_0 = \text{number of vertexes of 1-voxels in } \mathcal{S}(V) \text{ which share } V. \quad (4.37)$$

$$\Delta n_1 = (\text{number of edges of 1-voxels in } \mathcal{S}(V)$$
$$\text{containing the vertex } V) \times 1/2. \quad (4.38)$$

$$\Delta n_2 = (\text{number of faces of 1-voxels in } \mathcal{S}(V)$$
$$\text{containing the vertex } V) \times 1/4. \quad (4.39)$$

$$\Delta n_3 = (\text{number of 1-vowels in } \mathcal{S}(V)$$
$$\text{containing the vertex } V) \times 1/8. \quad (4.40)$$

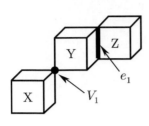

	6-c	18-c	18'-c	26-c
n_0	24	22	24	21
n_1	36	35	36	35
n_2	18	18	18	18
n_3	3	3	3	3
$\mathcal{E}$	3	2	3	1

Fig. 4.11. Example of the triangulation method for calculating Euler number. Let us consider a figure consisting of three voxels X, Y and Z shown here. Their values of n_ks in 4.7.1 are given as the table above corresponding to each type of connectivity. For example, n_0 is the number of vertices in this figure. Each voxel (a cube) has eight vertices. Therefore, the number of vertices in this figure n_0 is 24 $(= 8 \times 3)$ for the 6-c case. In the 26-c case, voxels X and Y are connected and the vertex V_1 is not a vertex of this figure. The edge e_1 is not the edge of the figure, because V_1 and e_1 are inside the figure in the 26-c case. For details, see [Gray71, Toriwaki02a].

Then, the amount of the contribution $\Delta \mathcal{E}(V)$ to the Euler number $\mathcal{E}$ at the vertex V is given by,

$$\Delta \mathcal{E}(V) = \Delta n_0 - \Delta n_1 + \Delta n_2 - \Delta n_3. \tag{4.41}$$

The Euler number $\mathcal{E}$ is obtained by adding $\Delta \mathcal{E}(V)$ of all vertexes in a 3D object, that is,

$$\mathcal{E} = \sum_V \Delta \mathcal{E}(V). \tag{4.42}$$

The type of connectivity should be taken into consideration again in the similar way as was presented in Fig. 4.11. An example is shown in Fig. 4.12.

The value of $\Delta \mathcal{E}(V)$ defined above is uniquely determined by the configuration of 1-voxels in $\mathcal{S}(V)$. Since there are 256 possible configurations and by considering various symmetric relations it is known that only 22 among them are different patterns, the value of $\Delta \mathcal{E}(V)$ for each configuration can be calculated beforehand and stored in the form of a table. Thus, the computation of the Euler number is reduced to the iterative table searches and additions. All of possible $2 \times 2 \times 2$ configurations are shown in Table 4.4 with values of $\Delta \mathcal{E}(V)$.

An efficient algorithm to find which pattern among these 22 cases a given $2 \times 2 \times 2$ subpattern corresponds to is given as follows.

Algorithm 4.1. Denote the number of 1-voxels in $\mathcal{S}(V)$ by n_0. Then the value of the contribution to the Euler number $\mathcal{E}(V)$ at the vertex V is determined by the flowchart in Fig. 4.13 and Table 4.4.

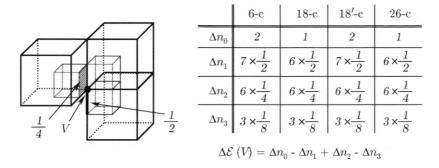

	6-c	18-c	18'-c	26-c
Δn_0	2	1	2	1
Δn_1	$7 \times \dfrac{1}{2}$	$6 \times \dfrac{1}{2}$	$7 \times \dfrac{1}{2}$	$6 \times \dfrac{1}{2}$
Δn_2	$6 \times \dfrac{1}{4}$	$6 \times \dfrac{1}{4}$	$6 \times \dfrac{1}{4}$	$6 \times \dfrac{1}{4}$
Δn_3	$3 \times \dfrac{1}{8}$	$3 \times \dfrac{1}{8}$	$3 \times \dfrac{1}{8}$	$3 \times \dfrac{1}{8}$

$$\Delta \mathcal{E}\,(V) = \Delta n_0 - \Delta n_1 + \Delta n_2 - \Delta n_3$$

Fig. 4.12. The number of simplexes counted as in Fig. 4.11 is totaled up for each vertex V. In the case of this figure, for example, Δn_0, Δn_1, Δn_2, and Δn_3 are added up as in the above table.

Note that this algorithm does not depend on the type of the connectivity. The value of $\mathcal{E}(V)$ for the desired type of connectivity can be found from the table prepared beforehand.

This method to calculate the Euler number is an extension of the method for 2D figures given by [Gray71]. A similar method was reported in [Lobregt80] for only the 6-c and 26-c cases based upon a closed netted surface model and Eq. 4.8.

4.7.2 Simplex counting method

The Euler number is calculated by counting simplexes of each dimension contained in a 3D object and substituting the results for n_rs in Eq. 4.5. In the 6-c case, for example, the Euler number $\mathcal{E}$ is calculated as shown in Fig. 4.14.

The counting of simplexes as presented above may be performed by local template matching over a $2 \times 2 \times 2$ local area or equivalently by calculating a value of a pseudo-Boolean expression defined over the $2 \times 2 \times 2$ local area. The latter procedure is presented in the following theorem.

Theorem 4.4. Let $x_0, x_1, \ldots, x_6$ and x_7 denote density values (0 or 1) of voxels $P = (i, j, k)$ and its neighbors $(i+1, j, k), \ldots,$ and $(i+1, j+1, k+1)$ in the $2 \times 2 \times 2$ local area as shown in Fig. 4.14 ($1 \le i \le L, 1 \le j \le M, 1 \le k \le N$). Then the Euler number $\mathcal{E}(k)$ (k represents the type of the connectivity ($k = 6, 18, 18'$, or 26)) of a binary image with the size $L \times M \times N$ is given by the following equations. Here we assume that the edge of an input image is filled with 0-voxels [Toriwaki02a, Toriwaki02b].

$$\mathcal{E}^{[6]} = \sum_{i=2}^{L-1} \sum_{j=2}^{M-1} \sum_{k=2}^{N-1} \{x_0[1 - x_1(1 - x_4 \cdot x_5)$$

n_0 = Number of 1-voxels which share the vertex V in $S(V)$

$$n_0 = \begin{cases} 0 \rightarrow Q_{01} \\ 1 \rightarrow Q_{11} \\ 2 \rightarrow (\text{Number of } \boxplus) = \begin{cases} 1 \rightarrow Q_{21} \\ 0 \rightarrow (\text{Number of } \boxed{?}) = \begin{cases} 0 \rightarrow Q_{23} \\ 1 \rightarrow Q_{22} \end{cases} \end{cases} \\ 3 \rightarrow (\text{Number of } \boxplus) = \begin{cases} 0 \rightarrow Q_{33} \\ 1 \rightarrow Q_{32} \\ 2 \rightarrow Q_{31} \end{cases} \\ 4 \rightarrow (\text{Number of } \boxplus) = \begin{cases} 0 \rightarrow Q_{46} \\ 2 \rightarrow (\text{Number of } \boxed{?}) = \begin{cases} 2 \rightarrow Q_{45} \\ 3 \rightarrow Q_{44} \end{cases} \\ 3 \rightarrow (\text{Number of } \boxed{?}) = \begin{cases} 2 \rightarrow Q_{43} \\ 3 \rightarrow Q_{42} \end{cases} \\ 0 \rightarrow Q_{41} \end{cases} \\ 5 \rightarrow (\text{Interchange 0 and 1}) \rightarrow (\text{Number of } \boxplus) = \begin{cases} 0 \rightarrow Q_{53} \\ 1 \rightarrow Q_{52} \\ 2 \rightarrow Q_{51} \end{cases} \\ 6 \rightarrow (\text{Interchange 0 and 1}) \rightarrow (\text{Number of } \boxplus) = \begin{cases} 0 \rightarrow (\text{Number of } \boxed{?}) = \begin{cases} 0 \rightarrow Q_{63} \\ 1 \rightarrow Q_{62} \end{cases} \\ 1 \rightarrow Q_{61} \end{cases} \\ 7 \rightarrow Q_{71} \\ 8 \rightarrow Q_{81} \end{cases}$$

Q_{ij} = see Table 4.4

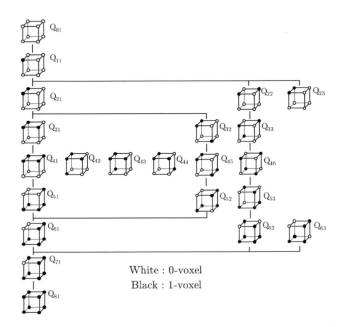

White : 0-voxel

Black : 1-voxel

Fig. 4.13. Flowchart of Algorithm 4.1 (pattern matching for calculating the Euler number).

Table 4.4. Possible $2 \times 2 \times 2$ subpatterns and their contributions to the Euler number.

Connectivity * subpattern **	vertex Δn_0			edge $-\Delta n_1 \cdot 2$			face $\Delta n_2 \cdot 4$			volume $-\Delta n_3 8$			Euler differential $\Delta \mathcal{E}(V)$ ***		
	6	18	26	6	18	26	6	18	26	6	18	26	6	18	26
Q_{01}	0	0	0	0	0	0	0	0	0	0	0	0	0	0	0
Q_{11}	1	1	1	-3	-3	-3	3	3	3	-1	-1	-1	1	1	1
Q_{21}	1	1	1	-4	-4	-4	5	5	5	-2	-2	-2	0	0	0
Q_{22}	2	1	1	-6	-5	-5	6	6	6	-2	-2	-2	2	-2	-2
Q_{23}	2	2	1	-6	-6	-6	6	6	6	-2	-2	-2	2	2	-6
Q_{31}	1	1	1	-5	-5	-5	7	7	7	-3	-3	-3	-1	-1	-1
Q_{32}	2	1	1	-7	-6	-6	8	8	8	-3	-3	-3	1	-3	-3
Q_{33}	3	1	1	-9	-6	-6	9	9	9	-3	-3	-3	3	-1	-1
Q_{41}	1	1	1	-5	-5	-5	8	8	8	-4	-4	-4	0	0	0
Q_{42}	1	1	1	-6	-6	-6	9	9	9	-4	-4	-4	-2	-2	-2
Q_{43}	1	1	1	-6	-6	-6	9	9	9	-4	-4	-4	-2	-2	-2
Q_{44}	2	1	1	-8	-6	-6	10	10	10	-4	-4	-4	0	0	0
Q_{45}	2	1	1	-8	-6	-6	10	10	10	-4	-4	-4	0	0	0
Q_{46}	4	1	1	-12	-6	-6	12	12	12	-4	-4	-4	4	4	4
Q_{51}	1	1	1	-6	-6	-6	10	10	10	-5	-5	-5	-1	-1	-1
Q_{52}	1	1	1	-7	-6	-6	11	11	11	-5	-5	-5	-3	1	1
Q_{53}	2	1	1	-9	-6	-6	12	12	12	-5	-5	-5	-1	3	3
Q_{61}	1	1	1	-6	-6	-6	11	11	11	-6	-6	-6	0	0	0
Q_{62}	1	1	1	-7	-6	-6	12	12	12	-6	-6	-6	-2	2	2
Q_{63}	0	1	1	-6	-6	-6	12	12	12	-6	-6	-6	-6	2	2
Q_{71}	1	1	1	-6	-6	-6	12	12	12	-7	-7	-7	1	1	1
Q_{81}	1	1	1	-6	-6	-6	12	12	12	-8	-8	-8	0	0	0
Q_{63} (18'-c)	1	1	1	-6	-6	-6	12	12	12	-6	-6	-6	2	2	2

* For the 18'-c, all except Q_{63} is the same as the 6-c.
** Codes of subpatterns are shown in Fig.4.13.   *** $\Delta \mathcal{E}(V) = \Delta n_0 - \Delta n_1 + \Delta n_2 - \Delta n_3$

$$-\boldsymbol{x}_2(1 - \boldsymbol{x}_1 \cdot \boldsymbol{x}_3) - \boldsymbol{x}_4(1 - \boldsymbol{x}_2 \cdot \boldsymbol{x}_6) - \prod_{i=0}^{7} \boldsymbol{x}_i]\}. \tag{4.43}$$

$$\mathcal{E}^{[18]} = \sum_{i=2}^{L-1} \sum_{j=2}^{M-1} \sum_{k=2}^{N-1} \{\underline{\boldsymbol{x}}_0[1 - \underline{\boldsymbol{x}}_1(1 - \underline{\boldsymbol{x}}_4 \cdot \underline{\boldsymbol{x}}_5)$$

$$-\underline{\boldsymbol{x}}_2(1 - \underline{\boldsymbol{x}}_1 \cdot \underline{\boldsymbol{x}}_3) - \underline{\boldsymbol{x}}_4(1 - \underline{\boldsymbol{x}}_2 \cdot \underline{\boldsymbol{x}}_6) - \prod_{i=0}^{7} \underline{\boldsymbol{x}}_i]\}$$

$$+ \sum_{m=0}^{3} [\boldsymbol{x}_m \cdot \boldsymbol{x}_{7-m} \cdot \underline{\boldsymbol{x}}_{else}^6]. \tag{4.44}$$

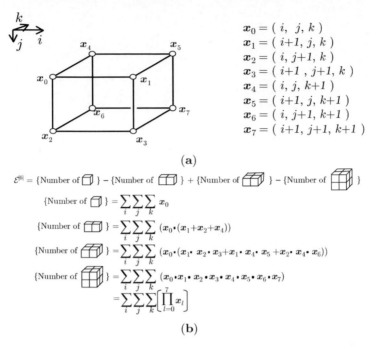

$$x_0 = (\ i, \ j, \ k \ )$$
$$x_1 = (\ i+1, \ j, \ k \ )$$
$$x_2 = (\ i, \ j+1, \ k \ )$$
$$x_3 = (\ i+1 \ , \ j+1, \ k \ )$$
$$x_4 = (\ i, \ j, \ k+1 \ )$$
$$x_5 = (\ i+1, \ j, \ k+1 \ )$$
$$x_6 = (\ i, \ j+1, \ k+1 \ )$$
$$x_7 = (\ i+1, \ j+1, \ k+1 \ )$$

(a)

$\mathcal{E}^{[6]} = \{\text{Number of } \square \} - \{\text{Number of } \square \} + \{\text{Number of } \square \} - \{\text{Number of } \square \}$

$\{\text{Number of } \square \} = \sum_i \sum_j \sum_k x_0$

$\{\text{Number of } \square \} = \sum_i \sum_j \sum_k (x_0 \cdot (x_1 + x_2 + x_4))$

$\{\text{Number of } \square \} = \sum_i \sum_j \sum_k (x_0 \cdot (x_1 \cdot x_2 \cdot x_3 + x_1 \cdot x_4 \cdot x_5 + x_2 \cdot x_4 \cdot x_6))$

$\{\text{Number of } \square \} = \sum_i \sum_j \sum_k (x_0 \cdot x_1 \cdot x_2 \cdot x_3 \cdot x_4 \cdot x_5 \cdot x_6 \cdot x_7)$
$$= \sum_i \sum_j \sum_k \left[\prod_{l=0}^{7} x_l \right]$$

(b)

Fig. 4.14. Computation of Euler Number: (a) variables; (b) equations.

$$\mathcal{E}^{[18']} = \sum_{i=2}^{L-1} \sum_{j=2}^{M-1} \sum_{k=2}^{N-1} \{x_0[1 - x_1(1 - x_4 \cdot x_5)$$

$$-x_2(1 - x_1 \cdot x_3) - x_4(1 - x_2 \cdot x_6) - \prod_{i=0}^{7} x_i]\}$$

$$+ \sum_{m=0}^{3} [\underline{x}_m \cdot \underline{x}_{7-m} \cdot x_{else}^6]. \tag{4.45}$$

$$\mathcal{E}^{[26]} = \sum_{i=2}^{L-1} \sum_{j=2}^{M-1} \sum_{k=2}^{N-1} \{\underline{x}_0[1 - \underline{x}_1(1 - \underline{x}_4 \cdot \underline{x}_5)$$

$$-\underline{x}_2(1 - \underline{x}_1 \cdot \underline{x}_3) - \underline{x}_4(1 - \underline{x}_2 \cdot \underline{x}_6) - \prod_{i=0}^{7} \underline{x}_i]\}, \tag{4.46}$$

where $\underline{x}_i = 1 - x_i$ and x_{else}^6 ($\underline{x}_{else}^6$) means the product of all six values x_is ($\underline{x}_i$s) such that $i = 0, 1, \ldots, 7, i \neq m, i \neq 7 - m$.

(Proof)[6-c case] Considering simplexes in Fig. 4.5,

$$\text{Number of 0-simplex} = \sum_i \sum_j \sum_k x_0$$

$$\text{Number of 1-simplex} = \sum_i \sum_j \sum_k \boldsymbol{x}_0(\boldsymbol{x}_1 + \boldsymbol{x}_2 + \boldsymbol{x}_4)$$

$$\text{Number of 2-simplex} = \sum_i \sum_j \sum_k \boldsymbol{x}_0(\boldsymbol{x}_1\boldsymbol{x}_2\boldsymbol{x}_3 + \boldsymbol{x}_2\boldsymbol{x}_4\boldsymbol{x}_6 + \boldsymbol{x}_1\boldsymbol{x}_4\boldsymbol{x}_5)$$

$$\text{Number of 3-simplex} = \sum_i \sum_j \sum_k [\prod_{l=0}^{7} \boldsymbol{x}_l], \tag{4.47}$$

where $\sum_i \sum_j \sum_k$ means the summation over the whole of a given image. Substituting them into Eq. 4.5, we obtain Eq. 4.43.

[26-c case] Let $\boldsymbol{F} = \{f_{ijk}\}$ and $\underline{\boldsymbol{F}} = \{\underline{f}_{ijk}\}$ denote an input image $\boldsymbol{F}$ and its inversion, that is, $\underline{\boldsymbol{F}} = \{1 - f_{ijk}\}$. Denoting the Euler number of an image $\boldsymbol{F}$ for the m-c case ($m = 6, 18, 18', 26$) by $\mathcal{E}^{(m)}(\boldsymbol{F})$, following relations hold:

$$\mathcal{E}^{(6)}(\boldsymbol{F}) = \mathcal{E}^{(26)}(\underline{\boldsymbol{F}}), \ \mathcal{E}^{(26)}(\boldsymbol{F}) = \mathcal{E}^{(6)}(\underline{\boldsymbol{F}}) \tag{4.48}$$

$$\mathcal{E}^{(18)}(\boldsymbol{F}) = \mathcal{E}^{(18')}(\underline{\boldsymbol{F}}), \ \mathcal{E}^{(18')}(\boldsymbol{F}) = \mathcal{E}^{(18)}(\underline{\boldsymbol{F}}). \tag{4.49}$$

These are proved by calculating $\varDelta\mathcal{E}(V)$ of Eq. 4.41 for all $2 \times 2 \times 2$ or $3 \times 3 \times 3$ configurations given in Table 4.4. Eq. 4.46 is derived immediately from Eq. 4.48.

[18'-c case] From the definition of the 18'-connectivity, $\mathcal{E}^{(18')}$ (Eq. 4.45) is obtained by adding to the $\mathcal{E}^{(6)}$ (Eq. 4.43) the contribution of the configuration shown in Fig. 4.4 which is a 2-simplex for the 18'-c case.

[18-c case] Eq. 4.44 is immediately derived from Eqs. 4.45 and 4.49.

4.8 Algorithm of deletability test

A deletability test is performed by examining conditions in Theorem 4.2 or Corollary 4.1 and is implemented as follows.

(a) Calculation of connectivity number and connectivity index by pseudo-Boolean expression (Theorem 4.3).
(b) Local pattern matching on a $2 \times 2 \times 2$ or a $3 \times 3 \times 3$ local subarea.
(c) Test of shape features in the projection graph.
(d) Calculation of the adjacency matrix corresponding to the projection graph [Yonekura80b, Yonekura80c, Yonekura82c].

Different combinations of these are used for different objectives. Rough guidelines will be given as follows.

(i) Enumeration of $3 \times 3 \times 3$ local patterns are used to derive a new procedure. Reduction of a 3D arrangement of voxels to a 2D image by the use of the projection graph can be used for convenience [Yonekura82c].

(ii) Pattern matching can be used if the number of relating local patterns is low (one or two, for example) and their structure is simple.

(iii) If the conditions match as in (ii) and are expressed in a well-defined mathematical form, pseudo-Boolean equations will be effectively used in (i) and (ii).

(iv) Tests for features of a projection graph are realized effectively by examining logical expressions such as a kind of a decision tree or pseudo-Boolean expressions, if features are simple (e.g., existence of an isolated point).

(v) The adjacency matrix will be used if tests of complicated characteristics are necessary such as detection of a path of the given length.

Generation of a projection graph and its use for the deletability test are given in [Yonekura82b, Yonekura82c].

Algorithm 4.2 (Deletability test – 6-connectivity case).

(1) Calculate the connectivity number $Nc^{(6)}(\boldsymbol{x})$ at $\boldsymbol{x}$.
Go to (2), if $Nc^{(6)}(\boldsymbol{x}) = 1$. Otherwise, $\boldsymbol{x}$ is not deletable.

(2) Denoting by $n(\boldsymbol{x})$ the number of 1-voxels in the 6-neighborhood of $\boldsymbol{x}$,
   (i) $\boldsymbol{x}$ is not deletable, if $n(\boldsymbol{x}) \leq 3$
   (ii) Go to (3), if $n(\boldsymbol{x}) = 4$
   (iii) Go to (4), if $n(\boldsymbol{x}) = 5$
   (iv) Go to (5), if $n(\boldsymbol{x}) = 6$

(3) Calculate the following equation $s(\boldsymbol{x})$

$$s(\boldsymbol{x}) = \sum_{k \in S_1} \sum_{h=1,3} [\underline{\boldsymbol{x}}_{h,k+1} \cdot \boldsymbol{x}_{h,k} \cdot \boldsymbol{x}_{h,k+2} \cdot \boldsymbol{x}_{h,0} \cdot \boldsymbol{x}_{2,k} \cdot \boldsymbol{x}_{2,k+1} \cdot \boldsymbol{x}_{2,k+2}], \quad (4.50)$$

where $\underline{\boldsymbol{x}}_{a,b} = 1 - \boldsymbol{x}_{a,b}$, $S_1 = \{1, 3, 5, 7\}$.
$\boldsymbol{x}$ is not deletable, if $s(\boldsymbol{x}) = 1$; $\boldsymbol{x}$ is deletable, otherwise.

(4) Calculate the above $s(\boldsymbol{x})$.
$\boldsymbol{x}$ is not deletable, if $s(\boldsymbol{x}) = 1$; otherwise generate the projection graph [Yonekura80b, Yonekura80c, Yonekura82a] of $\boldsymbol{x}$. Then, $\boldsymbol{x}$ is not deletable, if the graph has an isolated node (a node connected to no other node next to an edge), $\boldsymbol{x}$ is deletable otherwise.

(5) Generate the projection graph $G(\boldsymbol{x})$ of $\boldsymbol{x}$. Then $\boldsymbol{x}$ is deletable, if the graph $G(\boldsymbol{x})$ is connected; $\boldsymbol{x}$ is not deletable, otherwise. Whether the graph $G(\boldsymbol{x})$ is connected or not is known using the following: Denoting the adjacency matrix (6×6) of a graph $G(\boldsymbol{x})$ by $\mathbf{M}$, calculate

$$\mathbf{N} = \mathbf{M}(\mathbf{I} + \mathbf{M}(\mathbf{I} + \mathbf{M}(\mathbf{I} + \mathbf{M}(\mathbf{I} + \mathbf{M})))), \quad (4.51)$$

where $\mathbf{I}$ is the identity matrix.
Then $\boldsymbol{x}$ is not deletable ($G(\boldsymbol{x})$ is not connected), if any element of the value 0 exists in $\mathbf{N}$. Otherwise $\boldsymbol{x}$ is deletable [Yonekura80a, Yonekura80b, Yonekura80c, Yonekura82c].

Correctness of this algorithm is shown by enumerating all possible projection graphs for $Nc(\boldsymbol{x}) = 1$ [Yonekura82a, Yonekura82c]. Examples of a projection graph are also included in [Yonekura80b, Yonekura80c].

The test as given in Algorithm 4.3 is obtained for the 26-connectivity case by noting that

$$R^{[26]}(X, \boldsymbol{x}) = 1, \text{ and } H^{[26]}(X, \boldsymbol{x}) = Y^{[26]}(X, \boldsymbol{x}) = 0, \qquad (4.52)$$

are equivalent to the following:

$$R^{[6]}(\underline{X}, \boldsymbol{x}) = 1, \text{ and } H^{[6]}(\underline{X}, \boldsymbol{x}) = Y^{[6]}(\underline{X}, \boldsymbol{x}) = 0. \qquad (4.53)$$

Algorithm 4.3 (Deletability test – 26-connectivity case).

(1) Calculate the connectivity number $Nc^{[26]}(\boldsymbol{x})$ at $\boldsymbol{x}$. Go to (2), if $Nc^{[26]}(\boldsymbol{x}) = 1$. Otherwise, $\boldsymbol{x}$ is not deletable.
(2) After inverting 1 and 0 of all voxels in the 26-neighborhood, apply the step (2) and all steps following that of Algorithm 4.2.

For the 18-connectivity case, see [Yonekura80c].

4.9 Path and distance functions

In this section we introduce how to define a distance measure on a digitized image. We need to understand two concepts, path and distance function. A path is a sequence of voxels and a distance function is a digital version of the Euclidean distance in the continuous space.

4.9.1 Path

We will begin with a formal definition of a path.

Definition 4.12 (Path). A sequence of voxels $\boldsymbol{x}_0(= \boldsymbol{u}), \boldsymbol{x}_1, \ldots, \boldsymbol{x}_K(= \boldsymbol{v})$ such that

$$\boldsymbol{x}_{i+1} \in \mathcal{N}^{(m)}(\boldsymbol{x}_i), \ i = 0, 1, \ldots, K - 1, \ m = 6, 18, 18', 26 \qquad (4.54)$$

is called a *path* from a voxel $\boldsymbol{u}$ to a voxel $\boldsymbol{v}$, or more strictly an *m-connected path* ($m = 6, 18, 18', 26$). The number of voxels K contained in a path is called *length* of a path. Given two voxels $\boldsymbol{u}$ and $\boldsymbol{v}$, a path of the specified connectivity with the minimum length from $\boldsymbol{u}$ to $\boldsymbol{v}$ is called *minimal path*. Note here that the length of a path defined above does not always give the distance between two voxels. Even the length of the minimal path does not always become a distance measure in the ordinary sense.

Before proceeding to the distance function, we will extend a path to a more general one called a variable neighborhood path.

Definition 4.13 (Variable neighborhood path). Let

$$\beta_M = \{b_0, b_1, \ldots, b_{M-1}\} \tag{4.55}$$

denote a sequence of neighborhoods, where b_i is a suitable symbol showing the kind of the neighborhood. Then a sequence of voxels

$$\boldsymbol{x}_0(=\boldsymbol{u}),\ \boldsymbol{x}_1, \boldsymbol{x}_2, \ldots, \boldsymbol{x}_{K-1}, \boldsymbol{x}_K(=\boldsymbol{v}), \tag{4.56}$$

where $\boldsymbol{x}_{i+1} \in \mathcal{N}^{[b_i]}(\boldsymbol{x}_i)$, $i = 0, 1, \ldots, K - 1$, is called a *variable neighborhood path* from $\boldsymbol{u}$ to $\boldsymbol{v}$ with the neighborhood sequence β_M. Here $\boldsymbol{x}_{i+1} \in \mathcal{N}^{[b_i]}(\boldsymbol{x}_i)$ means that $\boldsymbol{x}_{i+1}$ is in the b_i-neighborhood of $\boldsymbol{x}_i$. Neighborhoods are employed according to the order of the given neighborhood sequence β_M. If $M < K$, the entire sequence β_M is employed repeatedly. In practice we use the following three types most frequently:

$\beta_M = \{6\}$ (6-connected path),
$\beta_M = \{18\}$ (18-connected path),
$\beta_M = \{26\}$ (26-connected path).

As these examples show, a variable neighborhood path includes the path of Def. 4.12 as its special case. That is, if the neighborhood sequence β_M includes only one element, the variable neighborhood path reduces to the path in Def. 4.12. This case we call *fixed neighborhood path* if we need to distinguish it from the path in Def. 4.13. The minimal path is also defined for a variable neighborhood path in the same way as Def. 4.12.

To find the length of the variable neighborhood minimal path from an arbitrary voxel $\boldsymbol{u}$ to another voxel $\boldsymbol{v}$ for a given neighborhood sequence is not simple. We show here an algorithm to obtain this for a neighborhood sequence consisting of only the 6-, 18-, and the 26-neighborhoods [Okabe83a, Okabe83b].

Theorem 4.5. Suppose that two voxels $\boldsymbol{u} = (i, j, k)$ and $\boldsymbol{v} = (p, q, r)$, and the neighborhood sequence $\beta_M = \{b_0, b_1, \ldots, b_{M-1}\}$ (where $b_i = 6, 18, 26$ for all is) are given. Then the length of the variable neighborhood minimal path $d(\boldsymbol{u}, \boldsymbol{v}; \beta_M)$ is calculated by the following equations:

$$d(\boldsymbol{u}, \boldsymbol{v}; \beta_M) = \max\{d_1(\boldsymbol{u}, \boldsymbol{v}), d_2(\boldsymbol{u}, \boldsymbol{v}), d_3(\boldsymbol{u}, \boldsymbol{v})\}, \tag{4.57}$$

where

$$
\begin{aligned}
d_1(\boldsymbol{u}, \boldsymbol{v}) &= P[\alpha_1/Q_1] + h(z_1, \beta_M) \\
\alpha_1(\boldsymbol{u}, \boldsymbol{v}) &= |p - i| + |q - j| + |r - k| \\
Q_1 &= F_6 + 2F_{18} + 3F_{26} \\
z_1(\boldsymbol{u}, \boldsymbol{v}) &= \mathrm{mod}(\alpha_1, Q_1) \\
d_2(\boldsymbol{u}, \boldsymbol{v}) &= P[\alpha_2/Q_2] + h(z_2, \beta'_M)
\end{aligned}
\tag{4.58}
$$

Table 4.5. Examples of values of the function $h(z, \beta_M)$.

β	F_6	F_{18}	F_{26}	Q_1	z 0 1 2 3 4 5
{ 6 }	1	0	0	1	0 ——————
{ 18 }	0	1	0	2	0 1 —————
{ 26 }	0	0	1	3	0 1 1 ————
{ 6, 18 }	1	1	0	3	0 1 2 ————
{ 6, 26 }	1	0	1	4	0 1 2 2———
{ 18, 26 }	0	1	1	5	0 1 1 2 2—
{ 6, 18, 18 }	1	2	0	5	0 1 2 2 3—
{ 6, 18, 26 }	1	1	1	6	0 1 2 2 3 3

$$\alpha_2(\boldsymbol{u}, \boldsymbol{v}) = \max\{|p - i| + |q - j|, |q - j| + |r - k|, |r - k| + |p - i|\}$$
$$Q_2 = F_6 + 2F_{18} + 3F_{26} \tag{4.59}$$
$$z_2(\boldsymbol{u}, \boldsymbol{v}) = \mathrm{mod}(\alpha_2, Q_2)$$
$$d_3(\boldsymbol{u}, \boldsymbol{v}) = \alpha_3(\boldsymbol{u}, \boldsymbol{v}) = \max\{|p - i|, |q - j|, |r - k|\}, \tag{4.60}$$

where $P = F_6 + F_{18} + F_{26}$, F_m is the number of m-neighborhoods in β_M, $[\ ]$ represents the ceiling function, β'_M is the neighborhood sequence derived by replacing all 26-neighborhoods in β_M by the 18-neighborhood, and $h(z, \beta_M)$ is the function calculated by the following Algorithm 4.4.

Algorithm 4.4 (Calculation of the function $h(z, \beta_M)$). Calculate a value of the function $h(z, \beta_M)$ for a given z and β_M.
$\beta_M = \{b_0, b_1, \ldots, b_M\}$: neighborhood sequence, z: integer variable

(1) Initialization: $\beta(0) \leftarrow z, t \leftarrow 0$, Go to (2)
(2) Test of the terminating condition: If $\beta(t) > 0$, then Go to (3), else
$h(z, \beta_M) \leftarrow t$ and Stop.
(3) $\beta(t + 1) = \begin{cases} \beta(t) - 1 \text{ if } b_t = 6 \\ \beta(t) - 2 \text{ if } b_t = 18 \\ \beta(t) - 3 \text{ if } b_t = 26 \end{cases}$
$t \leftarrow t + 1$. Go to (2).

Note here that for a given neighborhood sequence β, z satisfies $0 \le z < Q_1$, where Q_1 is given in Eq. 4.58, and also $0 \le h(z, \beta_M) < P$. Therefore, we can avoid execution of the algorithm for each $\boldsymbol{u}$ and $\boldsymbol{v}$ by calculating the values of $h(z, \beta_M)$ for all possible values of z and tabulating them beforehand. Several examples are shown in Table 4.5.

4.9.2 Distance function

As was stated in the last section, the length of the minimal path is not always the same as the distance measure. A different way to describe the distance between two voxels is required so that we may use the concept of distance in the same way as the Euclidean distance in the continuous space. Pay attention to the distance measure that is only applicable to a pair of voxels ordered on a cubic array. Noting that each voxel is defined by an integer triad that represents the number of a row, a column, and that of a plane, we can obtain the definition below:

Definition 4.14 (Distance function). If a mapping

$$d(\boldsymbol{x}, \boldsymbol{y}): \ \boldsymbol{A} \times \boldsymbol{A} \rightarrow \boldsymbol{R}' \tag{4.61}$$

where $\boldsymbol{A}$ is the set of all of integer triads (i, j, k) and $\boldsymbol{R}'$ is the set of non-negative real numbers, satisfies all of the following relations, the mapping (function) $d(\boldsymbol{x}, \boldsymbol{y})$ is called a *distance function* (or *distance measure*) on a 3D image.

$$\text{reflective law:} \ \ d(\boldsymbol{x}, \boldsymbol{y}) = 0 \Leftrightarrow x = y, \ \forall \boldsymbol{x} \in \boldsymbol{A}, \forall \boldsymbol{y} \in \boldsymbol{A}. \tag{4.62}$$

$$\text{symmetric law:} \ \ d(\boldsymbol{x}, \boldsymbol{y}) = d(\boldsymbol{y}, \boldsymbol{x}), \ \forall \boldsymbol{x} \in \boldsymbol{A}, \forall \boldsymbol{y} \in \boldsymbol{A}. \tag{4.63}$$

$$\text{triangle law:} \ \ \ \ d(\boldsymbol{x}, \boldsymbol{y}) < d(\boldsymbol{x}, \boldsymbol{z}) + d(\boldsymbol{z}, \boldsymbol{y}),$$

$$\forall \boldsymbol{x} \in \boldsymbol{A}, \forall \boldsymbol{y} \in \boldsymbol{A}, \forall \boldsymbol{z} \in \boldsymbol{A}. \tag{4.64}$$

This is the digital version of the axiom of the distance metric. A number of distance functions have been defined in past literatures. Important ones among them are shown in Table 4.6. Several examples are given in Fig. 4.15 [Kuwabara82]. Note here the shapes of equidistance (contour) surfaces. Table 4.6 also shows clear expressions of the distance values between two arbitrary voxels.

Remark 4.16 (Euclidean distance). The well known Euclidean distance $d_E(\boldsymbol{u}, \boldsymbol{v})$ between $\boldsymbol{u} = (u_x, u_y, u_z)$ and $\boldsymbol{v} = (v_x, v_y, v_z)$, is given as follows and also utilized anytime if necessary:

$$d_E(\boldsymbol{u}, \boldsymbol{v}) = [(u_x - v_x)^2 + (u_y - v_y)^2 + (u_z - v_z)^2]^{1/2}. \tag{4.65}$$

Remark 4.17. Distance functions in Table 4.6 have their own advantages and disadvantages. The 6-neighbor distance and the 26-neighbor distance have been used most frequently in practical applications, because they are calculated most easily. As is found by Fig. 4.15, however, the bias from the Euclidean distance is rather large, and their contours are quite different from those of the Euclidean distance, that is, a group of concentric circles. The use of the neighborhood sequence $\{6, 18\}$ or $\{6, 26\}$ somewhat compensates for this defect. In this case, contours become closer to circles. The major reasons for such errors are that the ratio of the distance to a 6-adjacent voxel to that of a diagonal-adjacent one is assumed to be $1 : 1$ instead of $1 : \sqrt{2}$ or , $1 : \sqrt{3}$, only integers are accepted as the distance values, and only local operations are employed in the calculation of distance values to save time. Therefore, improvement is achieved in several different ways.

Table 4.6. Examples of distance functions on 3D space ([ ] means the ceiling function).

	Neighborhood sequence β	$d_c(P, Q; \beta) =$ Distance between P and Q, where P $= (i, j, k)$, Q $= (l, m, n)$, and $\beta = $ neighborhood sequence
1	$\{6\}$	$d_1 = \|i - l\| + \|j - m\| + \|k - n\|$
2	$\{18\}$	$d_2 = \max(\max(\|i - l\|, \|j - m\|, \|k - n\|),$ $[(\|i - l\| + \|j - m\| + \|k - n\| + 1)/2])$
3	$\{26\}$	$d_3 = \max(\|i - l\|, \|j - m\|, \|k - n\|)$
4	$\{6, 18\}$	$d_4 = \max(\max(\|i - l\|, \|j - m\|, \|k - n\|),$ $[2(\|i - l\| + \|j - m\| + \|k - n\| + 1)/3])$
5	$\{18, 26\}$	$d_5 = \max(\max(\|i - l\|, \|j - m\|, \|k - n\|),$ $[2(\|i - l\| + \|j - m\| + \|k - n\| + 2)/5])$
6	$\{6, 26\}$	$d_6 = \max(\max(\|i - l\|, \|j - m\|, \|k - n\|),$ $[(\|i - l\| + \|j - m\| + \|k - n\| + 2)/4]+$ $[(\|i - l\| + \|j - m\| + \|k - n\| + 3)/4],$ $[2\{\max(\|i - l\| + \|j - m\|, \|i - l\|+$ $\|k - n\|, \|j - m\| + \|k - n\|) + 1\}/3])$
7	$\{6, 18, 26\}$	$d_7 = \max(\max(\|i - l\|, \|j - m\|, \|k - n\|),$ $[(\|i - l\| + \|j - m\| + \|k - n\| + 2)/3]+$ $[(\|i - l\| + \|j - m\| + \|k - n\| + 4)/6],$ $[3\{\max(\|i - l\| + \|j - m\|, \|i - l\|+$ $\|k - n\|, \|j - m\| + \|k - n\|) + 4\}/5])$

Remark 4.18. The length of the minimal path for a variable neighborhood path stated in Def. 4.13 becomes the distance measure if an appropriate neighborhood sequence is adopted. In 2D images, for example, the lengths of the minimal paths for the 4-connected, the 8-connected, and the octagonal path reduce to the 4-neighbor, the 8-neighbor, and the octagonal distance, respectively. Then what condition should a neighborhood sequence satisfy in order that the corresponding minimal path length becomes a distance measure? The following two theorems provide solutions to this problem for a 2D image [Yamashita84].

Theorem 4.6. If a neighborhood sequence $\beta_M = \{b_0, b_1, \ldots, b_{M-1}\}$ satisfies the equation

$$\mathcal{N}^{b_i} \subseteq \mathcal{N}^{b_i+1}, \; \forall i, i = 1, 2, \ldots, M - 1, \qquad (4.66)$$

then the length of the minimal path for the variable neighborhood path with the above neighborhood sequence becomes a distance measure.

Theorem 4.7. Given the neighborhood sequence $\beta_M = \{b_0, b_1, \ldots, b_{M-1}\}$ consisting of the 4- and the 8-neighborhood, that is, $b_i = 4$ or 8 for all is, consider an arbitrary cyclic permutation of the sequence β_M, that is,

$$\beta'_M = b_K, b_{K-1}, \ldots, b_{M-1}, b_0, b_{K-1}. \qquad (4.67)$$

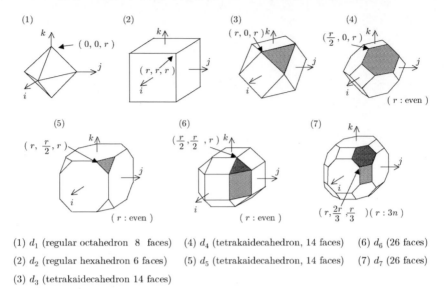

(1) d_1 (regular octahedron 8 faces) (4) d_4 (tetrakaidecahedron, 14 faces) (6) d_6 (26 faces)

(2) d_2 (regular hexahedron 6 faces) (5) d_5 (tetrakaidecahedron, 14 faces) (7) d_7 (26 faces)

(3) d_3 (tetrakaidecahedron 14 faces)

Fig. 4.15. Examples of equidistance surfaces (surfaces for the distance values $d_s = r, r =$ integer are shown for distance functions $d_s, s = 1, 2, \ldots, 7$, in Table 4.6). In d_3 of (3), slash line = double structure. In d_4 of (4), slash line = double structure for $r =$ even. In d_5 of (5), slash line = triple structure for $r =$ even, double structure for $r =$ odd. In d_6 of (6), slash line = double structure for $r =$ even, dark = triple structure for $r =$ even. In d_7 of (7), slash line = double except for $r = 3n - 2$, dark = double structure for $r = 3n - 1$, triple for $r = 3n$. Here n-fold structure means that n equidistance surfaces exist on the plane perpendicular to the coordinate axis such as $k - j$ plane.

Then, for an arbitrary β'_M and arbitrary pairs of pixels, if and only if the length of the minimal path for the variable neighborhood path between two pixels with the neighborhood sequence β'_M is never longer than that with β_M, the length of the variable neighborhood minimal path with β_M becomes a distance measure.

Furthermore, for an arbitrarily given constant c, the relative error of the distance according to the above minimal path length to the Euclidean distance can be kept smaller than c by finding a suitable neighborhood sequence. However, the absolute difference between such distance and the Euclidean distance cannot necessarily become smaller than c. In other words, there exists a pair of pixels such that the distance between them measured by the minimal path length with the neighborhood sequence differs from the Euclidean distance by the amount larger than c. For proof of these theorems, see [Yamashita84]. The similar results may be expected to be correct for a 3D image, but have not been reported yet.

Remark 4.19. Distance measures on a digitized space have been studied in many papers including [Borgefors84, Borgefors86a, Borgefors86b, Coquin95, Klette98, Kuwabara82, Okabe83a, Okabe83b, Ragnemalm90, Saito94a, Toriwaki01, Verwer91, Yamashita84, Yamashita86]. Furthermore, if a domain in which a path exists is limited, the distance between two pixels and the distance transformation from a subset of pixels should be significantly modified.

4.9.3 Distance function in applications

The distance function can be discussed from at least two different viewpoints.

(1) *Digital space viewpoint*: If we consider that a digitized image is defined only by voxels (or sample points), then it is enough that the distance between arbitrary two voxels is defined.
(2) *Approximation viewpoint*: We may consider that a digitized image is an approximation of a continuous image. From this viewpoint, it is desirable that a distance value on a digitized image is as close as possible to that on a continuous image.

The relative weight of two viewpoints varies in different applications. Thus, various research has been performed theoretically and experimentally. Examples of requirements in applications are as follows:

(i) *Difference from the Euclidean metric*: For the measurement of quantities such as the distance, area, and volume, the distance function nearer to the Euclidean distance is better (approximation view point).
(ii) *Computation cost (computational complexity)*: An explicit form of expression for a distance value is more convenient than an algorithmic procedure to calculate the distance between two points of given coordinates. For example, the formula to calculate the Euclidean distance between two given points is well known. Only an algorithm to find the minimum distance between two points is known for a variable neighbor distance on a digitized image (Theorem 4.5).
(iii) *Distance measure*: Is a distance measure required in the strict sense? In some applications the axiom of the distance metric is not always necessary.
(iv) *Distance from a point set*: To calculate the distance between a point and a point set (= figure), the definition and the algorithm are needed. For example, given a set of voxels S' and a voxel x_1 existing outside of S', the distance between a set S' and a voxel $x_1(d(x_1, S'))$ may be given as

$$d(x_1, S') \equiv \min\{d(x_1, y); \ y \in S'\}. \tag{4.68}$$

In this case, the algorithm to calculate effectively the distance between x and y for all ys in S' is more important than a formula to obtain the distance between two given voxels. See distance transformation in Section 5.4 (digital space viewpoint).

(v) *Necessity of distance values*: Distance values themselves are not always required in some applications. If we want to know the distance value that maximizes or minimizes a given object function, then other functions increasing (or decreasing) with the distance value will be enough. For example, if we want to find the closest point to a given point, the square distance will be useful instead of the distance value itself.

(iv) *Path and constraint*: The minimal path or voxels (points) to be considered may exist only in the limited area of the space. For instance, it may be needed to detect the closest point from a given point, or to find the shortest path between two given points both on a specific curved surface. In such cases, direct calculation of the distance is difficult. Such a procedure is useful in execution of path generation and calculation of the path length simultaneously. Concrete examples are derivation of the shortest path along the surface of a 3D object and detection of the shortest route to reach a goal avoiding obstacles.

4.9.4 Improvement in distance metric

Various research has been reported concerning the improvement of distance functions. We will summarize some of them below.

(1) *Extension of the neighborhood*: Use of a neighborhood larger than the 26-neighborhood was tried in several applications. This means that we can move to further voxels in one step when proceeding along a path. In other words, a direct path to a current voxel P from outside of the 26-neighborhood of P is acceptable. In this case, real distance values from P to voxels adjacent to P may differ among all adjacent voxels. Therefore, adjustment of distance values to adjacent voxels may become necessary. This point will be referred to in the next subsection.

(2) *Diversifying distance values*: We assume implicitly that the distance to adjacent voxels is a unit. This simplifies some algorithms in calculating distance values. A typical example is the distance transformation presented in the next chapter. However, in some of distance measures this simplification causes severe bias from the Euclidean distance metric. To overcome this defect, weights are multiplied to parts of distance values to adjacent voxels in the calculation of path lengths. Several examples are shown in Fig. 4.16. If we employ weight values that are equal to exact Euclidean distance, the computation load heavily increases because calculation of square roots of integers is required. Therefore, integer weights were developed so that ratios among them are kept closer to those of Euclidean distance values. This type of metric was called chamfer distance in various literatures regarding 2D and 3D image processing [Verwer91, Borgefors84, Borgefors86a, Borgefors86b].

(3) *Distance transformation*: Distance transformation gives all 1-voxels in an input image the distance to the nearest 0-voxel. The 0-voxels of an input

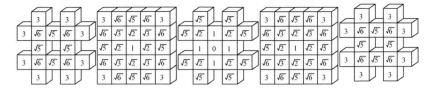

Fig. 4.16. An example of a weighted mask for calculation of distance using the $5 \times 5 \times 5$ neighborhood.

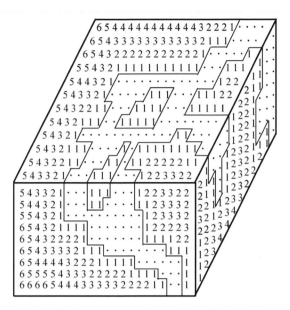

Fig. 4.17. Example of 3D distance transformation. (The 26-neighbor distance was employed. Figure shows only a part of a large 3D image.)

image are kept unchanged. In this transformation, distance values are calculated at all 1-voxels (Fig. 4.17). The use of Euclidean distance is most preferable, but computation load is heavy. Squared Euclidean distance is often employed. Various types of algorithms have been developed as will be presented in Chapter 5.

Remark 4.20. Many reports have been published concerning a distance function and a distance metric. Most of them, however, have treated a 2D image, and have discussed properties of metric theoretically [Borgefors84, Borgefors86a, Borgefors86b, Klette98, Okabe83a, Okabe83b, Ragnemalm90, Toriwaki92, Verwer91]. Discussion about their effectiveness in practical image processing is limited. Still some of them contain useful lists of literatures for related research. Furthermore, recent progress in technology such as decrease of memory cost, increase in computation speed, and development of the algorithm to calculate squared Euclidean distance have changed the significance of specific distance functions and various devices relating to them.

Remark 4.21 (Weighting in distance functions). One important problem in calculating distance on a digitized image is how to give weights to distances to adjacent voxels. For example, $w_{111} = \sqrt{3}$, $w_{112} = \sqrt{2}$, $w_{122} = 1$, if we employ weights equal to the Euclidean distance to voxels in the 26-neighborhood. Suffixes here show the locations according to Fig. 4.2 U. We will present below a mathematical formulation to optimize these weights[Verwer91].

Let us consider a set of fundamental vectors $U = \{r_1, r_2, \ldots, r_e\}$, and assign a distance (weight) d_i to a vector r_i. Consider next a path P_i as a sequence of basic vectors $\{r_{i1}, r_{i2}, \ldots, r_{im}\}$, where m is the length of the sequence and we define the weight $|P_i|$ of the path P_i as

$$|P_i| = \sum_{k=1}^{m} d_{ik} \quad (= \text{sum of distances assigned to} \qquad (4.69)$$
$$\text{fundamental vectors included in the path } P_i)$$

The distance between two grid points (or voxels) u and v is obtained as

$$d_{gc}(u, v) = \min\{|P_i|\} \quad (= \text{the minimum of the above weight of} \quad (4.70)$$
$$\text{a path between } u \text{ and } v)$$

Then let us find the set of weights $\{d_1, d_2, \ldots, d_e\}$ that minimizes the difference (error) of $d_{gc}(u, v)$ from the Euclidean distance between u and v. Results will depend on the selection of the fundamental vector set. Let us assume first a suitable set of fundamental vectors such as vectors from a point P to its 26-neighborhood or to its $5 \times 5 \times 5$ neighborhood. Following are examples of integer weights recommended in [Verwer91] as realizing relatively small errors.

$3 \times 3 \times 3$ neighborhood: $d_{100} = 4, d_{110} = 6, d_{111} = 7, d_{100} = 14,$
   $d_{110} = 21, d_{111} = 25$
$5 \times 5 \times 5$ neighborhood: $d_{100} = 9, d_{110} = 13, d_{111} = 16, d_{210} = 20,$
   $d_{211} = 22, d_{221} = 27$ or $d_{100} = 17, d_{110} = 25, d_{111} = 31, d_{210} = 39,$
   $d_{211} = 43, d_{221} = 53$

where suffixes show the locations of voxels in the neighborhood (Fig. 4.2 U) and numerical values mean recommended values of weights.

The margin for error will be reduced if fractions or large values are employed. If squared Euclidean distance is acceptable, this type of complicated distance may be not necessary.

4.10 Border surface

In a 2D continuous image, a border line (outline) of a region (or a figure) will be intuitively obvious if a figure is well formed. In a continuous 3D figure, the counterpart of a borderline is a border surface of a 3D object (3D figure). For a 3D digitized figure, the definition (or the concept) of a border surface is not as clear. There are several ways of defining a border surface of a 3D object in the 3D digitized space as follows.

(a) *A set of border voxels*: For the definition of a border voxel, see Section 4.5.3 (a). In this case, a border surface of an object (a 3D connected component) P always belongs to P, that is, the border surface of a 3D figure (connected component) P is a set of the outermost layer of voxels in P.

(b) *Continuous surface*: The surface of a 3D figure (a 3D connected component) P is the surface of a 3D continuous figure corresponding to a digitized figure P (see Definition 4.5). Here the border surface of P is also a continuous figure consisting of parts of faces of cubes corresponding to border voxels.

(c) *A set of border voxels (outside)*: A set of 0-voxels such that there exists at least one 1-voxel of a k-connected component P in their k-neighborhood. In this case a border surface of a 3D object P consists of 0-voxels and belongs to the background.

(d) *Border voxels (outside and inside of a figure)*: This is the set sum of (a) and (c) above.

In the discussion concerning border surfaces and their processing, we should express explicitly which one of the above (a) ∼ (d) or others is treated.

In this book we define a border surface as follows.

Definition 4.15 (Border surface). Let us consider an m-connected component of 1-voxels P and an $\underline{m}$-connected component of 0-voxels Q. Then a *border surface* of P to Q, $B(P,Q)$ is a set of all voxels in P that have at least one voxel of Q in their $\underline{m}$-neighborhood. Here the $\underline{m}$-connectivity means the admissible type of the connectivity of 0-voxels when the m-connectivity is employed for 1-voxels. We call the remainder of P after removing $B(P,Q)$ from P the *inside* of the component P.

Let us give again the definition of a border voxel for the convenience of explanation.

Definition 4.16 (Border voxel). A border voxel of an m-connected component P of the value f $(= 0$ or $1)$ is a voxel in P that has at least one voxel of the value $1 - f$ in the $\underline{m}$-neighborhood.

Remark 4.22. For a connected component with a cavity, more than one border surface exists; one of them is the outside surface and the rest are on cavities. In other words, a border surface consists of more than one component. Therefore, in order to specify one of them, we need to designate a 1-component and a 0-component that are located on both sides of the border surface. This is the reason that two components P and Q are included in Definition 4.15. We need to describe explicitly a border surface of a 1-component P that faces on a 0-component Q or a border surface between a 1-component P and a 0-component Q.

Property 4.7. A border surface $B(P, Q)$ in Definition 4.15 (more strictly, a border surface of a 1-component P to a 0-component Q) has the following properties.
(i) $B(P, Q)$ is a set of border voxels of a connected component P. A border voxel here is defined as Definition 4.16.
(ii) A set of voxels in the inside of P contains no voxel of a connected component Q in the m-neighborhood. In this sense, two components P and Q are separated by the border surface $B(P, Q)$.
(iii) A border surface $B(P, Q)$ is the minimum figure (in the sense that the number of voxels is minimum) satisfying (i) and (ii) above.

Proof of these properties are given in [Matsumoto84].

In this section we explained only the outline of the approach to study properties of a border surface of a 3D figure and parts of basic properties of a border surface. Further study will be needed in order to obtain a method to distinguish individual surfaces of each connected component. For instance, we need a method to give different marks to different components. Details of such algorithms will be presented in the next chapter.

Remark 4.23. Image processing algorithms and the digital geometry of 3D images were first reported in [Park71]. They discussed the labeling of connected components and gave a definition of the Euler number of a 3D figure. Only the 6- and the 26-connectivity was treated there. Three-dimensional image processing began to be studied around 1980. For example, detection and following of border surfaces by Herman et al. [Artzy85, Herman78, Liu77], connectivity index and topology preservation by T.Yonekura et al. [Yonekura80a, Yonekura80b, Yonekura80c, Yonekura82a, Yonekura82b, Yonekura82c, Yonekura82d], and other areas of study was researched. Research reports are collected in [Kong85, Kong89, Toriwaki85a, Toriwaki85b]. [Kong85, Kong89] mainly pointing out many problems requiring study, but references are limited and research from Japan is not included. [Toriwaki02a, Toriwaki02b, Toriwaki85a, Toriwaki85b] will complement this. More recent research is included in [Toriwaki02a, Toriwaki02b, Toriwaki04, Klette98, Nikolaridis01, Rogalla01, Bertland01]. A border surface and related topics including border following algorithms were presented in detail in [Artzy85, Udupa94, Herman98].

5

ALGORITHM OF BINARY IMAGE PROCESSING

5.1 Introduction

In this chapter we present several algorithms for processing 3D images, in particular for treating connected components and figures in a 3D image. Aims of this chapter are:

(1) to understand processes essential in proceeding to the analysis of a 3D figure in a 3D gray-tone image
(2) to learn the structure of algorithms through examples

In order to extract significant information from an input 3D gray-tone image, we first need to segment a 3D figure that is likely to correspond to a 3D object in the real world. Next, we extract features that have more condensed information and derive from this a description of the figure. A binary image is produced as a result of distinguishing figures from the background. Each connected component corresponds to a 3D figure. If this segmentation of a figure has been performed correctly, every connected component represents a 3D object meaningful in the real 3D world. This may not always be true in practical image processing, but this is not currently important.

Information carried by a binary image is mainly in the *shape* of a figure. Hence most algorithms presented here relate to processes based on the geometrical properties of a 3D figure. Essential features of those algorithms are transformations preserving connectivity or topology, extraction of the inside, outside, and the border surface of a figure, and calculation of the distance on a digitized image.

From the viewpoint of information concentration, we transform a massive figure (a 3D figure) to a planar figure (the center plane and/or the border surface), and transform a planar figure further to a linear figure (or a curve). In another type of algorithm, we calculate the shortest distance from a voxel inside of a figure to the background. We then concentrate the information to local maximum points in the distribution of such distance values. Axis/surface thinning, border surface following, and distance transformation are explained as examples of algorithms realizing such information concentration.

Algorithms used to execute those processes are also given. Through the explanation of algorithms, we intend to provide algorithms that can be used for practical applications, and at the same time we expect readers to understand various characteristics of algorithms and methods to design algorithms by themselves. As examples, detailed sequential and parallel algorithms, concentration and restoration of figures, serial composition, and 1D decomposition are presented.

Although most algorithms in this chapter are described by program-like expressions, they are neither programs themselves nor definitions of algorithms in their strict meanings. Our aim is to give readers the most essential parts of algorithms while avoiding ambiguity. We omit some parts of procedures that might be necessary for correct behavior of a program, but are less important in the definition of such algorithms as detection of the overflow in numerical calculation and exceptional processing for the frame of an input image. The descriptions of some algorithms may vary. This is to avoid errors in rewriting descriptions from original papers.

All algorithms presented in this chapter have been coded and executed at least once in the authors' laboratory and their expected performance has been confirmed.

5.2 Labeling of a connected component

A connected component was defined already in Def. 4.3. Roughly speaking, each connected component corresponds to an individual 3D figure. Hence extraction of a connected component is useful as a tool to find the topological properties of a figure, such as the Euler number. Connected component extraction is very useful also for practical applications of image processing.

Procedures to extract a connected component (= labeling) are basically the same as those of a 2D image [Rosenfeld82, Watt98]. Here we will present concrete algorithms for all of four types of connectivity [Yonekura82a]. The $18'$-connectivity case is neglected because it is the same as the 6-connectivity case. We will use positive integers as labels as was stated in Section 4.2.

Algorithm 5.1 (Labeling of connected components).

$F = \{f_{ijk}\}$: input image (binary image).

$L = \{l_{ijk}\}$: label image: l_{ijk} is a positive integer representing a label of each connected component, (The value 0 is reserved for the background and so the value of a 0-voxel is not changed.)

λ: variable representing the number of a connected component.

$T(i)$: label table (1D array).

(1) Initialization: $\lambda \leftarrow 0$. Start the raster scan from a voxel $(2, 2, 2)$.

(2) Denote a current voxel by (i, j, k).

If $f_{ijk} = 1$, then go to (3). If $f_{ijk} = 0$, then $l_{ijk} \leftarrow 0$, and go to (4).

(3) Let us use the scanning method given in the left figure of Fig. 5.1 (b) and denote a current voxel by $x_0 = (i, j, k)$. Denote voxels that were already scanned in its neighborhood as in the right figure of Fig. 5.1 (b) and assume that the label of x_p (= the value of an image L) is l_p (= positive integer) $(p = 0, 1, 2, \ldots, 13)$.

(3-1) If there are n kinds of different positive values in $\{T(l_p),\ p = 0, 1, 2, \ldots, 13\}$, let us express those integers by $L_1, L_2, \ldots, L_n$ in the increasing order.

If $n = 0$ (no positive value exists), then go to (3-2); go to (3-3) if $n = 1$. Otherwise go to (3-4).

(3-2) $\lambda \leftarrow \lambda + 1$, $T(\lambda) \leftarrow \lambda$, $l_{ijk} \leftarrow \lambda$. Go to (4).

(3-3) $l_{ijk} \leftarrow L_1$. Go to (4).

(3-4) $l_{ijk} \leftarrow L_1$. For all $T(\gamma)$ such that $T(\gamma) = L_p$ $(2 \leq p \leq P, 1 \leq \gamma \leq \lambda)$, $T(\gamma) \leftarrow L_1$. Go to (4).

(4) If all voxels have been processed, go to (5). Otherwise proceed to the next voxel. Then go to (2).

(5) Rewrite all integers (labels) in the table $T(\lambda)$ to the serial number integers. Denote the maximum value (of the label) by b_0. Go to (6).

(6) Rewriting labels: For all (i, j, k)'s, if $l_{ijk} > 0$, $l_{ijk} \leftarrow T(l_{ijk})$.

In step (3) of the above procedure, $p \leq 3$ for both the 6-connectivity case and the 18'-connectivity case, $p \leq 9$ for the 18-connectivity case, and $p \leq 13$ for the 26-connectivity case. It is obvious from the definition of the connectivity that $n \leq 4$ for the 26-connectivity case, and otherwise $n \leq 3$.

This algorithm is a straightforward extension of a method that has been widely used in 2D image processing. Although it may seem complicated, the performance will be good if only a conventional sequential computer with a single processor is employed, because scanning the whole of an input image is required only twice.

In an output label image, serial numbers of integers starting by unit are given to each connected component as its label. Therefore, the maximum label means the number of connected components included in an input image. By extracting voxels storing a specified integer value, we can extract individual connected components separately. Due to these properties, labeling is frequently utilized as a preprocessing in object counting or feature measurement of images including many objects.

5.3 Shrinking

Shrinking is a processing that replaces a deletable 1-voxel by a 0-voxel while preserving topology. When shrinking is complete, a simply connected component becomes a single isolated voxel (= only one 1-voxel). Results cannot be

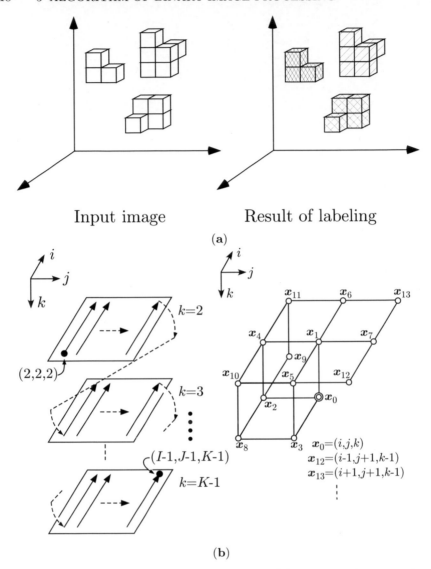

Fig. 5.1. Labeling of 3D connected components : (a) Labeling of connected components -basic idea ; (b) illustration of Algorithm 5.1.

predicted for a multiconnected component, because it depends on the shapes of each component. The topology of each connected component (the number of holes and cavities, etc.) is preserved through the shrinking procedure because only a deletable 1-voxel is changed into a 0-voxel. Thus, if an input image includes only simply connected component, shrinking can be used for counting the number of figures (connected components). Shrinking is more useful as the base for deriving the surface or axis thinning algorithms which will be presented in the following section.

By using procedures of deletability determination given in the previous chapter, an algorithm for shrinking is obtained as stated below:

Algorithm 5.2 (Shrinking).

Input: $F = \{f_{ijk}\}$. Binary image of the size $I \times J \times K$. 1-Voxels represent figures and 0-voxels represent the background.

(1) Repeat (2) $\sim$ (4) for $k = 1, 2, \ldots, K$.
(2) Repeat (3) for $j = 1, 2, \ldots, J$.
(3) Repeat the following for $i = 1, 2, \ldots, I$.

   If x_{ijk} is a 1-voxel and deletable, then replace x_{ijk} by a 0-voxel (delete x_{ijk}) and proceed to the next voxel.

   If otherwise, proceed to the next voxel with doing nothing.
(4) If at least one 1-voxel was deleted in (1) $\sim$ (3) above, then go to (1). Stop if no deletion occurred in (1) $\sim$ (3).

This algorithm can be executed only on the memory area storing an input image, that is, only one 3D array is needed. Only an input image is referred to during execution, that is, one 3D array is enough for execution. As soon as a deletable voxel is found, it is deleted at once. Only a 1-voxel in an input image is changed, and a 0-voxel is never changed. Thus, this algorithm is a sequential type according to the classification given in Chapter 2. According to the classification of algorithms for a 2D image [Yokoi79], this is classified into the type I below and sequential. An output image (a result) of the shrinking algorithm applied to an input image F is called the *shrunk skeleton* of an image F.

Remark 5.1. A shrinking algorithm for a 2D image is classified as follows:

(Type I algorithm) Only a 1-voxel can be deleted. A shrunk skeleton of a simply connected component is a single 1-voxel included in an input connected component.

(Type II algorithm) Both a 1-voxel and a 0-voxel can be rewritten. A shrunk skeleton of a simply connected component is a single voxel. This shrunk skeleton may be either inside or outside of an input connected component. Details are presented in [Yokoi79].

Many of these properties will be extended to a 3D image, although a detailed report has not yet been published.

Property 5.1. A shrunk skeleton of Algorithm 5.2 is always contained in an input figure. Topological properties of a shrunk skeleton (numbers of cavities, holes, and components) are the same as those of an input figure.

(Proof) The former half is obvious from that only 1-voxels are changed, and 0-voxels are kept unchanged. The latter half is immediately known from the fact that only a deletable voxel is deleted.

The following property is expected to hold and has been confirmed experimentally, although it has not been proved theoretically.

Property 5.2. (1) A shrunk skeleton of a simply connected figure (a figure that has neither a hole nor a cavity) is an isolated voxel (a single 1-voxel).
(2) A shrunk skeleton of a figure having one hole and no cavity (torus) consists of only such voxels as $(R, H, Y) = (2, 0, 0)$ (= connecting voxel). Intuitively it is a loop-like line figure in 3D space.
(3) A shrunk skeleton of a figure having only one cavity and no hole (sphere shell) consists of only such voxels as $(R, H, Y) = (1, 1, 0)$ (inner voxel on a 2D surface). Intuitively it is a sphere shell with one voxel thickness.

Concerning (1) above, it is expected that a simply connected component consisting of three or more voxels contains at least two deletable voxels. By deleting a deletable voxel one by one a simply connected figure will be reduced to an isolated voxel.

5.4 Surface thinning and axis thinning

5.4.1 Definition

In 2D image processing a process that extracts a center line of a figure with the finite width is called *thinning* (or *skeletonization*). This is a very important procedure widely used in practical applications of 2D pattern recognition such as character recognition and document analysis. It is also employed in processing of a gray-tone image in extraction of borders and edges.

The meaning of *thinning* in 2D image processing seems to be clear. However, it is not so easy to define *thinning* exactly. The word *thinning* expresses the concept of a centerline of a *natural* or a *reasonable* shape located at the *reasonable* position. This depends on the subjective judgment of the observer, however, and cannot be specified theoretically.

A new problem occurs in the extension of the thinning to 3D image processing even in subjective description. For example, the concept of a center line is naturally acceptable for an elongated long figure such as a wire. In such a case thinning is easily understood. On the other hand, some problems still remain for a figure like a plate which is of a finite thickness. Imagine that we have a wide plate with the unit thickness after shaving an input figure iteratively from both sides. Then should we shave (thin) it until a *centerline* is reached or should we stop a thinning procedure because we have already reached a center *surface*?

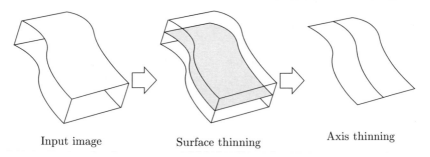

Input image   Surface thinning   Axis thinning

Fig. 5.2. Concept of surface/axis thinning.

For the moment we will take into consideration both cases above, and we call the former case *surface thinning* and the latter case *axis thinning* (Fig. 5.2). Thus, we will define or specify surface/axis thinning as follows.

Definition 5.1 (Surface thinning). *Surface thinning* is a process that transforms a 3D figure with a finite thickness to the center surface (a figure of the unit thickness located at the center of an input figure) while keeping the topology unchanged. In this sense, a surface figure means a figure such that all voxels x in it satisfy at least one of (i) and (ii) below.

(i) No 3D simplex (= arrangements of voxels shown in Fig. 5.3) is contained in the *3 × 3 × 3* neighborhood of x.

(ii) x is not deletable.

Definition 5.2 (Axis thinning). *Axis thinning* is a process that transforms a figure with a finite thickness and/or a finite width into a line figure with the unit thickness being located at the center of the figure without changing the topology. By a line figure we mean a figure that does not contain a deletable voxel except for at the end points.

These are conceptually straightforward extensions of those in 2D image processing to a 3D image. As was stated above, there are two cases of thinning: transformation into a center surface or into a centerline. This is a problem specific to 3D image processing.

However, an output of the axis thinning still may not become a line figure due to topology preservation requirement. An example is an input figure which has a cavity. Therefore, the difference between the axis thinning and the surface thinning may not always be clear for some kinds of input figures. For a long plate-like figure of the unit thickness, there are clearly two possibilities: whether it is further unchanged (surface thinning or medial surface extraction) or is transformed until it becomes a line figure (axis thinning or medial axis extraction) (Fig. 5.2). Either of them may be desired according to each application. We will present both types of algorithms here.

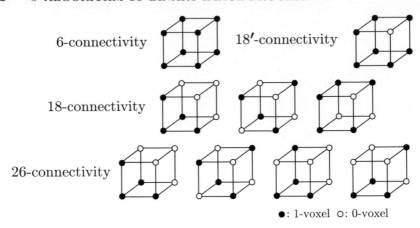

6-connectivity   18′-connectivity

18-connectivity

26-connectivity

● : 1-voxel ○: 0-voxel

Fig. 5.3. Voxel arrangements to be deleted in surface thinning (3D simplex).

5.4.2 Requirements of thinning

We will summarize the requirements of surface/axis thinning. An output of these algorithms should also have these features.

(*Requirement (R) 1*) Topological features of an input figure should be preserved in an output figure.

(*R2*) A resultant figure should be a surface figure of the unit thickness for surface thinning or a line figure of the unit thickness for axis thinning except for an exceptional local shape such as a cross point.

(*R3*) A resultant figure should be located on the center surface/center line of an input figure.

(*R4*) A resultant figure does not degenerate excessively.

(*R5*) The shape of an output figure should be a reasonable one in respect to crossing parts of an input figure.

(*R6*) The result is not affected by the rotation of an input figure. In other words, a result of thinning of a rotated figure is not too different from the rotation by the same angle after thinning an original input figure.

Several of these requirements are not always compatible with each other. Theoretically strict statements cannot be given for all of them except *R1*. Therefore, the performance of a thinning algorithm cannot help being evaluated intuitively and subjectively to some extent by a human observer. *R1* and *R2* are more essential than others, and the rest are guidelines.

5.4.3 Realization - the sequential type

Let us explain here how those requirements are realized in a concrete algorithm.

(1) *Topology preservation*: Scan the whole of an input image in the prespec-
ified scanning mode, and test the deletability of every 1-voxel. Delete a
1-voxel (replace by a 0-voxel), if the voxel is deletable. Only one voxel is
deleted at any one time (simultaneous deletion of more than one voxel
never occurs). A deletable 1-voxel is deleted as soon as it is detected. Further processes are applied to the image from which voxels were deleted.
That is, the algorithm is a sequential algorithm shown in Chapter 2.

The deletability test at each voxel is performed by testing whether local
features (connectivity index) satisfy the condition of Corollary 4.1 (component index = *1* and connectivity number = *1*) or Theorem 4.2 in the
3 × *3* × *3* neighborhood of the current voxel. The procedure to execute
this was presented in Section 4.8.

(2) *Surface thinning*: If a figure contains any of the voxel arrangements shown
in Def. 5.1 (Fig. 5.3), then a deletable voxel in such an arrangement is
eliminated (replaced by a 0-voxel). Unless a deletable voxel exists, no
deletion is required.

(3) *Keeping central position*: We shave a figure in the equal rate from the left
side, the right side, the up side, the down side, the front side, and the back
side. This is realized by applying the deletability test to only a 1-voxel that
has a 0-voxel in the specified side of the 6-neighborhood. For example, first
a 1-voxel that has a 0-voxel in the right is tested, second a 1-voxel having
a 0-voxel in the up side is tested, and so on. Thus, one time of scanning
the whole input image is achieved by scanning an image six times. These
six times of scanning are called a *subcycle*. This subcycle system has been
widely used in 2D image processing. Final results of thinning are affected
a little by the order of subcycles, although the effect is not extreme in
most cases. This effect is unavoidable in this type of algorithm.

(4) *Suppression of degeneration*: Subcycles are useful for suppressing degeneration, too.

(5) *Other features*: Only a local processing of the *3* × *3* × *3* neighborhood
is employed in an algorithm. The state of voxel values in the *3* × *3* × *3*
neighborhood is classified by the calculation of local features such as the
connectivity index and the deletability test using them. Pattern matching
is used only for at most the *2* × *2* × *2* neighborhood.

Remark 5.2. In 2D image processing, it is not difficult to list all possible arrangements of 0-and 1-pixels in the *3* × *3* neighborhood (*51* patterns
exist with excluding symmetrical patterns each other). Then, we may derive an algorithm by assigning a suitable output value to each of input
local patterns. Many thinning algorithms were designed by this procedure
[Toriwaki81, Stefanelli71, Tamura78, Tamura83]. On the other hand, for a 3D
image, there are *1,426,144* patterns of 0- and 1-voxels in the *3* × *3* × *3*
neighborhood even if mutually symmetric patterns have been excluded. Then
it is almost impossible to design an ad hoc algorithm while taking into consideration all of those patterns.

Remark 5.3. In shrinking and thinning algorithms, only deletable voxels are permitted to be deleted to preserve the topology of an input image. In a shrinking algorithm all deletable voxels are deleted as was explained in Section 5.3. In a thinning algorithm only parts of deletable voxels are really deleted because additional requirements stated in Section 5.4.2 have to be satisfied.

In order that the results of thinning are located at the center of an input figure, thinning algorithms shave deletable voxels by one layer from a border of a figure. This *shaving* must be executed at an equal rate in an upside border, downside border, left and right side border, and back and front side border, respectively. Intuitively, such *shaving of all deletable voxels on the surface of a figure* (*one-layer thinning*) is repeated around the number of times equal to half of the figure width. One main cycle is executed usually after being divided into six times of the *partial thinning* (*subcycle*) as follows, in order to keep a thinned result near the center of an original figure.

For example, all upside border voxels are tested for deletability first and replaced by a 0-voxel if deletable. Second, downside border voxels are tested and deleted if deletable. The same procedure is applied to left border voxels, right border voxels, front border voxels, and back border voxels in this order.

Thus, one main cycle consists of six subcycles of shaving. Each subcycle scans the whole of an input image one time and tests deletability of border voxels. The total number of subcycles is *the number of times of iteration* of an algorithm and is the most important factor to determine the computation time of the algorithm. Some of algorithms employ 12 subcycles and some others avoid subcycles by using larger neighborhoods and different types of the deletability test [Saito96, Saito01, Palagyi99, Ragnemalm90].

5.4.4 Examples of surface/axis thinning algorithms (sequential type)

Let us show an example of a surface-thinning algorithm basing upon the principle described above.

Algorithm 5.3 (Surface thinning).

Input: $F = \{f_{ijk}\}$ = input binary image.
    f_{ijk} = density value of a voxel (i, j, k) which takes *0* or *1*. A set of 1-voxels is considered to be a figure.
    m = type of the connectivity ($m = 6, 18, 18', 26$).
Output: $F = \{f_{ijk}\}$ = result of surface thinning is stored when the algorithm finishes. Physically the same array as the one storing an input image is assigned.
Conditions for *a finally preserved voxel* (*FPV*): A border voxel (i, j, k) satisfying at least one of the following $C1$ and $C2$ is called *FPV* and is never deleted in the subsequent procedure.

$C1$: None of arrangements in Fig. 5.3 (3D simplex) exists in the $3 \times 3 \times 3$ neighborhood of a voxel (i, j, k).

$C2$: A voxel (i, j, k) is not deletable in the m-connectivity.

(Main cycle processing)

[**STEP 1**] (Extraction and classification of border voxels)

Here a *border voxel* means a 1-voxel that has at least one 0-voxel in its 6-neighborhood. Classify each border voxel as follows according to the location of a 0-voxel in its 6-neighborhood.

for all (i, j, k)s **do** (See Note)

  if $f_{ijk} = 1$, **then**

    if $f_{i,j,k+1} = 0$, **then** $f_{ijk} \leftarrow 7$

    if $f_{i,j+1,k} = 0$, **then** $f_{ijk} \leftarrow 6$

    if $f_{i+1,j,k} = 0$, **then** $f_{ijk} \leftarrow 5$

    if $f_{i-1,j,k} = 0$, **then** $f_{ijk} \leftarrow 4$

    if $f_{i,j-1,k} = 0$, **then** $f_{ijk} \leftarrow 3$

    if $f_{i,j,k-1} = 0$, **then** $f_{ijk} \leftarrow 2$

  else no operation is performed

  endif

enddo

(Subcycle processing)

[**STEP 2**] (Deletion of a voxel)

for bordertype $= 2$ **to** 7 **do**

  [**STEP 2.1**] (Detection of *finally preserved voxel* (*FPV*))

  Detect a voxel that is regarded as the unit thickness (surface voxel) and give it a mark of *FPV*.

  for all (i, j, k)s **do**

    if $f_{ijk} = $ bordertype $\wedge (C1 \vee C2)$

    then $f_{ijk} \leftarrow 10$ (*FPV*)

    else no operation is performed

    endif

  enddo

enddo

[**STEP 2.2**] (Deletion of a 1-voxel)

Delete a deletable voxel.

for all (i, j, k)s **do**

  if $f_{ijk} = $ bordertype

  then

    if (i, j, k) is deletable $(\neg(C1 \vee C2) \wedge (\text{not } FPV))$

    then $f_{ijk} \leftarrow 0$ (deletion)

Note: Here "for all (i, j, k)s do" means that each voxel is processed in the order as shown in Fig. 2.13, and Fig. 5.1 (according to a raster scan given in the above figures). This is the same in other algorithms presented in the following sections.

Note: $\neg C1$ means logical negation of $C1$.

    else $f_{ijk} \leftarrow 10$ *(FPV)*
   endif
  else no operation is performed
  endif
enddo

[**STEP 3**] (Examine the terminating rule)
if no point changed through [**STEP 2**]
then stop
else go to [**STEP 1**] (repetition of the main cycle)
endif

Remark 5.4. In this type of algorithm, which includes deletion of voxels performed sequentially, a border voxel that was not deletable at one time of processing may become deletable afterwords due to the change in the local arrangement of voxels caused by the processing in the subsequent cycles. This fact is worth being taken into consideration when designing an algorithm. In Fig. 5.4 (a), for example, the voxel B satisfies the condition $C2$ (not deletable because a hole is generated by the deletion). After the voxel A was deleted, however, B is deletable because its state is the same as A before its deletion. As this situation is repeated, an unnatural result as shown in Fig. 5.4 (b) might occur. This is a typical example of the phenomenon called *degeneration*. In Algorithm 5.3, we prevent this type of excessive degeneration by employing the deletability test (=the preservation test) at a specified point in the execution and by preserving a voxel satisfying a given condition without testing deletability in sequent procedures. Such voxels are called a *finally preserved voxel (FPV)*. In [STEP 2] of Algorithm 5.3, *FPV* is first detected and given the mark in [STEP 2.1]. After that conditions $C1$ and $C2$ are tested only at a voxel having no *FPV* mark in [STEP 2.2] and a voxel is deleted, if deletable. In this step, a voxel that was deemed deletable was immediately replaced by a 0-voxel (deleted).

Let us show a property of Algorithm 5.3 below:

Property 5.3. (1) A line figure on a surface figure that is contained in a plane perpendicular to one of the coordinate axes is never deleted because any voxel in such a figure is regarded as either an inside pixel or a connecting pixel or an edge pixel of a 2D figure [Toriwaki85a, Toriwaki85b]. An inside voxel and a connecting voxel become a finally preserved voxel according to the condition $C1$ and $C2$. An edge voxel also becomes a finally preserved voxel according to the condition $C1$ (Fig. 5.5).
(2) When an input figure is a parallelepiped of the size (the number of voxels) $I \times J \times K$ $(I > J > K)$, and all edges are parallel to one of the coordinate axes, an output figure is a plane of the size $I' \times J' \times K'$ (voxels) where

$$(I - K + 1) \leq I' \leq (I - K + 2)$$

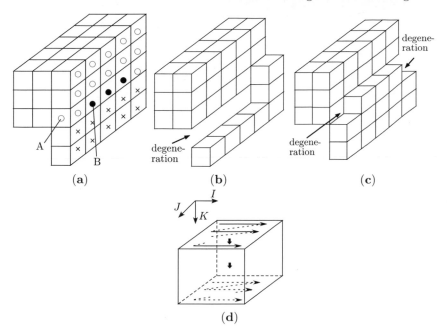

Fig. 5.4. Property of Algorithm 5.3 (surface/axis thinning). Condition of finally preserved voxel and degeneration (○: deletable, ×: preserved (not deletable) by the condition $C1$, ●: preserved by the condition $C2$).

$$(J - K + 1) \leq J' \leq (J - K + 2)$$
$$K' = 1.$$

The above algorithm is a prototype of a 3D surface-thinning algorithm, and has not been refined so much. In fact, it contains the surface thinning only. One may expect that an axis-thinning algorithm is obtained by excluding the condition $C1$ in this algorithm. However, the problem is not so simple. For example, a center line had to be obtained, even if a figure of the unit thickness is given as an input figure. If a parallelepiped figure is given as an input figure, it would be expected that the final result of a center line is obtained after an intermediate result of the same shape as a result of the surface thinning is reached. Let us give an example of such an algorithm in Algorithm 5.6.

5.4.5 Surface thinning algorithm accompanying the Euclidean distance transformation

Another problem of the above algorithm is that a thinned result is affected significantly by the rotation of an input figure. One major reason for this lies in the order that the algorithm shaves surface voxels from an input figure. Voxels at the unit distance from the background is tested for deletability and

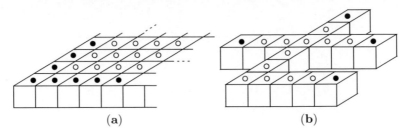

(a)   (b)

Fig. 5.5. Property of Algorithm 5.5 (surface thinning of a 2D plane figure in 3D space). ○: Preserved by the condition $C1$ and $C2$, ●: preserved by the condition $C1$.

replaced by a 0-voxel if deletable. The 6-neighbor distance used in the algorithm is significantly affected by the orientation of an input figure, although the distance is recalculated in each main cycle. This effect of the rotation will be reduced if the squared Euclidean distance is used instead of the 6-neighbor distance. Computation load will become too much, however, if the Euclidean distance is calculated directly according to its definition. One possible solution to overcome this difficulty is the application of the Euclidean distance transformation as a preprocess. Let us show an example of how to implement this idea [Saito95, Saito96]. The distance transformation will be explained in detail in the next Section 5.5.

Algorithm 5.4 (Surface thinning accompanied by squared Euclidean distance transformation).

Input: $\boldsymbol{F} = \{f_{ijk}\}$ = input binary image ($L \times M \times N$).
   f_{ijk} = density value of a voxel (i, j, k) which takes 0 or 1. A set of 1-voxels is considered as a figure.
   m = type of the connectivity ($m = 6, 18, 18', 26$).
Output: $\boldsymbol{F} = \{f_{ijk}\}$ = result of surface thinning is stored when the algorithm finishes. Also this is used to store intermediate results (values of distance transformation, labels, etc.) produced during execution. Physically the same array as the one that stores an input image is assigned.
Conditions for *a finally preserved voxel (FPV)*: A border voxel (i, j, k) satisfying at least one of the following $C1$ and $C2$ is called *FPV*, and is never deleted in the subsequent procedure (same as in Algorithm 5.3).
   $C1$: None of arrangements in Fig. 5.3 (3D simplex) exists in the $3 \times 3 \times 3$ neighborhood of a voxel (i, j, k).
   $C2$: A voxel (i, j, k) is not deletable in the m-connectivity.

[STEP 1] (Squared Euclidean distance transformation)
for all (i, j, k)s **do** (See Note)

Note: $de((i, j, k), (p, q, r))$ means the Euclidean distance between voxels (i, j, k) and (p, q, r). For squared Euclidean distance transformation and details of its algorithm, see Section 5.5

$$f_{ijk} \leftarrow \min_{(p,q,r)} \{(de(i,j,k),(p,q,r))^2;$$
$$f_{pqr} = 0,\ 1 \leq p \leq L, 1 \leq q \leq M, 1 \leq r \leq N\}$$

enddo

(Shift distance values by *20* for using integers *1* ∼ *19* as labels)

for all (i,j,k)s **do**

  if $(f_{ijk} \neq 0)$ **then** $f_{ijk} \leftarrow f_{ijk} + 20$

enddo

maxd ← (Maximum of the Euclidean distance transformation values in the
        image $\boldsymbol{F}$)

mind ← (Minimum of the nonzero values of the Euclidean distance
        transformation in the image $\boldsymbol{F}$)

(Main cycle processing)

[STEP 2]

for distance = mind to maxd **do**

  [STEP 3] (Extraction of *FPV* and classification of voxels to be tested the
  deletability)

  for all (i,j,k)s **do**

    if f_{ijk} = distance

    then

      if $(C1 \vee C2)$

      then $f_{ijk} \leftarrow 1$ (*FPV*)

      else

        $m \leftarrow$ (the number of non-0 voxels in the 26-neighborhood of (i,j,k))

        $f_{ijk} \leftarrow \mathrm{int}(m/3) + 7$ (give a label showing a group of the voxel. Label
        takes values *7* ∼ *15*)

      endif

    else no operation is performed

    endif

  enddo

  (Subcycle processing)

  [STEP 4] (Deletion of a voxel)

  for bordertype = *7* to *15* **do**

    for all (i,j,k)s **do**

      if f_{ijk} = bordertype

      then

        if $(C1 \vee C2)$

        then $f_{ijk} \leftarrow 1$ (*FPV*)

        else $f_{ijk} \leftarrow 0$ (Deletion of a 1-voxel)

        endif

      else no operation is performed

      endif

    enddo

  enddo

  [STEP 5] (Test of terminating rule)

enddo

[**STEP 6**] (Postprocessing)
for all (i, j, k)'s **do**
   if $f_{ijk} \neq 0$
   then $f_{ijk} \leftarrow 1$
   endif
enddo

Explanation of Algorithm 5.4. In this algorithm, we first apply the squared Euclidean distance transformation [Saito92, Saito93, Saito94a, Saito94b] to the whole of an input image. As a result, all 1-voxels of an input image are given the square of the shortest distance to the background. We now calculate the square of the distance instead of the exact distance value. Computation load is greatly reduced by doing this because the algorithm is simplified by avoiding the calculation of the square root and by using only the calculation of integers throughout the procedure. We need only the order of the distance value to the nearest 0-voxel, and need not use the absolute value of the distance.

Next we classify a voxel of the unit-squared distance into subgroups according to the number of nonzero voxels in the 26-neighborhood represented by m in the above description of the algorithm. For the sake of convenience, grouping is performed at every three of the value of m. The deletability test is applied to 1-voxels in the order of the value of m (a voxel of the smaller m is tested earlier). A border voxel in Algorithm 5.3 corresponds to a voxel of the unit (squared) distance value here. The deletability test and the relating procedure here are applied to the set of 1-voxels remaining at that point.

Classification of border voxels according to the locations of 0-voxels in their neighborhood is replaced here by the classification of voxels of the unit distance according to the number of nonzero voxels in the 26-neighborhood. The idea is basically the same in both algorithms. It is common to both algorithms that a deletable voxel is replaced by a 0-voxel when it is detected (sequential type of algorithm).

This algorithm proceeds to the processing of voxels with the (squared) distance value _2_, after all deletable voxels with the unit distance have been processed. The same procedure is repeated again to 1-voxels of the (squared) distance _2_. Thus, at the point that the processing of voxels of the (squared) distance d begins, all deletable voxels of the (squared) distance less than d have been deleted. Therefore, voxels of the (squared) distance d have become border voxels. Keeping a resultant figure at the center or in the vicinity and reducing the effect of the rotation of an input figure are both realized by executing procedures according to increasing order of the (squared) distance values.

The above procedure is performed repeatedly for voxels of all (squared) distance values.

The deletability test was applied earlier to voxels having more 0-voxels in the 26-neighborhood among voxels of the same distance values. Using this order, an isolated narrow protrusion tends to be shaved earlier. This tendency is desirable in that it prevents the generation of meaningless short branches in a thinned result from small irregularities of the surface of an input figure.

The meaning of [STEP 5] in the above algorithm may become clearer by writing as follows:

[**STEP 5**] (Test of terminating rule)
if no point changed through [**STEP 4**]
then
    if distance = maxd
    then stop (finishing the whole processing)
    else go to [**STEP 2**] (finishing a subcycle)
    endif
else go to [**STEP 3**]
endif

Remark 5.5 (Problems in realization). Major problems that should be considered in implementing and executing surface/axis thinning algorithms by computer are memory requirement and processing time (or computation load). Concerning the first problem, at least one 3D array is necessary for storing an input image. The above algorithm uses the same 3D array for not only storing the distance transformation, but also storing a label image produced at the intermediate step and storing the final result. This means the memory requirement is almost minimum, that is, only one 3D array of nearly the same size is required as an input image.

5.4.6 Use of a 1D list for auxiliary information

Processing time is, in principle, proportional to the number of iterations in the main cycle. This factor cannot be discussed in general because the number of iterations strongly depends on each individual image. Another factor that is important for practicality is the number of times each voxel is accessed (individual element of a 3D array). One possible way to reduce the number of times of access is the use of a 1D list that stores a 1-voxel to be processed and attributes of each voxel such as coordinates and labels. Subsequent procedures are executed according to the contents of this list.

It has been ascertained through experiments that this method could significantly reduce the processing time of the above algorithm, although algorithms become a little more complicated due to the list manipulation. The total amount of memory may increase a little by preparing the space for the list. The memory space for a list also depends on each input image. The size of the memory space for a list is usually not very big. In most cases it is small compared to the memory size required for an input 3D image. Roughly speaking, it will be enough to prepare a 1D memory of the size of a few times of the number of border voxels in an input image. An example of this type of algorithms is given below.

(a) Surface thinning

Algorithm 5.5 (Surface thinning accompanied by Euclidean distance transformation using list manipulation).

Input: $\boldsymbol{F} = \{f_{ijk}\}$ = input binary image is stored when the algorithm starts.
 f_{ijk} = density value of a voxel (i, j, k) that takes 0 or 1 when the algorithm starts. A set of 1-voxels is considered to be a figure.
 m = type of the connectivity ($m = 6, 18, 18', 26$).
Output: $\boldsymbol{F} = \{f_{ijk}\}$ = result of surface thinning is stored when the algorithm finishes.
Border voxel list: list = $\{e_n : (i_n, j_n, k_n, l_n)\}$: Each element in the list consists of 3D coordinate values of a voxel and its label.
Function int(x). Convert the value of an argument into an integer (omit the fractional part).

[STEP 1] (Squared Euclidean distance transformation (same as Algorithm 5.4))
for all (i, j, k)s **do**
 $f_{ijk} \leftarrow \min\limits_{(p,q,r)} \{de((i, j, k), (p, q, r))^2;$
 $f_{pqr} = 0, \ 1 \le p \le L, 1 \le q \le M, 1 \le r \le N\}$
enddo
(For details of algorithm of the Euclidean distance transformation, see Section 5.5)
(Shift distance values by 20 for using integers $1 \sim 19$ as labels)
for all (i, j, k)s **do**
 if $(f_{ijk} \ne 0)$, **then** $f_{ijk} \leftarrow f_{ijk} + 20$
enddo
maxd $\leftarrow$ (Maximum of the Euclidean distance transformation values in the image $\boldsymbol{F}$)
mind $\leftarrow$ (Minimum of the nonzero values of the Euclidean distance transformation in the image $\boldsymbol{F}$)

[STEP 2] (Detection of initial border voxels and write them into the list)
for all (i, j, k)s **do**
 if $f_{ijk} > 20$ and a 0-voxel exists in the 6-neighborhood of f_{ijk}
 then
 add(i, j, k, f_{ijk}) to the list
 (At this moment, the distance value of a voxel (i_n, j_n, k_n) is given to l_n of the list)
 $f_{ijk} \leftarrow 1$
 endif

enddo
$N \leftarrow$ length of the list

(Main cycle processing)
[STEP 3] (Detection of *FPV* ($l_n \leftarrow 0$ means *FPV*) and classification of border voxels)
for $n = 1$ to N **do**
  if $(l_n \leq$ mind)
  then
    if $C2$ is true $(= (i_n, j_n, k_n)$ is not deletable)
    then exclude an element e_n from the list (FPV)
    else
      if $C1$ is true $(=$ thickness of a figure at (i_n, j_n, k_n) is 1)
      then exclude e_n from the list (FPV)
      else
        $m \leftarrow$ (the number of non-0 voxels in the 26-neighborhood of (i_n, j_n, k_n))
        $l_n \leftarrow \text{int}(m/3) + 7$ (classification of border voxels)
      endif
    endif
  endif
enddo

(Subcycle processing)
[STEP 4] (Deletion of a voxel)
$N' \leftarrow$ length of the list
for bordertype $= 7$ to 15 **do**
  for $n = 1$ to N' **do**
    if $(l_n =$ bordertype)
    then
      if $C2$ is true $(= (i_n, j_n, k_n)$ is not deletable)
      then exclude e_n from the list (FPV)
      else
        if $C1$ is true $(=$ thickness of a figure at (i_n, j_n, k_n) is 1)
        then exclude e_n from the list (FPV)
        else
          $f_{i_n j_n k_n} \leftarrow 0$ (deletion of a voxel (i_n, j_n, k_n))
          exclude e_n from the list
          for (all voxels (i', j', k') in the 6-neighborhood of (i_n, j_n, k_n)) **do**
            if $(f_{i'j'k'} > 20)$
            then
              add $(i', j', k', f_{i'j'k'})$ to the list (addition of voxels to the list)
              $f_{i'j'k'} \leftarrow 1$
            endif
          enddo
        endif

```
      endif
    endif
  enddo
enddo
```

[**STEP 5**] (Test of the terminating rule)
$N \leftarrow$ length of the list
mind $\leftarrow$ the minimum of the distance values in the list (the minimum value
in all values over *20*)
if (mind < maxd or $N > 0$)
then go to [STEP 3]
endif

[**STEP 6**] (Postprocessing)
for all (i, j, k)s **do**
  if $(f_{ijk} \neq 0)$
  then $f_{ijk} \leftarrow 1$
  endif
enddo

Remark 5.6. A kind of trade-off exists in a surface/axis-thinning algorithm
between the appearance of false (undesired) branches and occurrence of degeneration. Here a false branch tends to appear in a thinned result due to
small irregularities on a border surface. Degeneration means that a thinned
result shrinks too much or becomes shorter than we naturally expect. An algorithm with a better performance concerning degeneration is likely to produce
more false branches and vice versa. Both of them are affected by the subject
in evaluation to some extent. In Algorithm 5.3 and 5.4, this trade-off is controlled only a little by the number of 1-voxels existing in the 26-neighborhood
of each 1-voxel. For example, the deletion is applied according to the order
of the number of 1-voxels in the 26-neighborhood. One method to control
this trade-off more successfully is given in [Saito01]. Prevention of degeneration is important in a thinning algorithm, but is not solved easily. Incorrect
strategies may cause the disappearance of the whole of a figure with the specific orientation. Many problems still remain to be solved in the prevention of
degeneration.

(b) Axis thinning

Let us show an example of the axis thinning algorithm. As was stated, it is
not always necessary to terminate the iteration procedures in an algorithm
concerning axis thinning at the moment that an input figure becomes a plane
of the unit thickness. A 1-voxel is given the mark of a *finally preserved voxel*

Note: Integers *0* ~ *20* are used as labels.

(*FPV*) only when the 1-voxel reached the state that the voxel is regarded as the end point of a 3D line figure. For example, voxels existing on a plane figure of the unit thickness cannot be deleted unless they are on a border of a figure because the topology is not preserved if they are deleted, even if the distance value is *1* on those voxels. However, even those voxels will become deletable at some point when they are shaved from a border according to the predetermined order until a centerline is obtained. Thus, some of voxels are in the state that they are kept in without deletion during only the same cycle as is currently executed. We call those voxels that should be preserved during only a specific one cycle currently being executed *temporary preservation state*. We give a specific mark showing the *temporary preservation state* to those voxels.

The following algorithm (Algorithm 5.6) was derived based on almost the same basic policy as Algorithm 5.4.

Algorithm 5.6 (Axis thinning accompanied by Euclidean distance transformation using list manipulation).
Explanation of input images, etc., is the same as Algorithm 5.5.

[**STEP 1**] (Squared Euclidean distance transformation) (Same as Algorithm 5.4 [STEP 1])

[**STEP 2**] (Detection of initial border voxels and write their coordinates into the list) (Same as Algorithm 5.5 [STEP 2])

(Main cycle processing)
[**STEP 3**] (Detection of FPV and classification of border voxels; $l_n \leftarrow 0$ means *FPV*.)
for $n = 1$ to N **do**
  if ($l_n \leq$ mind)
  then
    if $C2$ ($= (i_n, j_n, k_n)$ is not deletable)
    then $l_n \leftarrow 16$ (*temporal preservation voxel* (*TPV*))
    else
      if ((i_n, j_n, k_n) is an edge voxel) (See Note)
      then exclude an element e_n from the list (*FPV*)
      else
        $m \leftarrow$ the number of nonzero-voxels in the 26-neighborhood of (i_n, j_n, k_n)
        $l_n \leftarrow \text{int}(m/3) + 7$ (classification of border voxels)
      endif
    endif
  enddo

(Subcycle processing)
[**STEP 4**] (Deletion of a voxel)

Note: An edge voxel here means a voxel that has only one nonzero voxel in the 26-neighborhood.

$N' \leftarrow$ length of the list
for bordertype $= 7$ to 15 **do**
  for $n = 1$ to N' **do**
    if $(l_n = $ bordertype$)$
    then
      if $C2$ $(= (i_n, j_n, k_n)$ is not deletable$)$
      then $l_n \leftarrow 16$ (TPV)
      else
        if $((i_n, j_n, k_n)$ is an edge voxel$)$
        then exclude e_n from the list (FPV)
        else
          $f_{i_n j_n k_n} \leftarrow 0$ (Deletion of a voxel (i_n, j_n, k_n))
          exclude e_n from the list
          for (all voxels in the 6-neighborhood of (i_n, j_n, k_n)) **do**
            if $(f_{i'j'k'} > 20)$
            then
              add$(i', j', k', f_{i'j'k'})$ to the list
              $f_{i'j'k'} \leftarrow 1$
            endif
          enddo
        endif
      endif
    endif
  enddo
enddo

[**STEP 5**] (Test of the terminating rule)
$N \leftarrow$ length of the list
mind $\leftarrow$ minimum of the distance values in the list (the minimum value in the list over 20)
$m \leftarrow$ the number of nondeletable voxels ($l_n = 16$) in the list
if (mind $<$ maxd or $m > N$)
then go to [**STEP 3**]
endif

[**STEP 6**] (postprocessing)
Same as Algorithm 5.5 [STEP 6]

5.4.7 Examples of surface/axis thinning algorithm (parallel type)

The formal definition of the parallel type algorithm was already described in Chapter 2. In the context of the surface/axis thinning, it will be stated as follows:

    In every cycle of iteration the whole of an input image is examined to give a mark to all voxels that are deemed deletable and those which are to be preserved finally (*FPV*). However, deletable voxels are not actually deleted at the moment of detection. The deletion is executed simultaneously (all at once and in parallel) for all these voxels, when all voxels of an input image have finished being tested for deletability. A voxel is never deleted during any cycle of the iteration once it has been selected to be preserved.

The most difficult and the most critical problem is the prevention of the phenomenon that occurs when the whole of a figure with the two voxels width disappears as a result of deletion regardless of only a deletable voxel being deleted. This is a kind of degeneration. Let us show one example. Suppose that an input figure is a cube consisting of $2 \times 2 \times 2$ voxels. Then, any of these eight voxels satisfies the deletability condition if the deletability of each of them is tested independently from other voxels. Thus, if the deletion is performed simultaneously at all of those eight voxels, then the input figure will disappear.

The following three strategies have been known to avoid this type of degeneration:

(1) To develop a better algorithm for detecting a set of deletable voxels so that all of extracted voxels can be deleted all at once (*completely parallel-processing type*).
(2) To classify first all border voxels into suitable subgroups and the deletability test is applied to only one subgroup in one time of iteration. An example of the grouping is how many 0-voxels are adjacent and in which side of each border voxel. Each subgroup is processed according to the given order. All deletable voxels in the same subgroup are deleted simultaneously. Therefore, deletion is done in parallel within the same subgroup, and subgroups are processed sequentially (*subborder group type*).
(3) To divide all voxels in an input image into mutually exclusive subgroups beforehand, the same processing as (2) above is applied in parallel within the same subgroup. Each subgroup is processed sequentially according to the predetermined order (*subfield type*).

The first strategy leads to a parallel type of procedure. However, it cannot be realized by using a $3 \times 3 \times 3$ or smaller neighborhood. An algorithm using a $5 \times 5 \times 5$ neighborhood is shown in [Ma95, Ma96]. The second idea is essentially the same as the one employed in the subcycle system of thinning, which was introduced to keep a thinned result at or near the center of an input figure. This is a popular idea in the parallel type of algorithm used now. An example of the third idea is found in [Bertrand94a, Bertrand94b, Bertrand95, Saha94, Saha97], in which eight subfields are employed. Concrete algorithms are given in those papers.

5.4.8 Experimental results

Let us show experimental results of surface/axis thinning in Fig. 5.6 $\sim$ 5.9. Algorithms used here are Algorithm 5.3 and the algorithm in [Tsao81]. Input images were artificial figures (a sphere, a cube, connection of them), a hand, and a bronchus extracted from a CT image.

Figures 5.6 and 5.7 show thinned results of artificial figures. Input figures were put in parallel with coordinate axis in Fig. 5.6 and rotated in Fig. 5.7. Results from different thinning algorithms differ significantly from each other. The thinning algorithm accompanied by Euclidean distance transformation is affected less by the orientation and the rotation of an input figure and gives natural results. Results of Algorithms 5.4 and 5.5 applied to the same input image are shown in Fig. 5.8. By observing this carefully, the difference between the surface and axis thinning is clearly apparent. Finally, Fig. 5.9 is a result of axis thinning by Algorithm 5.6.

The generation of undesired branches (spurious branches) is controlled to some extent by two kinds of parameters as presented in [Saito01, Toriwaki01]. A result is shown in Fig. 5.10. An input figure here is a Y-shaped connection of three cylinders contaminated by random noise. A kind of trade-off between generation of spurious branches and degeneration of a figure will be confirmed in this example. Details of the method are presented in [Saito01, Toriwaki01].

5.4.9 Points in algorithm construction

Let us summarize in this section the important points in constructing thinning algorithms. They show a method to discover the requirements for thinning algorithms described in Section 5.4.2. How to integrate factors referred to in these points in individual algorithms also strongly depends on computer technologies available at the time. In fact, memory cost is much lower and speed is much faster now than in the 1980s.

(i) *Definition of functions*: What are the contents of "thinning" that we consider at the design of an algorithm. All of the following also relate to this, such as definitions of a line figure and a surface figure, intuitive understanding of them, and constraints of an input figure. Most input figures may be elongated figures in some applications. Topology preservation may not be so important in other applications. Algorithms will become much simpler in such cases.

(ii) *Topology preservation*: Did the topology of an input figure have to be preserved precisely or not? The shape of an input figure may be restricted in some applications.

(iii) *Deletability test*: The deletability test can be performed by either calculation of mathematical equations or local pattern matching. The former method was first reported in [Yonekura80b] for all four types of connectivity and the outline was explained in this book. Most other reports employ the latter method with template matching on the $3 \times 3 \times 3$ neighborhood except for completely parallel algorithms employing the $5 \times 5 \times 5$ neighborhood. Assuming the use of the $3 \times 3 \times 3$ neighborhood, at least six template patterns will be necessary which are symmetric to one particular template pattern, corresponding to six surfaces of a cubic voxel. When

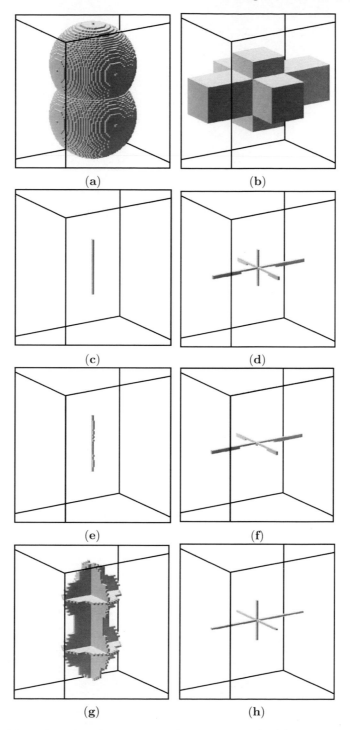

Fig. 5.6. Examples of surface thinning (artificial figure): (**a**) Input figure - connected balls; (**b**) input figure - connected cubes; (**c**), (**d**) Algorithm 5.4; (**e**), (**f**) Algorithm 5.3; (**g**), (**h**) method of [Tsao81].

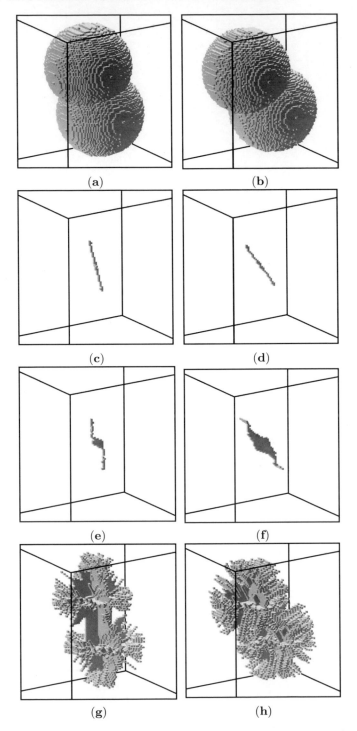

Fig. 5.7. Examples of surface thinning (artificial figure - rotated balls): (**a**) Input figure - the same figure as Fig. 5.6 (a) rotated by *15* degrees; (**b**) input figure - the same figure as Fig. 5.6 (a) rotated by *30* degrees; (**c**), (**d**) Algorithm 5.4; (**e**), (**f**) Algorithm 5.3; (**g**), (**h**) method of [Tsao81].

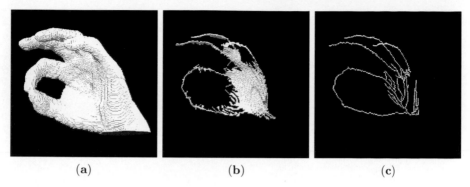

(a)   (b)   (c)

Fig. 5.8. Examples of thinning: **(b)** surface thinning by Algorithm 5.4; **(c)** axis thinning by algorithm; both applied to the same CT image of hand.

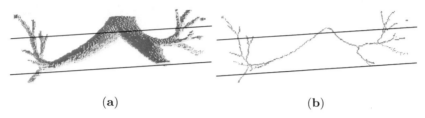

(a)   (b)

Fig. 5.9. Example of axis thinning. Algorithm 5.6 was applied to a CT image of bronchus and bronchus branches extracted from a 3D chest CT image.

we design a template based upon some heuristics, we first consider three horizontal arrangements of 3×3 voxels and then take into account the relationship between patterns on the upper and the lower planes. This is the typical way to obtain a 3D template for thinning.

In any algorithm, the deletability test, while keeping the topology of a figure unchanged, is the most essential part and the most time-consuming part of the procedure. In the algorithms presented in this section, the deletability test was completed directly. However, various other approaches and variations have been reported. For example, there is a method to detect the deletability by considering arrangements of 1-voxels on three orthogonal planes including the current voxel (called check planes) [Tsao81, Tsao82a, Tsao82b] (Fig. 5.11).

(iv) *Connectivity*: Only the deletability test presented in the previous chapter claims that it is applicable to all four connectivity types (6-, 18-, 18'-, and 26-connectivity). Most other methods only treat two types of connectivity, 6- and 26-connectivity. Some methods only treat the single type of connectivity (6- or 26-connectivity).

(v) *Mode of iteration*: Thinning algorithms are classified into two major types, the sequential type and the parallel type, according to the execution of

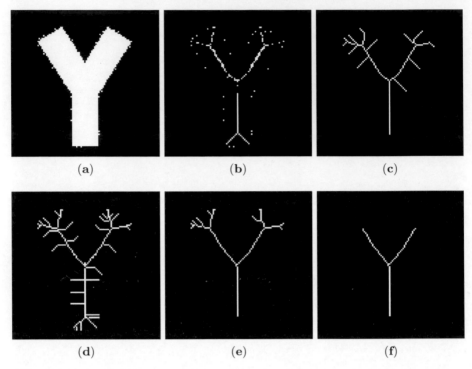

Fig. 5.10. Control by generation of spurious branches in the axis thinning by the method in [Saito01]. The α shows values of a control parameter in this method: (**a**) Input figure; (**b**) skeleton (See Section 5.5.5); (**c**) axis thinning by Algorithm 5.4; (**d**) thinning method by [Saito01] ($\alpha = 1.1$); (**e**) same as (**d**) ($\alpha = 1.5$); (**f**) same as (**d**) ($\alpha = 2.0$).

    deletion, that is, whether a deletable voxel is immediately replaced by a 0-voxel or not. The subcycle system (usually 6 subcycles) is adopted in order to keep results near the center of a figure. In the parallel type algorithm, the use of the subborder group system and the subfield system have been proposed. The total number of times of iteration differs in these different systems. In [Palagyi99], 12 times of iteration are performed in the subborder group system. The completely parallel type of algorithms will become really effective if one-to-one correspondence between processors and voxels is realized. This has not yet been realized.

(vi) *Surface and axis thinning*: Distinction between the surface thinning and the axis thinning defined in Definition 5.1 and 5.2 was discussed first by anchors with Algorithm 5.3 which made is possible for users to choose either of them. This problem has not been discussed much afterward [Bertrand95]. Differences between them may not have serious consequences in applications that treat slender figures.

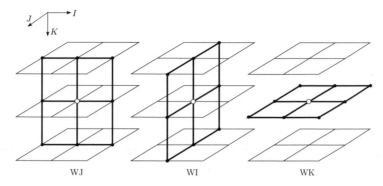

Fig. 5.11. An example of voxels used in deletability test in surface/axis thinning in [Tsao81, Tsao82a, Tsao82b]. A current voxel is denoted with ∘. Solid lines show check planes of *3 × 3* voxels.

(vii) *Subsidiary information*: Various subsidiary information is used to improve the quality of a thinned result and to achieve higher performance of algorithms. For example, the computation time can be significantly reduced by extracting border voxels and storing those coordinates in a list beforehand as in Algorithms 5.5 and 5.6. This is due to the fact that an object of deletion is only a border voxel. The use of distance transformation is also effective as in Algorithm 5.4. For example, a voxel of a smaller distance value may be deleted earlier, a skeleton voxel is considered as a candidate of a voxel to be deleted, and appearance of false branches in an output of thinning is controlled by using skeleton voxels [Saito01, Toriwaki01].

(viii) *Control of a finally preserved voxel (FPV)*: A user may wish that a specific voxel will remain in an output figure, or that a resulting line figure will pass specific voxels. These requirements are satisfied by giving a mark of *FPV* to those voxels beforehand.Thinning with an anchor point is an example of this and is effectively used for controlling the appearance of spurious branches. See Remark 5.7 [Ragnemalm90, Saito01, Toriwaki01].

Remark 5.7. Study of surface/axis thinning of a 3D image began in around 1980. Papers in those years are listed in [Toriwaki85a]. Papers [Tsao81, Kawase85] showed the conditions of topology preservation explicitly and provided a prototype of research in related fields. After these, a few papers have been published and are given in the reference list in the end of this book. Comparative studies have not been reported. A deletability test in [Kawase85, Saito95] is the one presented in Chapter 4, and those in other papers were similar to [Tsao81]. Comparative study on the quality of thinned results is very sparse. According to experimental results by the author's group, the method accompanied by Euclidean distance transformation seems to be better than others. The reason is perhaps that the deviation from the Euclidean distance is rather large in the 26-neighborhood and the 6-neighborhood distance and also that the directional inhomogeneity is more remarkable in 3D space than in 2D space.

Remark 5.8. For surface/axis thinning presented here the words *skeletonization* and *medial surface/axis thinning (extraction)* are also used, but an exact distinction among them has not been shown clearly. Skeleton extraction based upon the distance transformation stated in the following section is quite different from any others [Borgefors99]. Many papers concerning 3D thinning have seen published since around 2000. Examples are shown in Supplementary list in the reference list.

Remark 5.9. The surface/axis thinning stated here imposes the general and theoretically very strict requirement of *preserving the topology* of an input figure for an *arbitrary* binary image. In many practical applications, however, an input image or a resulting image may be restricted a little more. A thinning algorithm will be useful, even if it does not satisfy such a condition strictly. Many other algorithms have been developed for a wide range of practical problems. Following are examples of more moderate requirements and easier situations concerning thinning.

(a) Input figures are slender tubular figures extending in almost the same direction. The axis thinning will be achieved by connecting center points of their cross sections which are almost 2D circular figures.

(b) To connect center points of balls, inscribing an input 3D figure might give acceptable results. This is nearly equivalent to using skeleton voxels determined by the distance transformation presented in the following section.

(c) To extract a sequence of points (voxels) inside an input figure, which are as distant from a border of a figure as possible, and connect one and the other end of an input figure is discussed in [Bitter01]. A tree search algorithm and the minimization of weights of a tree are available for obtaining such a sequence of voxels.

(d) An input figure has no holes and cavities or they may be neglected even if they exist. One example of such cases is automated generation of paths for flying through colon and bronchus branches in virtual endoscopy [Saito00, Hayashi00, Hayashi03].

5.5 Distance transformation and skeleton

5.5.1 Definition

The distance transformation (DT) of a 3D figure is defined as follows.

Definition 5.3 (Distance transformation (DT)). A process to obtain an output image $D = \{d_{ijk}\}$ given below from an input image $F = \{f_{ijk}\}$ is called *distance transformation* of an image $F = \{f_{ijk}\}$.

3D distance transformation: $F = \{f_{ijk}\} \rightarrow D = \{d_{ijk}\}$

$$d_{ijk} = \min\{d((i,j,k),(p,q,r)); f_{pqr} = 0\}, \tag{5.1}$$

where $d(\times\times, \times\times) = $ distance between $\times\times$ and $\times\times$, if $f_{ijk} = 1$,
            $= 0$,   if $f_{ijk} = 0$.
An image D is also called *distance transformation* (sometimes it is called distance field and distance map).

The distance transformation is defined as follows.

(i) A process to give each 1-voxel of an input image the shortest distance (or the length of the shortest path) to the background (a set of 0-voxels).
(ii) A process to shave an input figure repeatedly by one layer in each iteration and to give a value k to a voxel shaved in the k times of iteration.

Contents of DT depend on the definition of the distance function $d(***, ***)$ in Eq. 5.1. Usually, the Euclidean distance and other suitable ones among those presented in Section 4.9 are employed. The use of the squared distance $d^2(***, ***)$ is acceptable instead of $d(***, ***)$ in some of applications. This is called *squared distance transformation*. Computation load is significantly reduced by using the squared distance in the Euclidean distance transformation. If the comparative relation in the size of the distance values is a main problem, results will be the same for using the distance value and the square of it. An example is the application for thinning presented in the previous section.

The use of the Euclidean distance is most natural in practical applications, but the algorithm is complicated. The distance transformation using the 6- and the 26-neighbor distance can be performed by much simpler algorithms. However, deviation from the Euclidean distance is large in these distance metrics, and results become unnatural in some cases. In subsequent sections we will introduce algorithms for both of them. Skeleton will be explained later in detail.

Distance transformations using variable and fixed neighborhood distances are called *variable* and *fixed neighborhood distance transformation*, respectively. The fixed neighborhood DT is called often by the name of the distance metric employed in it such as the 26-neighbor DT. In the case of the Euclidean metric, we need not consider a path if we want to calculate a distance between two points. A path was discussed in detail in Section 4.9.

Remark 5.10. An algorithm to perform DT closely relates to finding a shortest path. For instance, if we find the shortest 26-connected path from a set of all 0-voxels to a 1-voxel P, the length of this shortest path gives the value of the 26-neighborhood DT at the voxel P. On the other hand, this idea cannot be applied to the Euclidean DT. Thus a DT algorithm is classified into two groups: the Euclidean DT and the variable (or fixed) neighborhood DT. The latter group is classified further into *an ordinary type* and *a path extension type*. From the viewpoint of execution, they include the sequential type and the parallel type. Examples of algorithms in each class will be presented subsequently. Basic parts of algorithms of DT do not depend on the dimensionality (dimensionality-independent), and can be immediately extended to an *n*-dimensional DT.

5.5.2 Significance of DT and skeleton

Significance of the DT and the skeleton in image processing is summarized in (1) ~ (4) below [Toriwaki81]. (The skeleton will be explained later in Section 5.5.3. Although many reports referred to in this section treat 2D image processing, almost all of the contents presented there are immediately extendable to a 3D image.)

(1) *Distance value*: Values of the DT are used to discover the distance between two voxels, the distance from a voxel to a figure, and the distance between two figures. The Euclidean DT is the best for this.

(2) *Concentration of information*: Information that is stored, being scattered over subarea in the 3D space, is put together onto the lower dimensional subspace. For example, information distributed over a spherical region is collected on the center, which is extracted as a skeleton. Information distributed along a line figure is put together in specific points by the DT on a line pattern [Toriwaki82a]. This property of information propagation is made use of by applying the DT based upon the shortest path and the DT of a line pattern.

(3) *Shape feature*: Values of the DT and their distribution on a figure, the shape of equidistance surfaces, and skeletons are useful as shape features themselves and as tools of feature extraction. The DT is particularly effective in finding the distance from an arbitrary point to some 3D volumetric object. The DT is also effectively used in an ordinary image processing procedure as a tool of segmentation and as a similarity measure between 3D figures [Kitasaka02a, Kitasaka02b, Mori94a]. Detection of a narrow part in a figure is a good example and was applied to detecte a polyp in virtual colonoscopy.

(4) *Preprocessing*: DT is used as a preprocessing of other image processing such as in surface/axis thinning and calculation of Voronoi division [Saito92]. The Euclidean DT is best here, too.

(5) *Control information*: The process of performing the DT based upon the path length is available for controlling other kinds of processing and information propagation [Toriwaki79, Toriwaki81].

(6) *Theoretical analysis of algorithms*: DT of both a continuous image and a digitized image have interesting properties concerning shape feature analysis and formal description of algorithms. For example, parallel algorithms of DT are systematized in a beautiful form using image operations. Both a sequential type and a parallel type algorithm are most clearly correspondent with each other. The DT corresponds also to the morphology operation [Toriwaki81, Yokoi81, Serra82].

5.5.3 Classification of algorithms

Before proceeding to the introduction of concrete algorithms, let us summarize their basic principles.

The DT is a *process that gives each 1-voxel or a figure the distance to the nearest background voxel (0-voxel)*. Three ideas have been developed to perform this.

(i) Calculate directly at each 1-voxel the distance to the nearest 0-voxel (direct calculation method).
(ii) Propagate distance values to adjacent 1-voxels sequentially.
(iii) Shave a figure iteratively by one layer in one time of iteration from the outside. A voxel shaved in the k times of iteration is regarded as being at the distance k from the background.
(iv) Extend a path into the inside of a figure. The distance value at each voxel that the path passes through is found by calculating the path length when extended (path extension method).

The third and fourth methods cannot be used in the Euclidean DT. A voxel of the distance *1*, for example, is not always m-adjacent to a voxel of the distance *2* ($m = 6, 18, 26$). Thus the Euclidean DT is calculated via the first method or by the second method with a specific device. Other kinds of DT with the variable neighborhood or the fixed neighborhood are calculated mostly using the third and forth method due to ease of programming and computation.

5.5.4 Example of an algorithm – (1) squared Euclidean DT

First, we will show a basic concept [Saito92, Saito93, Saito94a].

Given an input image $\boldsymbol{F} = \{f_{ijk}\}$ ($L \times M \times N$), consider the following sequence of transformations.

$\boldsymbol{F} = \{f_{ijk}\} \rightarrow$ (transformation I) $\rightarrow \boldsymbol{G} = \{g_{ijk}\} \rightarrow$ (transformation II) $\rightarrow \boldsymbol{H} = \{h_{ijk}\} \rightarrow$ (transformation III) $\rightarrow \boldsymbol{S} = \{s_{ijk}\}$

(Transformation I) Apply the following transformation to an image $\boldsymbol{F}$ while referring to $\boldsymbol{F}$ only in the i-direction (1D weighted minimum filter). Denote an output image by $\boldsymbol{G} = \{g_{ijk}\}$ (Fig. 5.12 (a)).

$$g_{ijk} = \min_{x}\{(i - x)^2;\ f_{xjk} = 0,\ 1 \leq x \leq L\}. \tag{5.2}$$

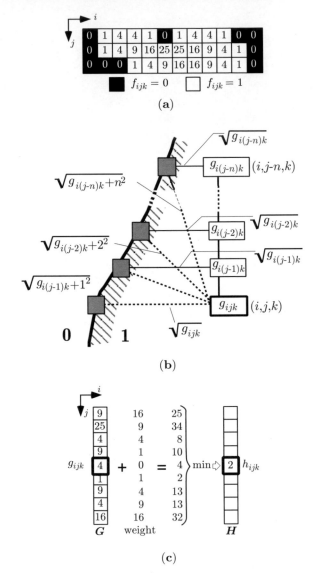

Fig. 5.12. Illustration of algorithm of squared Euclidean distance transformation:
(a) Example of Transformation I; (b) illustration of Transformation II; (c) example
of Transformation II.

(Transformation II) Perform the following transformation of the above image
$G = \{g_{ijk}\}$ referring G only in the j-direction (1D weighted minimum
filter). Denote an output image by $H = \{h_{ijk}\}$ (Fig. 5.12 (b), (c)).

$$h_{ijk} = \min_{y}\{g_{iyk} + (j - y)^2;\ 1 \le y \le M\}. \tag{5.3}$$

(Transformation III) Perform the following transformation of the above image $\boldsymbol{H}$ referring to $\boldsymbol{H}$ in the k-direction (1D weighted minimum filter). Denote an output image by $\boldsymbol{S} = \{s_{ijk}\}$ (Fig. 5.12 (c)).

$$s_{ijk} = \min_{z}\{h_{ijz} + (k - z)^2;\ 1 \le z \le N\}. \tag{5.4}$$

Then the following property holds true concerning an image $\boldsymbol{S}$.

Property 5.4. A value of a nonzero voxel in an image $\boldsymbol{S}$ obtained by Transformation III is equal to the square of the Euclidean distance from a nonzero voxel to the nearest 0-voxel. This is ascertained easily as follows [Saito93, Saito94a].

(Proof) From equation (5.2),

$$g_{ijk} = \min_{x}\{(i - x)^2;\ f_{ijk} = 0,\ 1 \le x \le L\} \tag{5.5}$$

$$= \text{the squared distance to the closest 0-voxel in the same row as } (i, j, k).$$

By substituting Eq. (5.5) with Eq. (5.3), we obtain

$$h_{ijk} = \min_{y}\{\min_{x}\{(i - x)^2;\ f_{xyk} = 0,\ 1 \le x \le L\} + (j - y)^2;\ 1 \le y \le M\}$$

$$= \min_{y}\{\min_{x}\{(i - x)^2 + (j - y)^2;\ f_{xyk} = 0,\ 1 \le x \le L;\ 1 \le y \le M\}$$

$$= \min_{(x,y)}\{(i - x)^2 + (j - y)^2;\ f_{xyk} = 0,\ 1 \le x \le L;\ 1 \le y \le M\} \tag{5.6}$$

$$= \text{the squared distance to the closest 0-voxel in the same plane as } (i, j, k).$$

By substituting the result to Eq. (5.4),

$$s_{ijk} = \min_{z}\{\min_{(x,y)}\{(i - x)^2 + (j - y)^2;$$

$$f_{xyk} = 0,\ 1 \le x \le L,\ 1 \le y \le M\} + (k - z)^2;\ 1 \le z \le N\}$$

$$= \min_{z}\{\min_{(x,y)}\{(i - x)^2 + (j - y)^2 + (k - z)^2;$$

$$f_{xyk} = 0,\ 1 \le x \le L,\ 1 \le y \le M;\ 1 \le z \le N\}$$

$$= \min_{(x,y,z)}\{(i - x)^2 + (j - y)^2 + (k - z)^2;$$

$$f_{xyk} = 0,\ 1 \le x \le L,\ 1 \le y \le M;\ 1 \le z \le N\}. \tag{5.7}$$

Thus it is shown that an image $\boldsymbol{S}$ is the squared EDT of an image $\boldsymbol{F}$.

If a voxel is not cubic but a parallelepiped, the above transformations should be modified as follows: assume here that the ratio among the lengths of three edges of a voxel is 1 (i-direction): α (j-direction): β (k-direction). Then, using the same notations as in the Transformations I $\sim$ III,

(Transformation II') Use the following equation instead of Eq. (5.3).

$$h_{ijk} = \min_{y}\{g_{iyk} + (\alpha(j - y))^2;\ 1 \le y \le M\}. \tag{5.8}$$

(Transformation III') Use the following equation instead of Eq. (5.4).

$$s_{ijk} = \min_{z}\{h_{ijz} + (\beta(k-z))^2; \; 1 \leq z \leq N\}. \tag{5.9}$$

The following algorithm is obtained by combining Transformations I $\sim$ III (or I, II', and III').

Algorithm 5.7 (Squared Euclidean distance transformation).

[**STEP 1**](Corresponds to Transformation I)
[**STEP 1.1**] Perform the following processing for each row.
Input image $\boldsymbol{F} = \{f_{ijk}\}(L \times M \times N)$,
Output image $\boldsymbol{G'} = \{g'_{ijk}\}$,
for all j, k **do**
  $d = 0$
  for $i = 1$ to L **do**
    if $f_{ijk} \neq 0$
    then $d \leftarrow d + 1$
    else $d \leftarrow 0$
    endif
    $g'_{ijk} \leftarrow d^2$
  enddo
enddo
i is changed from 1 to L (from left to right in each plane of an image (forward scan)).
[**STEP 1.2**] Perform the following processing for each row.
Input image $\boldsymbol{G'} = \{g'_{ijk}\}$,
Output image $\boldsymbol{G} = \{g_{ijk}\}$,
for all j, k **do**
  $d = 0$
  for $i = L$ to 1 **do**
    if $g'_{ijk} \neq 0$
    then $d \leftarrow d + 1$
    else $d \leftarrow 0$
    endif
    $g_{ijk} \leftarrow \min\{g'_{ijk}, d^2\}$
  enddo
enddo
i is changed from L to 1 (from right to left in each plane of an image (backward scan)).

[**STEP 2**](Corresponds to Transformation II)
Input image $\boldsymbol{G} = \{g_{ijk}\}$,
Output image $\boldsymbol{H} = \{h_{ijk}\}$
for all (i, j, k) **do** (Perform the following processing at each voxel)
  $h_{ijk} \leftarrow \min_{-r \leq n \leq r}\{g_{i(j+n)k} + n^2\}$ where $r = \sqrt{g_{ijk}}$

Search the minimum above by changing n sequentially over the range ($1 \leq j + n \leq M$) of an input image.
enddo

[**STEP 3**] (Corresponds to Transformation III)
Input image $\boldsymbol{H} = \{h_{ijk}\}$,
Output image $\boldsymbol{S} = \{s_{ijk}\}$
for all (i, j, k) **do** (Perform the following processing at each voxel)
$$s_{ijk} \leftarrow \min_{-r \leq n \leq r} \{h_{ij(k+n)} + n^2\} \text{ where } r = \sqrt{h_{ijk}}$$
Search area for the minimum the same as in [**STEP 2**].
enddo

If an input image $\boldsymbol{F}$ need not be preserved after the execution of the algorithm, images $\boldsymbol{F}$, $\boldsymbol{G'}$, $\boldsymbol{G}$, $\boldsymbol{H}$, and $\boldsymbol{S}$ may be assigned to the same array on the computer. In [STEP 2], after the values of i, j, and k are specified, a list (1D array) is necessary for storing $\{g_{ijk}; \ 1 \leq j \leq M\}$. This is the same in [STEP 3].

Details of the algorithm are shown in [Saito92, Saito93, Saito94a, Kato95] with the range of search in [STEP 2] and [STEP 3] and faster algorithms. Modifications for a parallelepiped voxel will be obvious.

Let us summarize properties of this algorithm:

(a) *Squared Euclidean distance*: This algorithm gives the squared Euclidean distance transformation. Exact values of distances are easily obtained by calculating the square root of suitable voxel values in the output image. Only calculation among integers is used in the algorithm (square roots appearing in the range of search in [STEP 2] and [STEP 3] are only for saving the computation time). Exact calculation of them is not always required.

(b) *Amount of computation*: Amount of computation in three transformations in the algorithm is estimated as follows.
(Transformation I) O (Num)
(Transformation II) O (average of square roots of voxel values in $\boldsymbol{G} \times$ Num)
(Transformation III) O (average of square roots of voxel values in $\boldsymbol{H} \times$ Num)
Here, O means the order and Num is the number of voxels in an input image. If averages of square roots of voxel values in images $\boldsymbol{G}$ and $\boldsymbol{H}$ are large compared with image sizes M and N, the above estimation may not be applicable, because the range of search is mostly determined by the image size.

Assuming that the total amount of computation is approximated by the sum of that of three transformation, and that square roots of voxel values in $\boldsymbol{G}$ and $\boldsymbol{H}$ are approximated by the square roots of the distance transformation $\boldsymbol{S}$ multiplied by a constant, the total amount of computation is given approximately as O (arrange of values of the DT $\times$ Num). This result is confirmed in experiments [Saito94a, Saito94b].

(c) *Memory requirement*: When an input image is preserved after the execution of the DT, two arrays of the same size as an input image are required for storing an output image and a work area. If an input image needs not be preserved after the transformation and it is desirable to minimize memory requirements, the algorithm can be executed using one 3D array of the same size as an input image and one 1D array of the size max (M, N). In this case, an input image, working area, and an output image are all assigned to the same 3D array. A 1D array is necessary also as a work area. This is one of the main advantages of this algorithm when a very large 3D input image has to be processed.

(d) *Type of algorithm*: This algorithm is sequential in an approximate sense, because it can be executed on one 3D array. However, this is not true, in a strict sense, because the processing of [STEP 2] and [STEP 3] (search of the minimum) is not always sequential. Since the range of search cannot be fixed beforehand and depends on input data, the algorithm is of the data-dependent type. Thus it cannot be regarded as the local processing. One-dimensional decomposition is achieved because it is represented as a serial composition of three 1D processing, each of which is performed in each coordinate axis direction. Thus this algorithm cannot be classified into a well-defined execution type. It is not yet clear how it is advantageous in hardware implementation. Implementation of the squared Euclidean DT on a parallel-type computer was discussed in [Miyazawa06, Hirata96].

Next let us introduce a parallel-type algorithm of the Euclidean DT.

Algorithm 5.8 (Euclidean distance transformation - parallel type).

Input image: $\boldsymbol{F} = \{f_{ijk}\}$
Output image: $\boldsymbol{G} = \{g_{ijk}\}$ (distance transformation)
for all (i, j, k) **do**

$$g_{ijk} \leftarrow \begin{cases} \text{radius of the maximum ball which has the center at } (i, j, k) \text{ and} \\ \text{does not contain a 0-voxel inside it, if } f_{ijk} = 1, \\ 0, \text{ if } f_{ijk} = 0, \end{cases}$$

enddo

In order to find the maximum radius of a ball we need to perform a kind of search procedure. Although various shortcuts may be possible in this process, much computation time is still necessary. If the width of a figure is small everywhere, this type of algorithm may be useful.

Remark 5.11. An algorithm has been developed in which a coordinate value of the nearest 0-voxel is propagated. This propagation does not always correspond to a path introduced in Section 4.9. The algorithm is implemented by a kind of iterative procedure. Examples of such algorithms for a 2D image were given in [Yamada84, Danielsson80], and the extension to a 3D image was briefly introduced in [Borgefors84]. Memory requirements in those algorithms are rather large for higher-dimensional images because n-dimensional arrays are necessary as work areas in performing the n-dimensional DT.

5.5.5 Example of algorithms − (2) variable neighborhood DT (parallel type)

Let us consider the distance transformation (DT) based on the length of the minimal path using the variable neighborhood sequence (= *variable neighborhood distance transformation* (*VNDT*)). Algorithms to perform VNDT of a 3D image are almost the same as those for 2D images. Let us explain here a parallel-type algorithm as a typical example [Toriwaki81, Yokoi81].

First, we define the minimum filter with the neighborhood $\mathcal{N}_b((i,j,k))$ as follows.

Definition 5.4 (Minimum filter).

$$\mathbf{MINF}\ (\mathcal{N}_b) : \boldsymbol{F} = \{f_{ijk}\} \to \boldsymbol{G} = \{g_{ijk}\}$$
$$g_{ijk} = \min\{f_{pqr};\ (p,q,r) \in \mathcal{N}_b((i,j,k))\} \tag{5.10}$$
$$\mathcal{N}_b((i,j,k)) = \text{set of voxels in the neighborhood of a voxel } (i,j,k).$$

The neighborhood is selected according to the rule given in the neighborhood sequence. By using this filter a parallel-type algorithm of the VNDT is given as follows.

Algorithm 5.9 (VNDT; parallel type).

$\boldsymbol{F} = \{f_{ijk}\}$: Input binary image
$\boldsymbol{G} = \{g_{ijk}\}$: Work array and output image
$\boldsymbol{B} = \{b_0, b_1, \ldots, b_n\}$: Neighborhood sequence (b_i is a suffix that represents the kind of neighborhood and the order it is employed)

[**STEP 1**] (Initialization)
for all (i,j,k) **do**
    if $f_{ijk} = 1$
    then $f_{ijk} \leftarrow M$ (= sufficiently large positive integer)
    else no operation
    endif
enddo
$\alpha \leftarrow 0$ (The number of a neighborhood)

[**STEP 2**]
for all (i,j,k) **do**
    if $f_{ijk} = 0$
    then $g_{ijk} \leftarrow 0$
    else

$d \leftarrow \min\{f_{pqr}, \ (p, q, r) \in \mathcal{N}_{b\alpha}((i, j, k))\}$
if $d \neq M$
then $g_{ijk} \leftarrow d + 1$
else $g_{ijk} \leftarrow M$
endif
  endif
  endif
enddo

[**STEP 3**]
if $F = G$ when [**STEP 2**] finishes,
then stop
else $F \leftarrow G$
endif
$\alpha \leftarrow (\alpha + 1) \bmod n$ (Neighborhood sequence is used repeatedly)
go to [**STEP 2**]

[**Explanation of the algorithm**]
    The basic idea of this algorithm is that we replace the value of each 1-voxel P in an input image by $\langle\langle$ 1 + the minimum in the neighborhood of the current neighborhood number $\mathcal{N}_{b\alpha}((i, j, k))$ of the 1-voxel P $\rangle\rangle$. Note here that in the initialization process we replace beforehand values of all 1-voxels P in an input image by a sufficiently large value M (at least not smaller than the expected maximum of the values of DT).

    Thus, in the first iteration of [STEP 2], any 1-voxel that has a 0-voxel in its neighborhood is given the value 1. In the next iteration step, all voxels that have at least one voxel of the value 1 in its neighborhood are given the value 2. The same procedure is iteratively performed until no voxel of the value M remains, that is, a voxel of which value is to be replaced does not exist.

    The order of execution concerning (i, j, k) in [STEP 2] may be arbitrary. In other words, calculation of g_{ijk} at each voxel may be performed in parallel, mutually independently at different voxels. However, an input image of the i-th iteration had to be kept unchanged until [STEP 2] finishes for all voxels. This means that an output image must be stored in an array different from an input image. The k-times of processing is applied to the output image of the $(k-1)$ times of processing. If there is no voxel for which the value is replaced, then the whole of processing terminates.

    [STEP 3] is not essential. The output image of the previous iteration is moved to an input image array for the convenience of the processing of the next iteration.

    Use of the value M and distinction of a voxel of a value M are only for the ease of understanding. If care is not taken to prevent the possibility of overflow, all voxels may be processed in the same way.

    Different types of neighborhoods given in the neighborhood sequence are used according to the order designated in the neighborhood sequence $\boldsymbol{B}$, starting from b_0 until b_n repeatedly. By doing this, the variable neighborhood distance determined by the length of the variable neighborhood minimal path is given to a voxel of an output image. Strictly speaking, this should be proved theoretically. For details see [Yokoi81, Toriwaki92].

Most of the process time is spent on the execution of [STEP 2]. Computation time primarily depends on how many times [STEP 2] is executed. It is dominated by the maximum of distance values and varies according to an individual input image. However, it is only voxels in the neighborhood of those updated in the previous iteration that a voxel value is replaceable during the current iteration. Therefore, it is possible to reduce the computation time by using a list in the same way as Algorithms 5.5 and 5.6. It is particularly effective in the fixed neighborhood DT.

Remark 5.12. Denoting the output image of the k times of iteration in the above algorithm by $\boldsymbol{F}^{(k)}$ and the operation to calculate it from $\boldsymbol{F}^{(k-1)}$ by $\boldsymbol{\Phi}^{(k)}$, then

$$\boldsymbol{F}^{(k)} = \boldsymbol{\Phi}^{(k)}(\boldsymbol{F}^{(k-1)}), \ k = 1, 2, \ldots \tag{5.11}$$

where $\boldsymbol{F}^{(0)} \equiv \boldsymbol{F}$ (input image)

Applying the serial composition of image operations presented in Section 2.3 to the above image operation,

$$\boldsymbol{F}^{(k)} = \boldsymbol{\Phi}^{(k)} \cdot \boldsymbol{\Phi}^{(k-1)} \cdot \boldsymbol{\Phi}^{(k-2)} \cdot \ldots \cdot \boldsymbol{\Phi}^{(1)}(\boldsymbol{F}). \tag{5.12}$$

Since $\boldsymbol{\Phi}^{(k)} = \boldsymbol{\Phi}$, $\forall k$ in the fixed neighborhood DT,

$$\boldsymbol{F}^{(k)} = \boldsymbol{\Phi}^k(\boldsymbol{F}). \tag{5.13}$$

However, it is not so easy to derive a theoretically clear form of representation for the contents of $\boldsymbol{\Phi}^k(\boldsymbol{F})$.

Let us consider the fixed neighborhood DT for the sake of simplicity, and let us perform always $g_{ijk} \leftarrow d + 1$ in [STEP 2] of Algorithm 5.9 and that two cases $d = M$ and $d \neq M$ are considered separately. The final result is the same as Algorithm 5.9. Denoted by $\boldsymbol{\Phi}$ the minimum filter of the neighborhood adopted there, the transformation from $\boldsymbol{F}^{(k-1)}$ to $\boldsymbol{F}^{(k)}$ is represented as $\boldsymbol{\Phi} + \mathrm{I}$, that is

$$\boldsymbol{F}^{(k)} = (\boldsymbol{\Phi} + \mathrm{I})(\boldsymbol{F}^{(k-1)}) = \boldsymbol{\Phi}(\boldsymbol{F}^{(k-1)}) + \boldsymbol{F}^{(k-1)}, \forall k. \tag{5.14}$$

Repeating this representation for all k, then

$$\boldsymbol{F}^{(k)} = (\boldsymbol{\Phi}^k + \boldsymbol{\Phi}^{k-1} + \ldots + \boldsymbol{\Phi}^2 + \boldsymbol{\Phi} + \mathrm{I})(\boldsymbol{F}). \tag{5.15}$$

This form of representation is common to both 2D images and 3D images.

Next, let us give the sequential type of algorithm for the fixed neighborhood DT [Kuwabara82].

Algorithm 5.10 (Fixed neighborhood (6, 18, 26-neighborhood) DT sequential type).

$\boldsymbol{F} = \{f_{ijk}\}$: Input binary image
$\boldsymbol{G}^{(2)} = \{g_{ijk}^{(2)}\}$: Output image (distance transformation)
$\boldsymbol{G}^{(0)} = \{g_{ijk}^{(0)}\}, \boldsymbol{G}^{(1)} = \{g_{ijk}^{(1)}\}$: Work array
Edges of these arrays are assumed to be filled with *0*.

[**STEP 1**] (Initialization)
Initial value image $\boldsymbol{G}^{(0)} = \{g_{ijk}^{(0)}\}$ is given as follows.
for all (i, j, k)s **do**
   if $f_{ijk} = 1$
   then $g_{ijk}^{(0)} \leftarrow M$ (M is a sufficiently large integer)
   else $g_{ijk}^{(0)} \leftarrow 0$
   endif
enddo

[**STEP 2**] (Forward scan)
for all (i, j, k)s **do**
   $g_{ijk}^{(1)} \leftarrow \min\{g_{ijk}^{(0)}, \min\{g_{pqr}^{(1)}; (p, q, r) \in S_1\} + 1\}$
enddo
Concerning (i, j, k), use the scan mode (I) in Fig. 5.13 (a). The S_1 is selected as shown in Fig. 5.13 (i), (ii), and (iii) according to the 6-, 18-, and 26-neighborhood.

[**STEP 3**] (Backward scan)
for all (i, j, k)s **do**
   $g_{ijk}^{(2)} \leftarrow \min\{g_{ijk}^{(1)}, \min\{g_{pqr}^{(2)}; (p, q, r) \in S_2\} + 1\}$
enddo
Concerning (i, j, k), use the scan mode (II) in Fig. 5.13 (a). The S_2 is selected as shown in Fig. 5.13 (i), (ii), and (iii) according to 6-, 18-, and 26-neighborhood.

5.5.6 Supplementary comments on algorithms of DT

Large numbers of papers and reports have been published on the DT of a 2D image, including various types of transformation and diversity of applications [Yokoi81, Toriwaki79, Toriwaki81, Toriwaki92, Jones06]. A chief motivation of different algorithms was that the difference from the Euclidean distance was significantly large in the DT using the simple 4-neighbor or 8-neighbor distance. Another reason was that a good algorithm of the Euclidean DT was not known. Although this situation has remarkably changed after the algorithm of the squared Euclidean DT had been developed about 1992 [Saito94a], such traditional algorithms are still useful to understand basic properties of DT. Let us briefly introduce here how those traditional algorithms are extended to a 3D image:

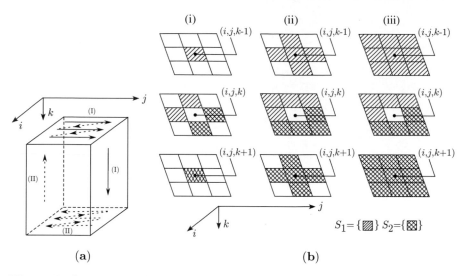

Fig. 5.13. Scanning mode and neighborhoods used for Algorithm 5.10 (fixed neighborhood DT): (**a**) Scanning mode; (**b**) definition of neighborhoods.

(1) *Introduction of variable neighborhood DT*: In the DT of a 2D image, an algorithm to use the 4-neighbor and the 8-neighbor alternately was proposed and called the octagonal DT because the form of equidistance contour line looks like an octagon. This idea was extended to a 3D image by using alternatively two of the 6-, 18-, and 26-neighborhood and called by the name of 6/26 octagonal DT, 18/26, and 6/18 octagonal DT [Borgefors84]. The sequential type algorithm is realized in the same way as Algorithm 5.10 except that eight times of iteration (scanning of the whole of an input image) are required.

(2) *Modification of the distance value*: The most important reason that the distance value is significantly different from the value of the Euclidean distance in any of the 6-, 18-, and 26-neighborhood distance is that the distance to adjacent voxels is regarded as a uniform unit. The effect of this uniform distance assumption is decreased by using another value that is closer to the true distance value. For instance, one possibility is to employ the Euclidean distance between center points of voxels that are adjacent to each other. That is, the distance to a 6-adjacent, 18-adjacent, and 26-adjacent voxels are regarded as 1, $\sqrt{2}$, and $\sqrt{3}$, respectively. However, even this type of algorithm still cannot give exact Euclidean distance values. Computation time will also increase because calculation among irrational numbers (or real numbers approximating them) is involved. Therefore weighting using only integers that provide better approximation have been studied. A triplet of integers $(3, 4, 5)$ instead of $(1, \sqrt{2}, \sqrt{3})$ is known as an example of relatively good

weights [Borgefors84, Borgefors86a, Borgefors86b, Danielsson80]. The distance measure weighted by them is called chamfer distance [Montanari68]. See also Chapter 4 [Jones06].

(3) *Enlargement of the neighborhood*: Euclidean DT is obtained with very high accuracy by employing an enlarged neighborhood except for small numbers of specific voxels. This was shown for a 2D image in [Danielsson80, Ragnemalm90]. By enlarging the neighborhood, the range of paths that can be searched is also extended, and eventually a minimal will be detected. This method may be extended to a 3D image, in principle. However, the number of paths to be searched increases rapidly according to the extension of the neighborhood ($5 \times 5 \times 5$, for example), and both computation time and memory requirement also increase rapidly. In fact, extension to a 3D image has not been reported.

(4) *Propagation of coordinate values*: See Remark 5.11.

(5) *Other variations*: Most variations of DT described in [Toriwaki81] will be extended in a straightforward manner to a 3D image. They include the directional DT [Yokoi81], the DT of a line figure [Toriwaki79, Toriwaki81, Toriwaki82a] and the max-type DT [Suzuki83]. The DT of the background (exoskeleton) and an application to the Voronoi division are also extended immediately to a 3D image at least in principle [Preston79, Mase81, Saito92]. It should be noted, however, that shapes of resulting line figures and surface figures will become complicated such as with a skeleton (see the next section) and a Voronoi division surface [Edelsbrunner94, Mase81, Toriwaki88, Yashima83].

5.5.7 Skeleton

One of the most useful features of DT G derived from an image F is that characteristic features of an image F are carried to a limited number of voxels, or that characteristics of an image F are condensed through the DT. Intuitively the result of condensation is represented by a set of voxels called a *skeleton*. A stricter definition of the skeleton is necessary for theoretical analysis of the skeleton and for deriving an algorithm to extract the skeleton. We will give here four types of definitions of the skeleton. They are each a little different from each other, and each of them has its own significance.

Definition 5.5 (Skeleton). Let us represent an input image by F and its DT by G.

(1) A set of voxels is called a *skeleton* of an image F or of a DT G, if an input image is restored exactly from coordinates of voxels of the skeleton and values of DT on them.

(2) A set of all local maximum points (voxels) of the DT of F is called a *skeleton* of an image F or of a DT G.

(3) Given a binary figure F, let us denote by ϕ a processing (image operation) to delete a 1-voxel which is at the unit distance from the background and

by μ a processing (image operation) to replace by a 1-voxel a 0-voxel which is at the unit distance from a figure. Then let us denote by $\phi^k(\boldsymbol{F})$ a figure obtained after k times of successive application of ϕ to an image $\boldsymbol{F}$, and denote by $\mu(\phi^k(\boldsymbol{F}))$ one time of application of μ to $\phi^k(\boldsymbol{F})$. Then if there exists a voxel which belongs to any figure in $\phi^{k-1}(\boldsymbol{F})$, but does not belong to $\mu(\phi^k(\boldsymbol{F}))$, such a voxel is called a *skeleton with the distance* k. The entire skeleton with all values of k is simply called a *skeleton* of an image $\boldsymbol{F}$.

(4) Let us call a set of all voxels within the distance r from a voxel P a *digital ball of the radius* r centered at P. Next, consider an image $\boldsymbol{F}$ and its distance transformation $\boldsymbol{G}$. Suppose that a suitable subset $\boldsymbol{Q}$ of 1-voxels in $\boldsymbol{F}$ and distance values on them are given. Let us imagine a set of digital balls centered at each voxel in the set $\boldsymbol{Q}$ and the radius of the same value as the distance value on each voxel. If a set sum of all such digital balls exactly coincides with the set of all 1-voxels in $\boldsymbol{F}$, then a set $\boldsymbol{Q}$ is called a *skeleton* of an image $\boldsymbol{F}$ or a *skeleton* of a distance transformation $\boldsymbol{G}$.

Definition 5.5 includes four kinds of definitions (1) ∼ (4) which are different from each other. Skeletons derived by those definitions are not exactly the same. For a given image $\boldsymbol{F}$, its skeleton is not always determined uniquely even if we adopt one of them.

The following are reasons for ambiguity in the definition of the skeleton.

(i) A local maximum point cannot be easily defined. For example, the type of neighborhood employed in the detection of local maxima and local minima cannot be fixed beforehand. In fact, a local maximum will be different according to which of the 6- and the 26-neighborhood is adopted. In the fixed neighborhood DT, we can select the same neighborhood as was used in the calculation of DT for the extraction of local maxima. This strategy will not be applied in the case of Euclidean DT. It is assumed that the second item of Definition 5.5 will satisfy (1) and (3) of Definition 5.5. This is not always true, however, when some specific types of the neighborhood are used in the definition of local maxima.

(ii) A set of voxels stated in Definition 5.5 (1), that is, a voxel set from which an original figure is restored exactly, is not determined uniquely. Even the minimum set of voxels needed for an original figure to be restored exactly from it is not always given uniquely. The algorithm to obtain such a minimal set of voxels may not always be derived easily [Borgefors97, Nilsson97].

(iii) This definition of the skeleton is less significant, unless a good algorithm to extract a skeleton and to restore an original figure from the skeleton is known. Only such a definition of the skeleton, if those algorithms exist, is acceptable from the viewpoint of practical applications.

(iv) The importance of each of the above factors varies depending on the kinds of DT, in particular, on the type of the distance function employed in DT.

It is not so easy to find a definition of the skeleton which is applicable to all kinds of DT.

The skeleton has been defined differently in papers published in the past. Here we employ the definition 5.5 (1) because we consider that the restoration of an original figure is the most important property of the skeleton.

Remark 5.13. Let us consider a definition of the skeleton from a different viewpoint from the above. The following properties were expected as desirable properties of the skeleton.

(a) An original figure is fully recovered from a skeleton and distance values on it (restorability).
(b) The number of voxels contained in a skeleton is minimum (minimality).
(c) A skeleton is close to a result of thinning. It is important that the skeleton has the same topological features (connectivity) as an input image (topology preservation).
(d) An efficient algorithm exists to extract the skeleton and to restore an input image (existence of an algorithm).

For any kind of DT known, no skeleton exists that satisfies all of the above four requirements. In this text, we consider, for the moment, that the first of the above is indispensable. In this case, it is easily known that there exists a figure that does satisfy (b) but does not satisfy (c). Therefore, we do not take into account the third requirement.

There has not been reported a skeleton that exactly satisfies both (b) and (d), although reasonable algorithms exist to extract such skeletons that meet both the restorability and the minimal requirements [Borgefors97, Nilsson97]. For example, let us assume that we extracted skeletons according to a suitable definition. Then we put on all the skeleton voxels digital balls of the radius which is equal to the distance value at each skeleton voxel. Then we eliminate a ball that is completely covered by other balls. By this algorithm we can reduce the number of skeleton voxels while keeping restorability of an original figure [Borgefors97, Nilsson97].

The first requirement in the above means that the skeleton consists of a relatively small number of voxels, although not always minimized. If we require the minimality condition too strictly, an effective algorithm to obtain it may not be found.

Let us assume that a skeleton S satisfying the restorability condition has been obtained. Then a set of voxels S^* that consists of S and one more 1-voxel selected arbitrarily from an input image still satisfies the above restorability condition. In other words, an arbitrary voxel set that includes any skeleton S satisfying the restorability will again satisfy the restorability requirement. Obviously such skeletons will be meaningless. Thus the minimality condition will be significant in the sense that such a meaningless skeleton is excluded.

Remark 5.14. Let us add several known results of algorithms to extract skeletons and to restore an original input figure.

First, the relationship between Def. 5.5 (1) and others in Def. 5.5 is presently not known exactly in the case of the Euclidean DT. Definition 5.5 (2) is not applicable to the Euclidean DT as was already stated in (i) concerning the ambiguity of the definition of the skeleton.

Second, Def. 5.5 (3) and 5.5 (4) are applicable to all types of DT, because they refer to algorithms to restore an input figure. Concerning extraction of the skeleton, however, they suggest only a trivial cut and try procedure, that is, extracting a suitable subset of voxels and testing whether an input figure is restored or not.

All of Def. 5.5 (1) ~ (4) are applicable to the fixed neighborhood DT employing the 6-, 18-, and 26-neighborhood and eventually coincident with each other, except for the ambiguity pointed out in (i) ~ (iv) above. The algorithm to extract skeletons will be obtained by Def. 5.5 (2), (3) and (4) will give procedures to restore an input figure from its skeleton.

For the variable neighborhood DT, a neighborhood sequence should be taken into consideration in all of Def. 5.5 (2) ~ (4). It is conjectured that Def. 5.5 (2) ~ (4) are eventually coincident also in the variable neighborhood DT, although it has not been proven theoretically.

5.5.8 Reverse distance transformation

The process to restore an input figure from its skeleton and distance values on it is called *reverse distance transformation*. Let us define this more clearly below.

Definition 5.6 (Reverse distance transformation (RDT)). Given a set of voxels $\boldsymbol{Q} = \{Q_1, Q_2, \ldots, Q_m\}$, where $Q_m = (i_m, j_m, k_m)$, and a density value $\{f_{i_m j_m k_m}\}$ on a voxel Q_m. Then consider a procedure to obtain a set of all voxels $\boldsymbol{P} = \{(i, j, k)\}$ such that

$$P = (i, j, k); \ \exists m, d(P, Q_m) < f_{i_m j_m k_m}, \ Q_m \in \boldsymbol{Q}. \qquad (5.16)$$

This procedure is called *reverse distance transformation* (*RDT*) by the distance function $d(***, ***)$.

The procedure is called *reverse squared distance transformation* (*RSDT*), if $d^2(P, Q_m)$ is used instead of $d(P, Q_m)$.

The voxel set $\boldsymbol{Q}$ in Def. 5.6 is the skeleton in the sense of Def. 5.5 (1). If the density value f_{ijk} is equal to the value of the DT, the result of RDT $\boldsymbol{P}$ coincides with an original input image.

The meaning of Eq. 5.16 is as follows. At every voxel P, let us represent by Q^* a voxel of $\boldsymbol{Q}$ which is nearest to P. Then, we make a voxel P' belong to P if the distance $d(P, Q^*)$ is smaller than the distance value of Q^*. This rule is applied to every voxel P.

The use of the squared RDT is more convenient in the case of Euclidean RDT. The following property holds in which $\boldsymbol{Q}$ is a skeleton and each voxel Q_m in $\boldsymbol{Q}$ has a density value $f_{i_m j_m k_m}$ which is equal to the value of the squared DT.

Property 5.5. Given an input image (skeleton image) $\boldsymbol{F} = \{f_{ijk}\}$,

$$f_{ijk} = \begin{cases} \text{the value of the squared DT, if } (i, j, k) \in \boldsymbol{Q}(\text{skeleton}), \\ 0, \qquad\qquad\qquad\qquad\qquad\qquad \text{otherwise,} \end{cases} \tag{5.17}$$

the set $\boldsymbol{P} = \{(i, j, k)\}$ given in Eq. 5.16 of Def. 5.6 is obtained by calculating the following image $\boldsymbol{H} = \{h_{ijk}\}$,

$$h_{ijk} = \max_{p,q,r}\{f_{pqr} - (i - p)^2 - (j - q)^2 - (k - r)^2\}. \tag{5.18}$$

The set $\boldsymbol{P}$ is obtained by extracting all voxels such that $h_{ijk} > 0$.

Property 5.6. The image $\boldsymbol{H} = \{h_{ijk}\}$ given in Property 5.5 is obtained by the following procedure including intermediate images $\boldsymbol{G}^{(1)} = \{g_{ijk}^{(1)}\}$ and $\boldsymbol{G}^{(2)} = \{g_{ijk}^{(2)}\}$.
(Transformation I)

$$\boldsymbol{F} \to \boldsymbol{G}^{(1)} = \{g_{ijk}^{(1)}\}; \ g_{ijk}^{(1)} = \max_{p}\{f_{pjk} - (i - p)^2\}. \tag{5.19}$$

(Transformation II)

$$\boldsymbol{G}^{(1)} \to \boldsymbol{G}^{(2)} = \{g_{ijk}^{(2)}\}; \ g_{ijk}^{(2)} = \max_{q}\{g_{iqk}^{(1)} - (j - q)^2\}. \tag{5.20}$$

(Transformation III)

$$\boldsymbol{G}^{(2)} \to \boldsymbol{H} = \{h_{ijk}\}; \ h_{ijk} = \max_{r}\{g_{ijr}^{(2)} - (k - r)^2\}. \tag{5.21}$$

This property is easily derived by successively substituting Eqs. (5.19) and (5.20) into Eq. (5.21).

5.5.9 Example of RDT algorithms – (1) Euclidean squared RDT

Property 5.6 is realized by performing three 1D transformations corresponding to i, j, and k axis directions which are executed consecutively and independently. This fact suggests that an RDT algorithm is constructed by a serial composition of 1D operations, each of which corresponds to an operation in each coordinate axis direction. The following algorithm is based on this idea [Saito94b].

Algorithm 5.11 (Reverse Euclidean squared distance transformation).

Input: skeleton image $\boldsymbol{F} = \{f_{ijk}\}$ $(1 \leq i \leq M, 1 \leq j \leq N, 1 \leq k \leq K)$.

$$f_{ijk} = \begin{cases} \text{squared distance value, if a voxel } (i, j, k) \text{ is a skeleton voxel} \\ 0, \qquad\qquad\qquad\qquad \text{otherwise} \end{cases}$$

Output: $\boldsymbol{G} = \{g_{ijk}\}$: squared reverse distance transformation image (all voxels are initialized as 0).

Work array: $\boldsymbol{G'} = \{g'_{ijk}\}$ (all voxels are initialized as 0).

(The outside of an input image is regarded as being filled with the value 0 during the processing. Arrays $\boldsymbol{G}$ and $\boldsymbol{G'}$ are assigned physically to the same memory area.)

[STEP 1](Fig. 5.14)

(1-1) Input image: $\boldsymbol{F} = \{f_{ijk}\}$,
Output image: $\boldsymbol{G} = \{g_{ijk}\}$
Perform the following procedure row by row, increasing the value of i from 1 to M (forward scan).

(a) If $f_{ijk} < f_{(i-1)jk}$ (Fig. 5.7 (a)), perform the following procedure for all n such as $0 \leq n \leq (f_{(i-1)jk} - f_{ijk} - 1)/2$ (See Note).

(a-1) If $f_{(i+n)jk} \geq f_{(i-1)jk} - (n + 1)^2$, go to the next i.

(a-2) If otherwise and $(g_{(i+n)jk} < f_{(i-1)jk} - (n + 1)^2)$, $g_{(i+n)jk} \leftarrow f_{(i-1)jk} - (n + 1)^2$, and go to the next n.

(a-3) Except the above (a-1) and (a-2), go to the next n.

(b) If $f_{ijk} \geq f_{(i-1)jk}$ (Fig. 5.7 (b)),

(b-1) If $g_{ijk} < f_{ijk}$, then $g_{ijk} \leftarrow f_{ijk}$ and go to the next i.

(b-2) If otherwise go to the next i.

(1-2) Input image: $\boldsymbol{G} = \{g_{ijk}\}$.
Output image: $\boldsymbol{G'} = \{g'_{ijk}\}$.
Perform for each row the following procedure, decreasing the value of the suffix i from M to 1 (backward scan).

(a) If $g_{ijk} < g_{(i+1)jk}$, perform the following procedure for all n such as $0 \leq n \leq (g_{(i+1)jk} - g_{ijk} - 1)/2$.

(a-1) If $g_{(i-n)jk} \leq g_{(i+1)jk} - (n + 1)^2$, go to the next i.

(a-2) If otherwise and $g'_{(i-n)jk} < g_{(i+1)jk} - (n + 1)^2$, then $g'_{(i-n)jk} \leftarrow g_{(i+1)jk} - (n + 1)^2$, and go to the next n.

(a-3) Except (a-1) and (a-2) go to the next n.

(b) If $(g_{ijk} \geq g_{(i+1)jk})$,

(b-1) If $(g'_{ijk} < g_{ijk})$,
$g'_{ijk} \leftarrow g_{ijk}$, and go to the next i.

(b-2) If otherwise, go to the next i.

[STEP 2]
Input image: $\boldsymbol{G'} = \{g'_{ijk}\}$.

Note: Here the value $n = (f_{(i-1)jk} - f_{ijk} - 1)/2$ is a crossing point of the square functions $C_1(n) = f_{ijk} - n^2$ and $C_2(n) = f_{(i-1)jk} - (n + 1)^2$ such as $n > 0$.

Output image: $G = \{g_{ijk}\}$.

Same as [**STEP 1**] except that the processing is applied to each column (the suffix i is replaced by the suffix j).

[**STEP 3**]

Input image: $G = \{g_{ijk}\}$.

Output image: $G' = \{g'_{ijk}\}$.

Same as [STEP 1] except that the processing is applied to each plane (the suffix j is replaced by the suffix k).

[**STEP 4**]

Input image: $G' = \{g'_{ijk}\}$.

Output image: $G = \{g_{ijk}\}$.

Binalize G, that is,

for all (i, j, k) **do**

  if $g'_{ijk} > 0$

  then $f_{ijk} \leftarrow 1$

  else $f_{ijk} \leftarrow 0$

  endif

enddo

[**Explanation of the algorithm**]

The basic idea is almost the same as that of DT, except that it is what is called a *reverse* operation. An input image is a skeleton image (although not described as such), in which a voxel of a skeleton has a distance value (a squared distance value in this case) and the other voxels are given the value *0*. Algorithm 5.11 is in principle a formal description of the procedure in Property 5.6. It is devised so that the range of the search for the maximum may be reduced as much as possible. For details, see [Saito94b].

Suppose that a voxel P in an input image F has the squared DT value f_p. Then the value of the squared RDT on a voxel at the distance d from P is at most $f_p - d^2$. This value is substituted subsequently to intermediate output images G and G'.

For more detailed explanation, let us put $d^2 = d_i^2 + d_j^2 + d_k^2$ where d_i, d_j, and d_k represent components of d^2 which are given by the difference between the coordinate components in the i, j, and k directions, respectively. Then the value of $f_p - d^2$ is not calculated directly. In this algorithm, it is obtained subsequently according to the following order: $f_p - d_i^2$ in [STEP 1], $(f_p - d_i^2) - d_j^2$ in [STEP 2], $(f_p - d_i^2 - d_j^2) - d_k^2$ in [STEP 3]. This part of the procedure is illustrated in Fig. 5.14 (c) $\sim$ (e). Circles in Fig. 5.14 (a) show skeleton voxels in an input image F. Processing in Algorithm 5.11 is considered to arrange parabolas so that their peaks come to the location of the mark $\bigcirc$ and to obtain their upper envelope.

Negative values may be substituted temporarily into an output image G as is known from this figure. Then an original input image is derived by replacing all positive values in G by *1* and all the other negative values in G' by *0*. However, density values stored in the output image G when the process is

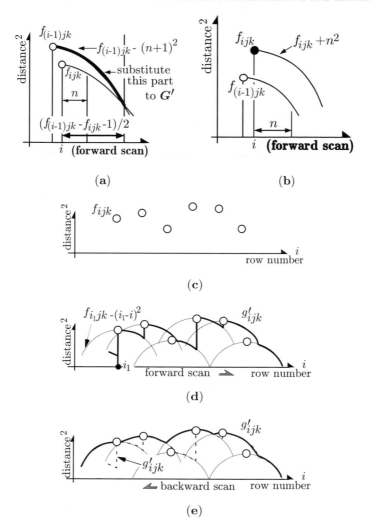

Fig. 5.14. Illustration of reverse squared Euclidean distance transformation (Algorithm 5.11) [Saito94b]: (a) $f_{ijk} < f_{(i-1)jk}$: substitute the part of ▬▬ for $\boldsymbol{G'}$; (b) $f_{ijk} \geq f_{(i-1)jk}$: substitute f_{ijk} for g'_{ijk}; (c) an input picture; (d) the forward scan; (e) the backward scan.

terminated are not the density values (or the squared density values) obtained by DT. In other words, a DT image is not restored by this algorithm.

We will summarize properties of this algorithm below.

(1) The amount and the time of computation are about the same as those of the squared DT realized by Algorithm 5.7.

(2) This algorithm can be broken down into three 1D processes, each of them correspondings to i, j, and k directions, respectively. This is advantageous to the execution by a conventional general purpose computer.

(3) This algorithm is applicable to an image of heterogeneous spatial resolution, that is, an image digitized by a cuboid voxel with little modification similar to that in the algorithm of the DT in Eqs. 5.8 and 5.9.

(4) Only two 3D arrays of the same size as an input image are required. Unless an input image is necessary to be preserved after finishing the algorithm, one 3D array for an input image and one 1D array of the length max (M, N, K) (= the maximum length of three edges of an input image) are enough for implementation of the algorithm.

(5) From the viewpoint of the algorithm type, this algorithm is the sequential type because it can be executed on an input array as was stated in (4) above. This is also able to be broken down into 1D processes as was pointed out in (2) above.

(6) By this reverse transformation, an input figure is restored, but distance values are not recovered. If distance values are needed, they are obtained by performing the DT again after an input figure was restored.

Next, let us present a parallel type algorithm executing of RDT.

Algorithm 5.12 (Reverse squared Euclidean distance transformation parallel type).

Input: skeleton image $\boldsymbol{F} = \{f_{ijk}\}$ ($1 \leq i \leq M, 1 \leq j \leq N, 1 \leq k \leq K$).

$$f_{ijk} = \begin{cases} \text{squared distance value, if a voxel } (i, j, k) \text{ is a skeleton voxel} \\ 0, \qquad\qquad\qquad\qquad\quad \text{otherwise} \end{cases}$$

Output: $\boldsymbol{G} = \{g_{ijk}\}$: squared reverse distance transformation image (all voxels are initialized as 0).

for all (i, j, k) **do**
  if $f_{ijk} > 0$
  then $g_{pqr} \leftarrow 1$ for all (p, q, r) included in a ball of the radius $\sqrt{f_{ijk}}$
  else no operation is performed
  endif
enddo
The order of execution concerning suffixes (i, j, k) is arbitrary.

This algorithm is simple and very clear, but not always effective for ordinary computers. In the execution by computer, the process of *filling the inside of a ball by the value 1* is repeated many times, and to do this access to a 3D array occurs. Thus computation time may become longer depending on the number of balls and the distance values (= the sizes of balls). More than one ball placed on different skeleton voxels may partially overlap each other. In the worse case two overlapping balls may differ in only a single voxel. In such cases the value *1* is written in the same voxel so many times. Deriving an algorithm to avoid such repetitive writing to the same voxel is not easy.

5.5.10 Example of RDT algorithm – (2) fixed neighborhood (6-, 18-, or 26-neighborhood) RDT (sequential type)

Algorithm 5.13 (Fixed neighborhood (6-, 18-, or 26-neighborhood) reverse distance transformation - sequential type).

Input: skeleton image $\boldsymbol{F} = \{f_{ijk}\}$ ($1 \leq i \leq M, 1 \leq j \leq N, 1 \leq k \leq K$).

$$f_{ijk} = \begin{cases} \text{distance value, if a voxel } (i,j,k) \text{ is a skeleton voxel,} \\ 0, \qquad\qquad\qquad \text{otherwise} \end{cases}$$

Output: $\boldsymbol{G}^{(2)} = \{g_{ijk}^{(2)}\}$: distance transformation image
Work array: $\boldsymbol{G}^{(0)} = \{g_{ijk}^{(0)}\}, \boldsymbol{G}^{(1)} = \{g_{ijk}^{(1)}\}$

[STEP 1] (Initialization)
initial image $\boldsymbol{G}^{(0)} = \{g_{ijk}^{(0)}\} \leftarrow \boldsymbol{F} = \{f_{ijk}\}$
[STEP 2] (Forward scan)
for all (i,j,k) **do**
$\quad g_{ijk}^{(1)} \leftarrow \max\{0, g_{ijk}^{(0)}, \max\{g_{pqr}^{(1)}; (p,q,r) \in S_1\} - 1\}$
enddo
Concerning (i,j,k), execute processing according to the scanning mode (I) in Fig. 5.13. Use as S_1 either of (a), (b), or (c) of Fig. 5.13 corresponding to the 6-, 18-, or 26-neighborhood, respectively.
[STEP 3] (Backward scan)
for all (i,j,k) **do**
$\quad g_{ijk}^{(2)} \leftarrow \max\{0, g_{ijk}^{(1)}, \max\{g_{pqr}^{(2)}; (p,q,r) \in S_2\} - 1\}$
enddo
Concerning (i,j,k), processing is executed according to the scanning mode (II) in Fig. 5.13. S_2 is selected from Fig. 5.13 (a), (b), or (c) according to the 6-, 18-, or 26-neighborhood, respectively.

[Explanation of the algorithm]
    Restoration of an original figure from its skeleton and distance values on it is achieved, in principle, by expanding regions from each voxel of the skeleton to all the adjacent voxels. Distance values that were given to each skeleton voxel are reduced by a predetermined value and handed to adjacent voxels after one expansion and the expansion is terminated when the distance value becomes 0. This means that each skeleton voxel can be expanded until the edge or the surface of a ball centered at each skeleton voxel and the radius of which is the same as the distance value at a skeleton voxel. Every voxel that receives a positive value during a repetitive expansion procedure can be expanded until the range of a ball with the radius of which is same as the value the voxel received.
    In the fixed neighborhood DT, a distance value given to a skeleton is reduced by a unit after one expansion of the neighborhood that is employed in the current DT. More than one different value may be written at more than

one expansion. In such cases, the propagation of distance values comes from more than one different skeleton voxel. Here, the largest of the arriving values should be stored and sent to adjacent voxels in the next propagation cycle.

The above algorithm executed this expansion or propagation by dividing the propagation twice into a different direction. One is the propagation toward the right and the downward (forward scan), and the other is toward the left and the upward (backward scan).

In this algorithm, a value of a voxel in an output image is written into the corresponding voxel as soon as it is fixed, and the updated value is used in the subsequent procedure. This is a typical style of the sequential algorithm. This execution of the algorithm makes it possible for this algorithm to be performed on a single 3D array. Thus this algorithm is regarded as a reversal version of Algorithm 5.10 both in its basic idea and in the type of an algorithm.

Next, we will give a parallel-type algorithm.

Algorithm 5.14 (Fixed neighborhood RDT - parallel type).

$\boldsymbol{F} = \{f_{ijk}\}$: Input image.

$$f_{ijk} = \begin{cases} \text{distance value, if a voxel } (i, j, k) \text{ is a skeleton voxel,} \\ 0, \qquad\qquad\qquad \text{otherwise} \end{cases}$$

$\boldsymbol{G} = \{g_{ijk}\}$: Work array, and output image. Initial value is 0 for all voxels.

[STEP 1]
for all (i, j, k) **do**
  if $f_{ijk} = 0$
  then $g_{ijk} \leftarrow 0$
  else
    $d \leftarrow \max\{f_{pqr}; (p, q, r) \in \mathcal{N}^{(k)}((i, j, k))\}$
    (The superscript k represents the type of neighborhood, $k = 6, 18, 26$)
    if $d \neq 0$
    then $g_{ijk} \leftarrow d - 1$
    else no operation
    endif
  endif
enddo
[STEP 2]
if $\boldsymbol{F} = \boldsymbol{G}$ when **[STEP 1]** finishes,
then stop
else $\boldsymbol{F} \leftarrow \boldsymbol{G}$
endif
go to [STEP 1]

[Explanation of the algorithm]
The meaning of each step of the algorithm will be understood from the explanation of the sequential-type algorithm. In fact, the description of the

algorithm is simple and clear. However, since conventional computers with single processors can manipulate one voxel at one time, this algorithm had to scan the whole of an input image as many times as the maximum distance value in an input DT image. Concerning the memory requirement, two 3D arrays are needed for storing an input image and an output image, separately.

When the algorithm is terminated, the result of the DT is restored exactly in an output image G. An original binary image is obtained at once by replacing all positive values in G by 1. These are the same as in Algorithm 5.10.

Remark 5.15. This idea is applicable to the variable neighborhood RDT, except that the neighborhood varies in every iteration and that the propagation is performed only inside that neighborhood. The neighborhoods in the given neighborhood sequence is used in the reverse order. The starting neighborhood of the neighborhood sequence is determined by the distance value. If the distance value on a skeleton voxel is k, for example, the entry of a given neighborhood sequence employed in the k-times of iteration is employed first. Details of the concrete algorithm are neglected here (an algorithm for a 2D image was given in [Toriwaki81, Yokoi81]). The same form of an algorithm will be possible for a 3D image. This way of analysis cannot be applied to the Euclidean DT, because the distance to an adjacent voxel is not always a unit. In other words, the length of a path defined by a sequence of voxels does not always correspond to the distance. By devising a neighborhood sequence in the variable neighborhood DT such as $\{6, 18, 26\}$, values of the DT will become closer to the Euclidean distance than those of the fixed neighborhood DT.

Remark 5.16. Algorithms of the fixed neighborhood DT using the 6-, 18-, and 26-neighborhood distances are obtained immediately from those of the 2D DT. Algorithms of the RDT were given here because they are useful for understanding restoration from a skeleton. The 26- and the 6-neighborhood DT (fixed neighborhood DT) are not so significant as the (squared) Euclidean DT in problems relating directly to the distance metric such as invariability to the rotation, utilization in thinning, and evaluation of the distance from a figure, because in such applications the squared Euclidean DT is much more advantageous. On the other hand, in the compression and deformation of a figure, the fixed neighborhood DT becomes more useful due to its merits, as follows:

(1) Both the DT and the RDT can be performed easily by simple algorithms.
(2) Relation between the DT and the RDT is very clear.

Remark 5.17. Image operator expressions similar to those presented in Remark 5.12 are derived as follows, corresponding to parallel algorithms of the fixed neighborhood DT. They are the same as those in a 2D image.

Definition 5.7. We call the following image operator $\mathbf{M}[\mathcal{N}^{(k)}]$ *maximum filter with the neighborhood $\mathcal{N}^{(k)}$*.

$$\mathbf{M}[\mathcal{N}^{(k)}] : \boldsymbol{F} = \{f_{ijk}\} \rightarrow \boldsymbol{G} = \{g_{ijk}\}$$

$$g_{ijk} = \max\{0, \max\{f_{pqr}; (p, q, r) \in \mathcal{N}^{(k)}((i, j, k)\} - 1\}$$

$$= \max\{0, f_{pqr} - 1; (p, q, r) \in \mathcal{N}^{(k)}((i, j, k))\}. \tag{5.22}$$

Representing by $\boldsymbol{F}^{(k)}$ an output image obtained after performing [STEP 1] in Algorithm 5.13,

$$\boldsymbol{F}^{(\alpha)} = \mathbf{M}[\mathcal{N}^{(k)}](\boldsymbol{F}^{(\alpha-1)}), \ \alpha = 1, 2, \ldots, k \tag{5.23}$$

$$\boldsymbol{F}^{(0)} \equiv \boldsymbol{F} \ (\text{input image}).$$

Hence an output image $\boldsymbol{G}$ is given as follows using a suitable finite value α :

$$\boldsymbol{G} = \mathbf{M}[\mathcal{N}^{(k)}]^{\alpha}(\boldsymbol{F}). \tag{5.24}$$

Here the constant α is determined, depending on an input image. A neighborhood $\mathcal{N}^{(k)}$ is any one of the 6-, 18-, and 26-neighborhoods. Neglecting $\mathcal{N}^{(k)}$ for the sake of simplicity of an expression,

$$\boldsymbol{G} = \mathbf{M}^{\alpha}(\boldsymbol{F}). \tag{5.25}$$

Representing a skeleton image (binary image) of the distance value α by $\boldsymbol{F}_{\alpha}$, that is, a binary image in which voxels of the skeleton with the distance value α are given the value 1 and other voxels are given 0, and an ordinary maximum filter by $\mathbf{M}$, the DT image $\boldsymbol{F}$ is expressed as

$$\boldsymbol{F} = \boldsymbol{F}_1 + \mathbf{M}(\boldsymbol{F}_2) + \mathbf{M}^2(\boldsymbol{F}_3) + \cdots + \mathbf{M}^{M-1}(\boldsymbol{F}_M). \tag{5.26}$$

5.5.11 Extraction of skeleton

A skeleton should be defined clearly before constructing an algorithm to extract it. A skeleton of a 2D image using the 4- and the 8-neighborhood has been studied in detail [Toriwaki81]. By extending it directly to a 3D image, a skeleton is defined clearly for the fixed neighborhood DT using the 6-, 18-, and 26-neighborhood. It has been known in this case that a resulting skeleton coincides exactly for all four ways of definition in Def. 5.5 (1) $\sim$ (4) except for some ambiguity pointed out there. Therefore, we can obtain a skeleton by simply extracting local maxima of the DT. That is, we extract a voxel (i, j, k) such that

$$f_{ijk} \geq f_{pqr}, \ \forall (p, q, r) \in \mathcal{N}^{(k)}((i, j, k)). \tag{5.27}$$

Note here that the type of the neighborhood should be the same as was used in the calculation of the DT.

These are almost the same, in principle, in the variable neighborhood DT. A neighborhood that was employed at the moment the DT value was fixed should be selected in Eq. (5.27). Thus, the neighborhood depends on a DT value of a voxel (i, j, k) as was shown in 5.5.5. The above discussion cannot be applied to the Euclidean DT.

Remark 5.18. Considering that the skeleton is defined as a set of voxels from which an original input figure is restored, it may be possible that the amount of memory can be reduced by storing coordinate values of a skeleton and the DT value (or the squared DT value) on it instead of an input image itself. That is, the skeleton may become a tool of image compression. From this viewpoint, the smaller number of voxels in a skeleton is desirable for saving memory space requirement. Therefore, it becomes more important that a skeleton extraction algorithm extracts a skeleton of a smaller number of voxels with reasonable computation time and that the skeleton satisfies the restoration requirement [Borgefors97, Nilsson97].

Let us assume that a cuboid of $5 \times 5 \times 100$ voxels was given. Consider that the fixed neighborhood DT of the 26-neighborhood was applied to this figure and then local maxima were extracted. If an extracted voxel set contains all voxels on the centerline of this cuboid except two voxels inside it from 5×5 faces of both sides, then such a set of voxels satisfies all conditions of the skeleton. All the known definitions of the skeleton will give such a result. However, the original cuboid will be recovered from a set of voxels extracted from the above skeleton every five voxels. Unfortunately such reduction of the skeleton is difficult without a prior knowledge of the shape of a figure.

Concerning image compression, we need not adhere to the Euclidean DT. Any of the fixed neighborhood DT, that is, the 6-, 18-, and 26-neighborhood DT will work reasonably well, although the performance may vary a little according to the shape of an input figure.

Next let us show an algorithm to extract a skeleton of the Euclidean DT [Saito94b]. We will first give two definitions of skeleton used here.

Definition 5.8 (Skeleton 1). Given a squared Euclidean DT image $\boldsymbol{F} = \{f_{ijk}\}$ (f_{ijk} = square of an Euclidean DT value), a set $\boldsymbol{S}$ of voxels (i, j, k) defined below is called a *Euclidean skeleton 1*.

$$\boldsymbol{S} = \{(i,j,k) | \exists (x,y,z), (i-x)^2 + (j-y)^2 + (k-z)^2 < f_{ijk} \text{ and}$$
$$\max_{(u,v,w)} \{f_{uvw} | (x-u)^2 + (y-v)^2 + (z-w)^2 < f_{ijk}\} = f_{ijk}\}. \quad (5.28)$$

Definition 5.9 (Skeleton 2). Assume that a squared Euclidean image $\boldsymbol{F} = \{f_{ijk}\}$ (f_{ijk} = square of an Euclidean DT value) is given, then a set $\boldsymbol{S}$ of voxels (i, j, k) defined below is called a *Euclidean skeleton 2*.

$$\boldsymbol{S} = \{(i,j,k) | \exists (x,y,z), (i-x)^2 + (j-y)^2 + (k-z)^2 < f_{ijk} \text{ and}$$
$$\max_{(u,v,w)} \{f_{uvw} - (x-u)^2 - (y-v)^2 - (z-w)^2\}$$
$$= f_{ijk} - (x-u)^2 - (y-v)^2 - (z-w)^2\}. \quad (5.29)$$

The above Skeleton 1 means as follows:

Put at each voxel (i, j, k) in an input figure a 3D maximum digital ball that is centered at (i, j, k) and that does not overflow an input figure. After

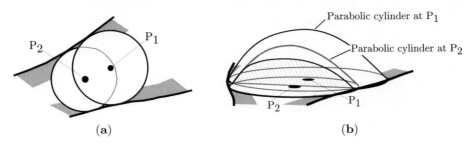

Fig. 5.15. Illustration of skeleton or Euclidean DT [Saito94b]: (**a**) Skeleton 1; (**b**) skeleton 2.

all such balls have been placed, select a ball that contains at least one voxel that is not covered by other balls. Then a set of centers of such balls gives a desired skeleton (Fig. 5.15 (a)). This skeleton corresponds to the skeleton in Def. 5.5 (1) and (4).

In the second case (Skeleton 2), a skeleton is generated by using a solid constructed by an image plane and a parabolic cylinder with the axis perpendicular to an image plane. This cylinder is placed on a figure so that its bottom surface (circle) does not surpass the border of an input figure. This circular bottom surface is centered at each voxel and its radius is equal to the distance value at the voxel. After all of such cylinders have been placed on possible voxels, select such parabolic cylinders that at least one point of the surface of the solid exists that is not covered by other cylinders (Fig. 5.15 (b)). Then a set of all center voxels on which the above selected parabolic cylinders were placed gives the Skeleton 2 defined in Def. 5.9. This skeleton satisfies the restorability requirement. The number of voxels in Skeleton 2 may become smaller than that of Skeleton 1. This point has not been discussed in depth.

The following algorithm has been developed to extract Skeleton 1 and Skeleton 2 [Saito93, Saito94b, Toriwaki01].

Algorithm 5.15 (Extraction of Skeleton 1 of Def. 5.8).

Input image $\boldsymbol{F} = \{f_{ijk}\}$: Squared Euclidean DT image.
Output image: $\boldsymbol{H} = \{h_{ijk}\}$: Skeleton image. Initial value is 0 for all voxels. In the output, the value 1 is given to skeleton voxels, and 0 is given to other voxels.
Work arrays: $\boldsymbol{X} = \{x_{ijk}\}$, $\boldsymbol{Y} = \{y_{ijk}\}$, $\boldsymbol{Z} = \{z_{ijk}\}$, and $\boldsymbol{R} = \{r_{ijk}\}$: Initial value is 0 for all voxels in all arrays.

for all (i, j, k) such that $f_{ijk} > 0$ **do**
   for all (p, q, r) such that $(p - i)^2 + (q - j)^2 + (r - k)^2 < f_{ijk}$ **do**
   if $r_{pqr} < f_{ijk}$
   then
      $x_{pqr} \leftarrow i$
      $y_{pqr} \leftarrow j$

$z_{pqr} \leftarrow k$
$r_{pqr} \leftarrow f_{ijk}$
  endif
 enddo
enddo
for all (i, j, k) such that $r_{ijk} > 0$ **do**
$h_{(x_{ijk})(y_{ijk})(z_{ijk})} \leftarrow 1$
enddo

Algorithm 5.16 (Extraction of Skeleton 2 of Def. 5.9).

Input image $\boldsymbol{F} = \{f_{ijk}\}$: Squared Euclidean DT image.
Output image: $\boldsymbol{H} = \{h_{ijk}\}$: Skeleton image. Initial value is 0 for all voxels.
   In the output, the value 1 is given to skeleton voxels, and 0 is given to
   other voxels.
Work arrays $\boldsymbol{G} = \{g_{ijk}\}$, $\boldsymbol{U} = \{u_{ijk}\}$, $\boldsymbol{V} = \{v_{ijk}\}$, $\boldsymbol{G'} = \{g'_{ijk}\}$, $\boldsymbol{V'} = \{v'_{ijk}\}$,
   and $\boldsymbol{T} = \{t_n\}$: Initial value is 0 for all voxels in all arrays.
During executing the program, all voxel values outside of an input image are
regarded as 0. Arrays $\boldsymbol{G}$ and $\boldsymbol{G'}$, and $\boldsymbol{V}$ and $\boldsymbol{V'}$ are assigned to the same
memory space, respectively.
[STEP 1] (Generation of a label image)
Input image: $\boldsymbol{F} = \{f_{ijk}\}$ squared Euclidean DT image
Output image: $\boldsymbol{U} = \{u_{ijk}\}$ (label image)
Scan an input image, and give labels represented by sequential positive num-
bers starting by 1 to a voxel of $\boldsymbol{F}$ having a positive value, that is, $f_{ijk} > 0$.
Labels are written into a corresponding voxel of a work array $\boldsymbol{U}$.

[STEP 2] (Reverse distance transformation with labels)
(1) Processing in the row direction (forward scan)
Input image: $\boldsymbol{F} = \{f_{ijk}\}$ Squared Euclidean distance transformation image,
$\boldsymbol{U} = \{u_{ijk}\}$ (label image).
Output image: $\boldsymbol{G} = \{g_{ijk}\}$ (Reverse Euclidean distance transformation image), $\boldsymbol{V} = \{v_{ijk}\}$ (label image).
Perform the following procedure in each row with increasing suffixes i from 1
until M.
(a) If $f_{ijk} < f_{(i-1)jk}$,
perform the following procedure for n such that $0 \leq n \leq (f_{(i-1)jk} - f_{ijk} -$
$1)/2$,
   (a-1) if $f_{(i+n)jk} \geq f_{(i-1)jk} - (n+1)^2$, go to the next i,
   (a-2) unless (a-1),
      (a-2-1) if $g_{(i+n)jk} < f_{(i-1)jk} - (n+1)^2$,
      $g_{(i+n)jk} \leftarrow f_{(i-1)jk} - (n+1)^2$,
      $v_{(i+n)jk} \leftarrow u_{(i-1)jk}$,
      go to the next n.
      (a-2-2) otherwise, go to the next n.
(b) If $f_{ijk} \geq f_{(i-1)jk}$,
   (b-1) if $g_{ijk} < f_{ijk}$,

$g_{ijk} \leftarrow f_{ijk}$,

$v_{ijk} \leftarrow u_{ijk}$,

go to the next i.

(b-2) Otherwise go to the next i.

Perform the following procedures (2) $\sim$ (7), which are the same as the above mentioned one, changing the directions of the coordinate axes and scanning "(1) in the direction of the row (forward scan)" as is indicated below.

(2) Row direction (direction of the suffix i) backward scan

  Input image: G, V

  Output image: G', V'

(3) Column direction (direction of the suffix j) forward scan

  Input image: G', V'

  Output image: G, V

(4) Column direction (direction of the suffix j) backward scan

  Input image: G, V

  Output image: G', V'

(5) Plane direction (direction of the suffix k) forward scan

  Input image: G', V'

  Output image: G, V

(6) Plane direction (direction of the suffix k) backward scan

  Input image: G, V

  Output image: G', V'

[**STEP 3**] (Skeleton extraction)

Read a label existing in a label image V'. Give a mark to a voxel of a label image U corresponding to the voxel readout here. Voxels marked here represent skeleton. A working table T is used for search and retrieval of labels in images U and V'.

(1) Generation of a work table for label retrieval.

Input image: $V' = \{v'_{ijk}\}$ (label image)

Output: $T = \{t_i\}$ (work table) (1D array)

for all (i, j, k) **do**

  $t_{(v_{ijk})} \leftarrow 1$

enddo

(2) Generation of a skeleton image.

Input image: $U = \{u_{ijk}\}$ (label image), T (work table)

Output image: $H = \{h_{ijk}\}$ (skeleton image)

for all (i, j, k) **do**

  if $t_{(u_{ijk})} = 1$

  then $h_{ijk} \leftarrow 1$

  else $h_{ijk} \leftarrow 0$

  endif

enddo

When this algorithm is executed, three 3D arrays F, G, and H can be assigned to physically the same memory space unless an input image needs to

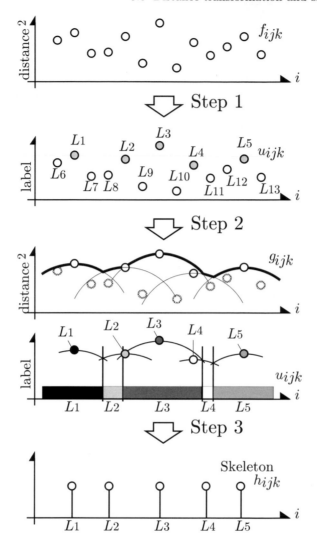

Fig. 5.16. Illustration of Algorithm 5.16 (extraction of Skeleton 2) [Saito94b].

be preserved. In [STEP 3], two 3D arrays U and V may also be allocated to the same place of the memory space if we perform labeling repeatedly using the array V, instead of referring to a label image U to find the location of a particular label.

In [STEP 2], two 1D arrays of the same size as a row and a column are needed as work areas. Thus, the minimum requirement for memory space for skeleton extraction includes two 3D arrays of the same size as an input image, two 1D arrays, and one table (1D array).

This algorithm consists of performing the squared DT and confirming that the restoration of an input figure is possible. It extracts voxels as the skeleton, which are effective for restoration of an input figure. Therefore, if skeleton extraction and restoration of an input figure are performed only once, skeleton extraction is not so significant. On the contrary, once we have extracted a skeleton, then an input figure can be restored from the skeleton and DT values on it at any time.

5.5.12 Distance transformation of a line figure

Distance transformation of a line figure is the process that gives the distance to each voxel of a line figure in turn starting at the edge point. It is defined both for a binary image and a grey-tone line image. Various algorithms to perform this have been studied in detail [Toriwaki79, Toriwaki82a, Toriwaki88, Suzuki85], and all of them can be extended to a 3D line pattern without significant modification. Practical applications including structure analysis of a figure is not studied in depth, although some properties specific to 3D images are expected to exist.

5.6 Border surface following

5.6.1 Outline

Border surface (boundary surface) following is a process to extract all border voxels in a 3D image by the methods satisfying a given set of requirements. The requirements include the following:

(i) All border voxels should be extracted. In other words, coordinates (the numbers of rows, columns, and planes) of each border voxels are recorded in a list.

(ii) Extracted voxels in a list are separated according to connected components that they belong to. According to the notation in Def. 4.15, border voxels are classified according to a component to which border voxels belong. That is, borders are classified according to each pair of figures P and Q in Def. 4.15.

(iii) Border voxels are recorded in the list according to the order specific to an individual algorithm utilized in border voxel extraction.

(iv) A border voxel belonging to each border surface is extracted only once except for exceptional cases such as voxels existing on a plane of one voxel width almost everywhere.

(v) The adjacency relation among border voxels are kept unchanged on the resulting list excluding a few exceptional cases.

Border following has been a well-known problem in the process of a 2D image. It is a processing to visit (follow) voxels on a boundary of a figure in the direction given by the predetermined rule and to store their coordinate values in the list [Rosenfeld82]. The borderline of a 2D figure is a 1D sequence of voxels. If we start the following of a border at a particular pixel and go forward clockwise (or counterclockwise), that is, seeing the inside of a figure on the right-hand side (or the left side), we always come back to the starting pixel after we have visited all border pixels. Thus, border following is a self-evident process except for the process at several exceptional pixels such as a crossing point and a branching point.

The situation is very different in a 3D figure. The border surface of a 3D figure is a 2D curved surface extending in 3D space, and a procedure to visit all voxels on it is not easily found. Therefore, we first need to know the method to visit all border voxels on a one border surface without missing any of the border voxel and without visiting the same voxel more than once. To achieve this, we use a kind of specific neighborhood relationship existing between border voxels and we extract border voxels utilizing this relationship.

Let us define this neighborhood relationship. For the sake of convenience of executing the algorithm, a special mark is given to a particular voxel. We call this *mark value* of a voxel P and denote it by $M(P)$. The explanation below is based on [Matsumoto84, Matsumoto85].

Definition 5.10 (Surface neighborhood). For a given voxel P_1 and an integer K, we call the set of all voxels P_2 satisfying the following conditions (i) and (ii) *surface neighborhood of P_1 with the value K*, and denote it by $NB_m(P_1, K)$ (Fig. 5.17).

(i) $P_2 \in \mathcal{N}^{[m]}(P_1)$, if P_1 is a 1-voxel, $P_2 \in \mathcal{N}^{[\underline{m}]}(P_1)$, if P_1 is a 0-voxel, where m denotes the type of connectivity shown in Table 4.1.

(ii) For two voxels q_1 and q_2 in positional relations shown in Fig. 5.17, q_1 and q_2 have density values different from P_1 and P_2, and either of the following (1) and (2) holds,

    (1) Density value of q_1 = density value of q_2 = K, where $K = 0$, or $K = 1$,

    (2) The mark value of q_1, $M(q_1)$ = the mark value of q_2, $M(q_2) = K$, where $K \neq 0$, and $K \neq 1$.

m and $\underline{m}$ denote a pair of the type of connectivity shown in Table 4.1.

Definition 5.11 (Border surface). Given a connected component of 1-voxels P (m-connected), and that of 0-voxels Q ($\underline{m}$-connected), *the border surface of P against Q*, denoted by $B(P, Q)$, is the set of all voxels in P such that at least one voxel of Q exists in the $\underline{m}$-neighborhood.

Definition 5.12 (Border voxel). A border voxel of an m-connected component consisting of voxels of the value f ($= 0$ or 1) is a voxel that has at least one voxel of the value $1 - f$ in its $\underline{m}$-neighborhood.

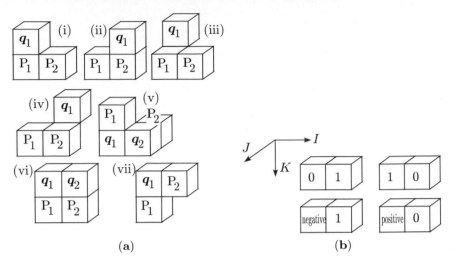

Fig. 5.17. Surface neighborhood and starting voxel pair: (**a**) Surface neighborhood. Assume the m-connectivity case. For $m = 6$, (i), (ii), (iii), and (iv); for $m = 18$, (v)and (vi); for $m = 18'$, (i) and (ii); and for $m = 26$, (v), (vi), and (vii) are used, respectively; (**b**) possible pattern of a starting voxel pair in Algorithm 5.17.

Following are important properties of the surface neighborhood defined in Def. 5.10.

Property 5.7. Assume that a mark value K is given to each voxel of a connected component Q of 0-voxels (assume that a voxel of $\bar{Q}$ (= set of voxels that do not belong to Q) does not have the value K). Then if X $\in B(P,Q)$ for a 1-voxel X and an arbitrary border surface $B(P,Q)$, then all voxels of the value K in the surface neighborhood of X belong to the border surface $B(P,Q)$.

Property 5.8. Assuming that each voxel in a connected component Q of 0-voxels has the mark value K ($K \neq 0, 1$), let us consider a graph as follows for a border surface $B(P,Q)$.

(1) Put a node at the center of each voxel in $B(P,Q)$.
(2) If two voxels in $B(P,Q)$ is in the surface neighborhood mutually, connect those two voxels with an edge.

Then this graph becomes a connected graph. Let us denote this graph by $\mathcal{G}\{B(P,Q), \varepsilon\}$, where ε is the set of all edges.

[Proofs of these properties were shown in [Matsumoto84]]

This property guarantees that we can extract all border voxels while keeping adjacency relations among them by searching the graph $\mathcal{G}\{B(P,Q), \varepsilon\}$ and extracting all nodes of the graph. Here each node corresponds to an individual border voxel. It should be noted that a mark K needs to be given to a connected component of border voxels beforehand in order that the surface neighborhood may be available. In this process it is enough that a border is given a mark. The extraction and storing of border voxels to a list while preserving the adjacency relation is not required here. This is performed by simply applying the same border surface-following algorithm to a set of 0-voxels.

5.6.2 Examples of algorithm

By integrating the above procedures, a border surface-following algorithm is derived, which consists of the following three steps:

(1) search of a starting voxel,
(2) border surface following of connected components of 0-voxels (marking),
(3) following of a border surface $B(P, Q)$.

Algorithm 5.17 (Border-surface following).

M_0, M_1: mark value for a 0-voxel and a 1-voxel.

(S_{01}, S_{02}): Starting voxel pair. A pair of a mutually 6-adjacent 0-voxel S_0 and a 1-voxel S_1 which are on the same scan line (on the same row). We assume that at least one of them has not been given a mark yet (Fig. 5.17).

TEMP: Work area. A cue or a stack that stores coordinate values of border voxels. (In the subsequent part, the expression *put a voxel into TEMP* simply means *write coordinate values (numbers of a row, a column and a plane) of a voxel into TEMP*.)

Output array: coordinate values of voxels belonging to the border surface are stored, being separated with a specific marker into each connected component.

P: Temporary variable representing a voxel.

Scanning of an image: Raster scan (Fig. 2.13).

Input: A 3D binary image. A set of 1-voxels is regarded as a figure. A figure is treated as an *m*-connected component (*m = 6, 18, 18'* or *26*).

[**STEP 1**] (Search of a starting voxel)
(1) $M_0 \leftarrow -1$, $M_1 \leftarrow 1$
(2) Scan an input image in the order shown in Fig. 2.13. Scan starts at the voxel next to the previous starting voxel. Search an input image for a starting voxel pair, that was shown in Fig. 5.17. Go to (3), if a starting pair was detected. Stop, if the whole of an input image has been scanned.
(3) $M_0 \leftarrow M_0 - 1$, $M_1 \leftarrow M_1 + 1$
If S_0 of the starting voxel pair (S_0, S_1) has a mark, go to [**STEP 3**]; otherwise go to [**STEP 2**]. Here S_0 is a 0-voxel and S_1 is a 1-voxel.

Note: Border following is reduced here to graph search. TEMP becomes a cue if we adopt the width-first search, and becomes a stack if the depth-first search is employed.

[**STEP 2**] (Trace of border voxels of the background)
(1) Put S_0 into the work area TEMP. Give the mark M_0 to S_0.
(2) Repeat the following until TEMP becomes empty.
Pull out one element P from TEMP. Extract from an input image all voxels
in the surface neighbor of P with the value 1 such that the mark has not been
given yet. Give them the mark M_0 and put them into TEMP.
(3) Go to [**STEP 3**]

[**STEP 3**] (Trace of voxels of a border surface)
(1) Put S_1 into the work area TEMP and the output array, and give a mark
M_1 to S_1.
(2) Repeat the following until TEMP becomes empty.
Pull out one element P from TEMP. Extract all voxels in the surface neighbor
of P with the value $M(S_0)$ such that they do not have the mark M_1; give them
the mark M_1, and put them into TEMP and an output array.
(3) Put a mark into the end of the output array in order to show the end of
border voxels sequence of one border surface. Go to (2) of [**STEP 1**].

This algorithm has the following property.

Property 5.9 (Property of Algorithm 5.17).

(1) Coordinate values of border voxels are output for all border surfaces. Con-
    tents of the output list are separated into individual border surfaces.
(2) One border voxel is output only once. If the same border voxel belongs to
    more than one border surface, that voxel is written into the list the same
    number of times as the number of border surfaces it belongs to.
(3) The adjacency relationship (connectivity relation) among voxels put into
    the output list is represented in the form of a graph (or a tree).
(4) The algorithm is applicable to all four types of connectivity (6, 18, 18',
    and 26 connectivity).
(5) An original input figure is restored exactly from the list of extracted border
    voxels and starting voxel pairs (see Section 5.6.3 also).

Remark 5.19. The reason that the marking process is applied to the set
of 0-voxels here, in spite of the following of borders of 1-components, is that
different border surfaces should be traced separately. In Fig. 5.18, for example,
let us consider a figure P with a cavity Q', and let us assume that the thickness
of the figure P is one (one voxel width) at a voxel X. Then, both the border
surface $B(P, Q)$ and $B(P, Q')$ share a voxel X. Unless a mark is given to 0-
voxels, two borders $B(P, Q)$ and $B(P, Q')$ are not separated at the voxel X.
Thus, those two borders are traced continuously without being separated into
two border surfaces. If a mark is given to 0-voxels of Q, $B(P, Q)$ and $B(P, Q')$
are followed separately as two border surfaces. The voxel X is visited and
output once for each border surface.

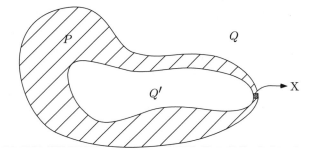

Fig. 5.18. Border surface of a 3D figure with the unit thickness.

5.6.3 Restoration of a figure

An original input figure is restored exactly from the result of border surface following. We will present below a concrete form of an algorithm to realize this.

Algorithm 5.18 (Restoration of a figure).

Input: One of the border voxels of the background (one voxel for each border surface)
   List of border voxels of a figure (output of Algorithm 5.17)
Output: Image F. (A 3D image. A restored binary image is stored after the execution of the algorithm. Initial values are 0 for all voxels.)
TEMP: Work array (1D, a queue, or a stack)

[STEP 1] (Restoration of a border surface)
Pull out in turn each element of the border voxel list, and put the value 1 into a correspondent voxel of an output image.

[STEP 2] (Marking of border voxels of the background)
Denote by (x, y) a starting voxel pair corresponding to each border surface, which is given as an output of Algorithm 5.17, and perform the following steps, by starting at the 0-voxel of the above starting voxel pair.
(1) Substitute -1 to a voxel of an output image corresponding to the starting voxel. Store the coordinate of the starting voxel to a work area TEMP (a queue or a stack).
(2) Repeat the following (i) ~ (iii) until TEMP becomes empty.
   (i) Read out the first element of TEMP.
   (ii) Extract all voxels of the surface neighborhood of the value 1.
   (iii) Store coordinate values of extracted voxels to TEMP, and substitute the value -1 to voxels of an output image corresponding to voxels extracted above.
(3) Go to **[STEP 3]**

[STEP 3] (Restoration of inner voxels and erasure of the mark)

Scan an output image with the raster scan (Fig. 2.13), and perform row by row the following restoration process.

(1) Substitute 0 to a work variable N.

(2) If the value of a voxel changes to 1 from -1, then set the value of N as 1, and substitute the value 1 to subsequent voxels on the same row in turn. If the voxel of the value -1 is met again on the same row, reset the value of N as 0, and stop substitution of the value 1 after that.

(3) Search the same row to detect change of the value from -1 to 1, and repeat the same procedure.

(4) If the end of the row is reached, go to the next row and go to (1). If the whole of an output image has been scanned, go to (5).

(5) Scan the output image again and erase all of -1 by replacing with 0.

Remark 5.20. Border surface following for a 3D image began to be studied actively in earlier days (1980s) in the history of 3D image processing chiefly by G. Hermam and his colleagues, and many papers have been published [Artzy85, Herman98]. Details are known from books and papers referred to in [Herman98, Kong85, Kong89, Toriwaki04]. That research is characterized, in particular, by the ideas that applications to simulate surgical operations were clearly intended, as well as authors' research [Artzy85, Herman78]. It should be noted that memory limitation was severe in computers in those days.

One example of applications in those days was fast processing of a 3D CT image of the skull. The border surface following algorithm was different from the one presented above and was studied in detail both theoretically and experimentally. For example, the basic idea is to trace the surface of a 3D figure consisting of cubes corresponding to voxels, that is, tracing the surface of a continuous figure defined in Def. 4.5, while in the above algorithm, border voxels themselves are followed. According to the former idea, the border surface becomes a continuous figure and is treated in a clear-cut way theoretically, although the number of voxels becomes much larger than the trace of voxel themselves.

Nowadays, memory has become much cheaper and a device with a much larger memory capacity is available even in portable computers, and the size of a 3D image data to be processed has also become much larger. A 3D CT image is becoming more precise and is required to be processed as a gray-tone image in many of applications. Thus the significance of border following is now changing.

5.7 Knot and link

5.7.1 Outline

One of the most important features specific to a 3D image is *knot* and *link* in a line figure (Fig. 5.19). In mathematics, a large amount of research work has been performed concerning the knot and the link. Almost all of the work treated an ideal form of a line figure in 3D continuous space [Kauffman87]. Reports on the processing of the knot and the link by computer were very few.

Past research of the knot can be roughly classified into two kinds. One is to transform a knotted line figure into a kind of symbolic representation, and replace the shape transformation of a continuous line figure by the symbol manipulation. This symbol manipulation is performed by computer. Examples are determination of the kind of a knot and decision on whether a line figure is knotted or not. This is performed by utilizing the transformation called *Reidemeister transformation* which is well known in mathematics.

The other is to study properties of a digitized knotted figure that correspond to those features that have been examined for a continuous knotted figure in mathematics. This type of study has been performed very little except for [Nakamura00, Saito90]. Let us introduce here basic properties of a digitized knot according to [Saito90].

Definition 5.13 (Digital knot). If a connected component C consists of four or more 1-voxels, and any of those 1-voxels has just two 1-voxels in its k-neighborhood ($k = 6, 18, 26$), that is, if a figure consists of connecting voxels only, a connected component (k-connected) is called a *digital simple closed curve* or (k-connected) *digital knot*. The number of 1-voxels contained in C is called *length* of this digital knot.

Consider then a line figure obtained by connecting center points of 1-voxels mutually adjacent on a digital knot with line segments. By doing this a polygonal knot in 3D continuous space is obtained. We call this a *continuous knot* C_C *corresponding to a digital knot* C. A continuous knot C_C corresponding to a digital knot C becomes a continuous knot in the continuous space. Results in the knot theory of mathematics can be applied to the above C_C.

First a knot of a continuous figure is defined as follows in mathematics.

Let us denote by C_p a figure derived by projecting the above continuous knot (a polygonal knot) onto a suitable plane P (more strictly an orthogonal projection of C_C presented in Chapter 7). Then, if n points of C_C are projected to the same point of C_p, this point is called n-fold point (multiple point) ($n \geq 2$). If the number of n-fold points is definite and all of them are generated from only projections of points of C_C, the projection is called a *regular projection*. In particular, a double-fold point is called a *crossing point*. The number of a crossing point varies according to a projected plane. It may change by the transformation of a figure, even if the topological properties of a figure do not change. The minimum number of crossing points in all regular projections of all knots topologically equivalent to a knot C_C is called a *minimum crossing point number* of a knot C_C. For a stricter description, see the monograph and text of mathematics [Kauffman87].

Thus, properties of a continuous figure C_C as a knot are frequently discussed by using its regular projection on to a 2D plane. We also discuss characteristics of a digital knot C using the regular projection of a polygon C_C

corresponding to C. For example, the number of crossing points of C_C is regarded as that of a digital knot C.

Definition 5.14. A digital knot of which the number of crossing points is *0* is called a *trivial knot* or *unknot*.

Intuitively speaking, the *knot* is a property of a single 3D simple curve or a *string*. If it is knotted when we pull both ends of it, then a string is said to be *knotted* or called a *knot* in the mathematical sense. Otherwise such string is called a *trivial knot* or said to be *unknotted*. Here (in this section) a knot means a *knotted* knot (Fig. 5.19).

Remark 5.21. A set of more than one closed curve is called a *link*. There are two types of links, too. One is the case that two closed curves are linked each other, and the other is a pair of two curves that are separate from each other.

5.7.2 Reduction of a digital knot

In order to study properties of a digital knot by the same method as in mathematics, we need to generate a large number of continuous polygonal knots corresponding to a given digital knot and derive their regular projections. It is not always easy. Large parts of drawing regular projections closely relate to our intuition or heuristic decisions as a human. Algorithmic generation of regular projections is never a trivial procedure. Thus it becomes significant to transform directly a digital knot contained in a digitized line figure and study its features.

Let us present here an algorithm to shrink a digital knot.

Algorithm 5.19 (Shrinking of a knot - arc elimination). Assume a digital knot C is given. At an arbitrary pair of voxels P and Q on C, if the length (= the number of voxels) from P to Q along the curve C is longer than the 26-neighbor distance between P and Q, then the part of the knot C between P and Q is translated so that the length of C may become shorter. Unless the topology of the curve C is preserved, the translation is not performed. If a voxel becomes redundant in a result of translation, that voxel is eliminated at that moment (Figs. 5.20, 5.21).

Algorithm 5.20 (Shrinking of a knot - corner elimination). A bulge of a curve is deformed to be straight as shown in Fig. 5.22. The deformation is not applied if topological properties of a curve C change by the deformation.

The following property holds true:

Property 5.10. Any trivial knot (unknot) is reduced to any one of unknots of the length *4* shown in Fig. 5.23 by repetitive application of Algorithms 5.19 and 5.20. There does not exist a knotted knot of the length *4*.

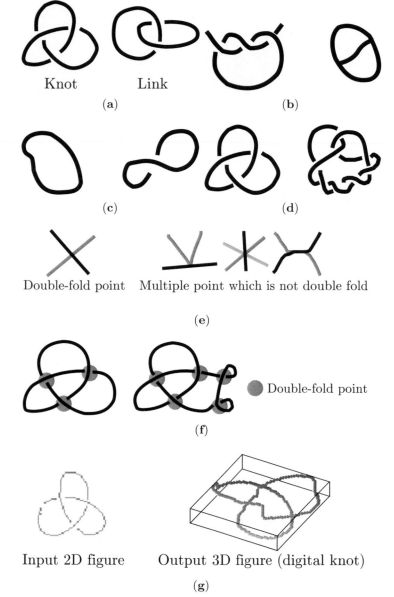

Double-fold point

Fig. 5.19. Illustration of a knot and link: (**a**) Knot and link; (**b**) unknotted line figure; (**c**) trivial (unknotted) knot; (**d**) knotted knot; (**e**)illustration of a double-fold point which determines a regular projection; (**f**) examples of knot with three points; (**g**) example of digital knot generated from a regular projection (2D figure).

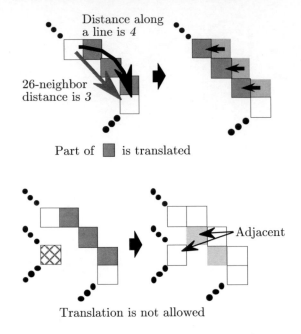

Fig. 5.20. Illustration of Algorithm 5.19 (arc elimination).

This is easily confirmed by noting that any trivial knot longer than *4* obviously includes the part that is reduced by Algorithms 5.19 and 5.20. The latter half is confirmed easily from Fig. 5.23.

The following is not proved, although it is expected empirically.

Conjecture 5.1. The minimum length of a knotted knot (nontrivial knot) is *26* and the number of crossing points is *3*.

[Explanation]
As an example, Fig. 5.25 shows a knot of the length *26* and the number of the crossing points *3*. As far as visual observation is concerned, this cannot be reduced to a knot shorter than *26*. A link consisting of two trivial knots requires two trivial knots of the length *12* (Fig. 5.24). By connecting them at two points, a knot of the number of the crossing points *3* is obtained. But it cannot be realized by a curve shorter than the length *25*.

Remark 5.22. Knottedness cannot be detected by features presented in the previous chapter such as the Euler number and the connectivity index.

5.8 Voronoi division of a digitized image

Voronoi division (Voronoi tessellation) was originally defined for a point set in continuous space, and has been studied extensively in the field of com-

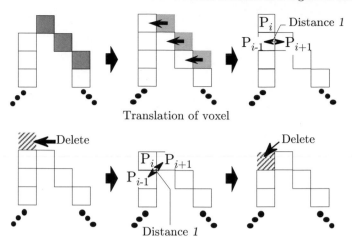

Translation of voxel

Fig. 5.21. Deletion of unnecessary or redundant voxels in a line figure (see Algorithms 5.19 and 5.20).

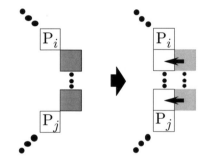

Fig. 5.22. Illustration of Algorithm 5.20 (corner elimination).

putational geometry (or digital geometry) [Goodman04]. It has been widely applied in a variety of areas including physics, biology, and geography. It has also become one of the inevitable tools in image pattern analysis and computer graphics. Thus, an enormous volume of papers and books have been published that referred to Voronoi tessellation and relating problems. Voronoi tessellation and its close relations have been called by different names, such as: Voronoi polygon, Dirichlet tessellation (division), Delaunay triangulation, Voronoi diagram.

Concepts of Voronoi tessellation and related topics are basically applicable to a digitized image. However, sometimes serious differences from the continuous space are found in procedures to solve concrete problems [Mase81, Toriwaki81, Toriwaki84, Toriwaki88]. Extension to a 3D image from a 2D image is not difficult in principle, but some complicated problems exist

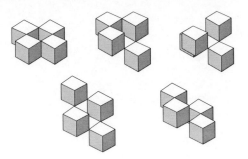

Fig. 5.23. Digital knots of the length *4*.

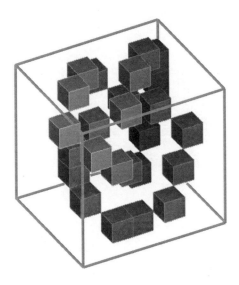

Fig. 5.24. Example of a link consisting of two digital knots of the length *12*.

in practical algorithms to calculate it. We will briefly introduce one idea to treat the Voronoi tessellation on a 3D image.

Let us consider a set of figures $S = \{F_1, F_2, \cdots, F_n\}$ on a 3D binary image F. Here F_i is an object (figure) in 3D space. Then, for an arbitrary voxel Q in the background of F, a set of voxels S_R defined by the following equation (5.30) is called a *dominance area* (or *Voronoi region*) of a figure F_i.

$$S_R = \{Q;\ \min_i d(Q, F_i) = d(Q, F_R),\ F_i \in S\} \qquad (5.30)$$

$$= \text{set of all background voxels such that the nearest figure in } S \text{ is } F_R$$

The result of division of all background voxels into dominance areas of figures F_is (Voronoi regions) is called *Voronoi tessellation*. In the case of a 2D image,

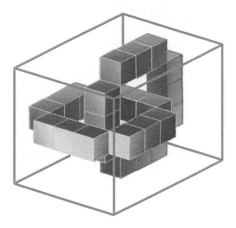

Fig. 5.25. Digital knot of the length *26* and three crossing points.

a diagram that shows border lines of all Voronoi regions is called a *Voronoi diagram*.

To calculate the Voronoi tessellation of a given 3D image, we first need to define $d(Q, F_i)$, the distance between a figure F_i and a voxel Q. The following is a widely employed example.

$$d(Q, F_i) = \min\{d(Q, P); \; P \in F_i\} \tag{5.31}$$
$$= \text{distance to the nearest voxel in } F_i$$

It is necessary to further determine the distance metric concretely. For more detail, see [Mase81, Yashima83].

Some additional problems, which were not caused in 2D continuous images, must be taken into consideration to calculate Voronoi tessellation of a 3D image.

(1) Voronoi division surface (borders of Voronoi regions) is, in general, a surface figure in 3D space. However, a large number of voxels may exist that are equally distant from two or more figures. Then a Voronoi division surface may become thick arbitrarily. The same situation may occur in a 2D digitized image [Mase81, Yashima83, Toriwaki84, Toriwaki88].

(2) A Voronoi division surface may have a hole, depending on the distance metric employed in its calculation.

(3) The shape of a Voronoi division surface (or dominate area) may become extraordinarily complicated.

Calculation of the Voronoi tessellation is not difficult in principle. One idea, for example, is to perform the labeling first, then to perform the distance transformation of the background with propagating labels synchronously or considering distance values if the 6-, 18-, or 26-neighborhood distance is employed. Different types of label propagation may be required in the case that the Euclidean distance is employed [Saito92]. However, good solutions have not been known for (1) and (2) above.

Concerning a Voronoi diagram of a 2D digitized image, see [Mase81, Yashima83, Toriwaki84, Toriwaki88]. Applications to feature extraction of tissue section 3D images is reported in [Saito92].

6

ALGORITHMS FOR PROCESSING CONNECTED COMPONENTS WITH GRAY VALUES

In this chapter we present algorithms processing a connected component in which each voxel has an arbitrary gray value (= a gray-tone connected component). We assume here that a gray value (= a density value) is positive inside a connected component and that a gray value outside a connected component is zero unless stated otherwise. Therefore, the image is a gray-tone image with a background.

A gray-tone connected component has the same topological features and general shape features as a binary connected component. Furthermore, it has additional density value features. The important characteristics of an algorithm processing a gray-tone connected component are a combination of those two types of information. The notice about the description of algorithms in the beginning of the previous chapter also concerns the description of algorithms in this chapter.

6.1 Distance transformation of a gray-tone image

6.1.1 Definition

The definition of the distance transformation (DT) of a gray-tone image is immediately derived from the extension of a 2D gray-tone image.

Definition 6.1 (DT of a gray-tone image). A process to calculate the following image $G = \{g_{ijk}\}$ from an input 3D gray-tone image $F = \{f_{ijk}\}$ with a background is called a *gray weighted distance transformation (GWDT)*.

$$\mathbf{GWDT} : F = \{f_{ijk}\} \rightarrow G = \{g_{ijk}\}$$

$$g_{ijk} = \begin{cases} \min\{|\pi|; \ \pi \text{ represents a path from a 0-voxel of} \\ \quad \text{an image } F = \{f_{ijk}\} \text{ to a voxel } (i,j,k), \\ \quad \text{and } |\pi| \text{ represents the sum of density values of} \\ \quad \text{voxels on a path } \pi \text{ in an input image,} \\ \quad \text{if } f_{ijk} > 0 \ ((i,j,k) \text{ is a voxel of a connected component}), \\ 0, \text{ if } f_{ijk} = 0 \ ((i,j,k) \text{ is on the background}) \end{cases} \quad (6.1)$$

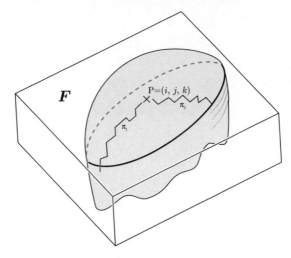

Fig. 6.1. Illustration of the gray weighted distance transformation of a gray-tone image with the background. Find a path to minimize the weight $|\pi|$ (= the sum of density values on a path) among paths $\{\pi_1, \pi_2, \ldots\}$ to a point P from a border surface and give the minimum weight to a point P.

$|\pi|$ is called *weight* of a path π. The name of *gray weighted* comes from this fact. A path that gives g_{ijk} is called a *minimal path* to (i, j, k) (Fig. 6.1).

Algorithms to calculate the 6-, 18-, and 26-neighborhood GWDT are obtained by straightforward extension of algorithms for a 2D image. The basic idea is the same as in a 2D image, that is, to find a path such that the total sum of distance values along a path (= the weight of a path) is minimized.

The extension of the Euclidean DT to a gray-tone image is not a complicated concept. That is, it is defined as the minimization of the total sum of density values along an arbitrary path in continuous space. This is not realized easily on a digitized image, because it is almost impossible to find a minimal path as a sequence of voxels. This is why an algorithm to perform the Euclidean GWDT has not been reported yet.

6.1.2 An example of algorithm

Let us discuss an example of the sequential algorithm of the 6-, 18-, and the 26-neighborhood GWDT.

Algorithm 6.1 (GWDT of a gray-tone image sequential type).

$\boldsymbol{F} = \{f_{ijk}\}$: Input image (gray-tone image with the background) (size $L \times M \times N$)

$\boldsymbol{G} = \{g_{ijk}\}$: Output image (= GWDT)

$\boldsymbol{W} = \{w_{ijk}\}$: Work array

L, M, N: Image size (numbers of rows, columns and planes of an image) (constant)

α: Weight coefficient

t: Work variable

[STEP 1] (Initialization)
for all (i, j, k)s **do**
   if $f_{ijk} = 0$
   then $g_{ijk} \leftarrow 0$;
   else $g_{ijk} \leftarrow$ Sufficiently large integer;
   endif
enddo

[STEP 2] (Iteration)
for all (i, j, k)s **do**
   if $f_{ijk} > 0$
     for all $(p, q, r) \in \mathcal{N}^{[26]}((i, j, k))$ **do**
       $\alpha \leftarrow \sqrt{3}$
       if $(p, q, r) \in \mathcal{N}^{[18]}((i, j, k))$
       then $\alpha \leftarrow \sqrt{2}$
       else
         if $(p, q, r) \in \mathcal{N}^{[6]}((i, j, k))$
         then $\alpha \leftarrow 1$
         endif
       endif
       $t \leftarrow \alpha \times g_{ijk} + f_{ijk}$, $(p, q, r) \in \mathcal{N}^{[26]}((i, j, k))$;
       if $t < g_{ijk}$
       then $g_{ijk} \leftarrow t$;
       endif
     enddo
   endif
enddo

[STEP 3] (Test of terminating rule)
if (no gray value in G changed) **stop**
else go to [STEP 2]
endif

Remark 6.1. The parallel processing of algorithms and operator expressions by use of the minimum filter [Yokoi81, Naruse77b] is immediately extended to a 3D image. See also Remarks 5.12, 5.17 in Chapter 5 concerning a binary image.

Note: In the calculation of the distance, the distance to a 18-adjacent voxel, and the distance to a 26-adjacent voxel are multiplied by $\sqrt{2}$ and $\sqrt{3}$, respectively, to reduce the amount of gap between the Euclidean distance.

Remark 6.2. The significance of the DT of a gray-tone image is not always clear in binary image processing. No specific applications have been reported other than the use in preprocessing of thinning images and the concept of the skeleton is unfamiliar.

6.2 Thinning of a gray-tone image

6.2.1 Basic idea

Information carried by a gray-tone image can be summarized as follows:

(1) The structure of line figures characterizing the spatial distribution of density values such as ridge lines and valley lines.
(2) The shape features of a figure (or of subspaces), determined by the spatial distribution of density values (for example, the shape of contour lines (or equidensity surfaces) of density values).
(3) Statistics concerning the distribution of density values (e.g., the histogram of density values, etc.).

The first and second items can be condensed in a line figure. The third item does not relate to shape information.

One way to concentrate the characteristics of a gray-tone image into a linear figure is to extend the concept by using a method extracting a centerline of a binary figure to a 3D gray-tone image. This process is called *thinning of a gray-tone image* with the analogy of the processing of a binary image, and we call an extracted linear figure the *centerline* or *core line*. This applies to the first and the second case discussed above . In the second case, we first segment a subimage (a figure containing gray values) from an input gray-tone image. We call this segmented figure a *gray-tone connected component* again by the analogy of a connected component in binary image processing. Thresholding is the most common method of segmentation. A segmented gray-tone connected component holds the details regarding the shape of a connected component as well as information concerning the distribution of density values inside it.

When considering shape features of a gray-tone connected component, the features common in the thinning process of a binary image become important, such as the location of a centerline (center surface) of a figure and the preservation of topological features. Many of the requirements (1) ∼ (7) described below relate to these.

On the other hand, the extraction of a borderline (or a border surface) of a gray-tone connected component (which may be substantially regarded as an equidensity surface) is not called surface thinning or axis thinning. In the example of a binary image, structural characteristics of density values may become *surface-like*. Another example is the surface thinning of a gray-tone image. For example, the part of a gray-tone image corresponding with a ridgeline of the density value distribution may become a curved surface with a constant density. There are no case studies of this as far as the author is aware. Here we will only discuss linear features such as a ridgeline and a valley line.

6.2.2 Requirements

The requirements for thinning are almost the same as those for thinning a binary image and we will summarize them again. Strictly speaking they are slightly different from those in binary image processing, because properties concerning the shape features of a connected component as well as the distribution of density values relate to the actual thinning process.

[Requirements for thinning a gray-tone image]

(1) *Connectivity*: A core line keeps topological properties of an input image without change.
(2) *Location*: A core line is located at the ridgeline of the density value distribution (in subsequent parts we simply write a *ridgeline*) of an input image, if a ridgeline exists.
(3) *Line width*: The width of the core line is one unit width (one-voxel width).
(4) *Degeneration*: The length of a core line is close enough to the value that a human observer recognizes as natural.
(5) *Branching part*: At the branching part and the crossing part of an input figure, the core line also becomes a branching part and a crossing part in the natural form.
(6) *Stability*: A core line is not affected excessively by noise irregularity in the shape of an input figure or by random variations in the density values of an input figure.
(7) *Rotation*: A core line is not affected by the rotation of an input figure.

It is extremely difficult to satisfy all of these. Some of them are not compatible with each other in principle.

Remark 6.3. Terms such as *centerline* and *core line* may not be suitable for structural lines such as a ridge line or a valley line, because they are not always located in the center of an input figure in the geometrical sense. A branching point (5) means both the branching as a shape feature and that of a ridgeline.

6.2.3 Principles of thinning

A 3D gray-tone image is, as stated in Chapter 1, a set of voxels accompanied by gray values (density values) in a 3D space. It seems that the thinning of such data has not been discussed much in past papers. Although basic ideas and methods of thinning 2D gray-tone images conceptually can be applied to a 3D image, their implementation and algorithms are not always obvious. We will summarize below the basic concepts of thinning 2D images and any important problems occurring when extending them to a 3D image.

(1) *Ridgeline extraction*: Thinning based on the ridgeline extraction of a curved surface of density values distributed on a 2D plane (= ridgeline extraction of a surface in 3D space) is extended to the extraction of ridge-lines of a curved surface in a 4D space [Enomoto75, Enomoto76, Yu90, Fritsch94, Pai94, Arcelli92, Niblack92, Monga95, Thirion95, Hirano00]. One problem here is the complexity in the shape of a ridgeline. The form of a ridgeline in a 3D gray-tone digital image may be difficult to define. It therefore will be difficult also to derive an algorithm to extract it based on heuristics. This type of idea can be applied to an arbitrary gray-tone image with no background. On the other hand, the shape features of a figure cannot be used in this type of method, and problems concerning the preservation of topology cannot be dealt with.

(2) *Classification of the state of a voxel*: In the processing of a 2D image, the state of each voxel is classified as *ridge-like*, *valley-like*, etc., according to the relation of density values of voxels in its neighborhood. Results are used for the extraction of a ridge line [Toriwaki75, Yokoi75]. This method has been applied to the analysis of terrain elevation data [Haralick83, O'Callaghan84, Johnston75, Peucker75]. However, a good quality ridgeline cannot be extracted when using only the local pattern features of a 3D image. This type of method cannot easily be extended to a 3D image. The classification of local patterns includes relations in density values that have not been discussed yet. Shape features cannot successfully be treated with this type of the method. In the case of a continuous image, the problem is treated using differential geometry [Enomoto75, Enomoto76].

(3) *Binarization of density values in a local area*: Methods of thinning a bi-nary image may be extended to a 3D gray-tone image by binarizing local subpatterns of a gray-tone image (with suitable thresholds and while ap-plying methods suitable for 3D binary images). For example, a method in [Toriwaki75, Yokoi75] can easily be extended to a 3D image. However, the quality of an obtained result is not always good because degeneration is likely to occur. Frequently parts of an input image remain without being converted to a linear figure.

(4) *Use of GWDT*: Methods described in (1), (2), or (3) above may be per-formed after GWDT has been applied to an input image. Information con-cerning the minimal paths obtained by performing GWDT is also available for thinning [Naruse77a, Naruse77b]. By the use of GWDT we can sup-press random noise in an input image, and we are able to utilize some of shape features. In combining GWDT with (1) ∼ (3) above, shortcomings are also inherited. The concept of a minimal path cannot be applied in the Euclidean DT. Therefore, the use of GWDT is affected significantly by the rotation of an input image. The topology of an input figure is not always preserved in the use of the minimal path.

(5) *Modification of a result by methods of thinning*: After binarizing an input image by an approximate threshold, any method of thinning a binary im-age can be applied to obtain an approximated result of thinning. Then

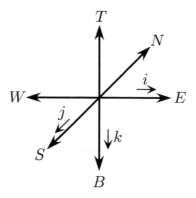

Fig. 6.2. Codes of direction for grouping border voxels in Algorithm 6.2.

we can modify results while considering the density values distribution of an input gray-tone image [Salari84]. Density values may be available in the process of thinning a binary image [Hilditch69, Saito95, Saito96]. The use of shape features and preservation of topology of an input image are realized immediately based on the discussion in Chapters 4 and 5. However, it is necessary to distinguish between the figures and the background beforehand. The modification of intermediate results using density values has eventually the same kind of disadvantages as in (1) and (2) above.

6.3 Examples of algorithms – (1) integration of information concerning density values

6.3.1 Algorithm

Algorithm 6.2 presented below is based on the concept of thinning of a 2D binary image [Hilditch69, Yokoi75], and was derived by adding to it a procedure to use density values. In principle, a voxel with a smaller density value is deleted earlier among deletable voxels. Deletable voxels of the same density value are deleted with an equal rate from six directions (T, B, W, E, N, S) (Fig. 6.2). The algorithm is as follows [Yasue96].

Algorithm 6.2 (Thinning of a gray-tone image).

$\boldsymbol{F} = \{f_{ijk}\}$: Input and output image. Input image (a positive image with the background) at the beginning of execution and output image at the end of execution. The size is $L \times M \times N$.
$\boldsymbol{W} = \{w_{ijk}\}$: Work array.
L, M, N: Numbers of rows, columns, and planes of an image.
min: Minimum of density values in an input image.
bordertype: Group number of border voxels.

[**STEP 1**] (Detection of positive border voxels and their grouping)
Extract all positive border voxels and group them according to the position of
0-voxels in their 6-neighborhood. Here a positive border voxel means a positive
voxel that has at least one 0-voxel in the 6-neighborhood. For example, a positive voxel that has a 0-voxel in the direction of T in Fig. 6.2 in the neighborhood is classified into the group BT. If more than one 0-voxels exists in the 6-
neighborhood, the priority is given in the order (T, B, W, E, N, S). Each group
of positive border voxels is represented as $\boldsymbol{B} = \{BT, BB, BW, BE, BN, BS\}$.
This process is written as follows.

for all (i, j, k)s **do**
  if $(f_{ijk} > 0) \cap ((i, j, k) \neq$ end voxel)
  then
    if $f_{i,j,k-1} = 0$ **then** $w_{ijk} \leftarrow 2$
    else if $f_{i,j,k+1} = 0$ **then** $wijk \leftarrow 3$
    else if $f_{i-1,j,k} = 0$ **then** $wijk \leftarrow 4$
    else if $f_{i+1,j,k} = 0$ **then** $wijk \leftarrow 5$
    else if $f_{i,j-1,k} = 0$ **then** $wijk \leftarrow 6$
    else if $f_{i,j+1,k} = 0$ **then** $wijk \leftarrow 7$
    endif
  endif
enddo

[**STEP 2**] (Extraction of a voxel that is of the minimum density value among
deletable voxels and that is not an end voxel) (See Note also)
Find a voxel in the set $\boldsymbol{B}$ that is deletable, not an edge voxel, and has the
minimum density value in $\boldsymbol{B}$. Denote the density value of a detected voxel by
min.

min $\leftarrow$ Sufficiently large integer;
for all (i, j, k)s **do**
  if $2 \leq w_{ijk} \leq 7$
    if $f_{ijk} <$ min $\cap ((i, j, k) =$ deletable and not an edge voxel)
    then min $\leftarrow f_{ijk}$;
    endif
  endif
enddo

[**STEP 3**] (Deletion)
(i) Search each group in $\boldsymbol{B}$ in the order of BT, BB, BW, BE, BN, BS.

Note: Deletability and a border voxel are defined in the same way as for a binary
image obtained by regarding all positive voxels as 1-voxels.
Note: If there is more than one deletable border voxel in some group, all of those
voxels are processed before moving to the processing of the next group. Deletion
of a voxel from an image $\boldsymbol{F}$ is executed at the moment when it is found to be
deletable. That is, the corresponding voxel is replaced by a 0-voxel (sequential
algorithm). Once a voxel is given a mark of an edge voxel, it is regarded as a
finally preserved voxel and will never be deleted in the subsequent procedure.

(ii) Find and remove from B an element satisfying all of the following conditions.
  (a) A density value is equal to min.
  (b) A voxel is deletable.
  (c) A voxel is not an edge voxel.
(iii) Delete a voxel of an image F corresponding to the element removed above. If the voxel is found to be not deletable in the above procedure, give a corresponding voxel the mark showing an edge voxel.
for bordertype = 2 to 7 **do**
  for all (i, j, k)s **do**
    if $(w_{ijk} = \text{bordertype}) \cap (f_{ijk} = \text{min})$
    then
      if $(i, j, k) \neq$ edge voxel
      then
        if $(i, j, k) =$ deletable
        then $f_{ijk} \leftarrow 0$
        endif
      else $(i, j, k) =$ edge voxel
      endif
    endif
  enddo
enddo

[**STEP 4**] (Test of the terminating rule)
if no voxel was deleted in [**STEP 3**]
then stop
else go to [**STEP 1**]
endif
The result of thinning is stored in an image F when the program finishes.

    This algorithm is a sequential type and repeatedly scans the whole of a input image (the procedure of [STEP 1] $\sim$ [STEP 3] is executed repeatedly). The number of times of iteration depends on the size (width) of an input figure (connected component).
    Next, let us present another algorithm, which is obtained by adding to the above Algorithm 6.2 a preprocessing consisting of 3D GWDT [Naruse77a]. As was stated in the previous section, GWDT is a processing that gives each voxel the minimum value of the sum of density values along a path (= the weight of a path) to that voxel from a background voxel. In this algorithm, we use the sum of density values weighted by the Euclidean distance between adjacent voxels instead of the simple sum of density values. Weight coefficients assume either of 1, $\sqrt{2}$, and $\sqrt{3}$ according to relative locations of an adjacent voxel. The outline of the algorithm is as follows [Yasue96].

Algorithm 6.3 (Thinning of a gray-tone image with GWDT − outline).

Input image: $\boldsymbol{F} = \{f_{ijk}\}$; 3D positive image with the background.
Output image : $\boldsymbol{G} = \{g_{ijk}\}$; result of thinning (binary image).

[**STEP 1**] (3D GWDT)
(Initialization)
for all (i, j, k)s **do**
  if $f_{ijk} > 0$
  then $g_{ijk} \leftarrow M$
  endif
  M is an integer that is sufficiently larger than the maximum distance value.
  if $f_{ijk} = 0$
  then $g_{ijk} \leftarrow 0$
  endif
enddo
(Iteration)
for all (i, j, k)s **do**
  $g_{ijk} \leftarrow \min\{g_{ijk},\ f_{ijk} + \pi_{pqrijk} \times g_{pqr};\ (p, q, r) \in \mathcal{N}^{[26]}(i, j, k)\}$:
  π_{pqrijk} is a coefficient, assuming either value of 1, $\sqrt{2}$, or $\sqrt{3}$ according to the
  location of (p, q, r) relative to (i, j, k). $\mathcal{N}^{[26]}(i, j, k)$ is the 26-neighborhood of
  (i, j, k).
  enddo
(Test of the terminating rule)
Stop the procedure and go to [**STEP 2**] if no change in a voxel value occurs
in the whole of an input image. Otherwise, go to (iteration).

[**STEP 2**] (Thinning)
Perform Algorithm 6.2, regarding the distance image $\boldsymbol{G}$ as an input positive
image. After finishing the procedure, the result of thinning of the image $\boldsymbol{F}$ is
stored in $\boldsymbol{G}$.

  This algorithm will be implemented easily by combining Algorithm 6.1
and 6.2.

6.3.2 Experimental results

An artificial 3D binary image including a geometrical figure was generated.
This figure (Object 1 and Object 2) consists of two or three cylinders in 3D
space (Figs. 6.3, 6.4). Density values inside these cylinders at the distance r
from the axis of a cylinder are determined by $[a \times (R + 1 - r)]$, where $[\ ]$
represents a ceiling function, $R =$ the radius of the cylinder, and $a =$ the
gradient of density distribution. In real experiments, $R = 10$ and $a = 10$.
Effects of the rotation of a figure, noise in density values, and noise in figure
shape were studied systematically. Parts of results are shown in Fig. 6.3.
  The same algorithms were also tested by a real CT image. A chest CT
image taken by helical CT was processed using thresholding operations to
obtain a positive image with the background. In this image figures roughly

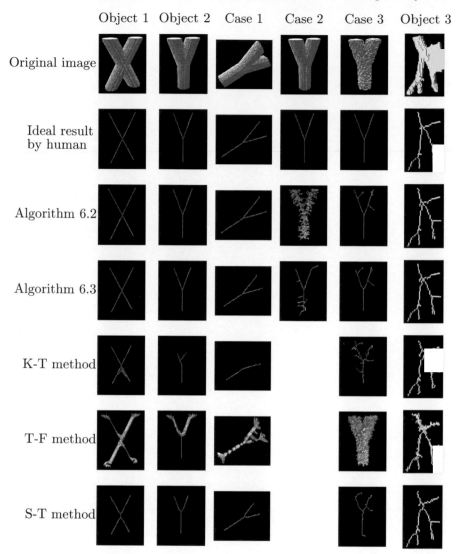

Fig. 6.3. Experimental results of Algorithm 6.2 [Yasue96] (applied to artificial images).

correspond to blood vessels. Voxels inside these figures keep original CT values which are likely to be higher in the vicinity of center lines. Parts of results are given in Fig. 6.3.

Thinned results created with the method mentioned above were compared with results obtained by algorithms for a binary image, because other methods for a 3D gray-tone image have not been reported. Three methods by [Kawase85] (K-T methods), by [Tsao81] (T-F method), and by [Saito95, Saito96] (S-T method) were used for experiments. Since all these methods were developed for a binary image, information concerning a density value is not used for thinning. An artificial image (presented above) was processed by these algorithms after an input image was binarized by thresholding with a suitable threshold value. A rough tendency was observed in the experiment using an artificial figure.

In Algorithm 6.2 the extracted center line is very close to an ideal core line except for in Case 2 of Fig. 6.3. The reason that many short branches appear in the result is that the local maxima of density value distribution inside a figure were erroneously regarded as edge points. The effect of the noise in a density value was suppressed to some extent in Algorithm 6.3 compared to Algorithm 6.2. This is due to the smoothing effect of GWDT. On the other hand, the result is affected more by the noise in the shape in Case 3 of Fig. 6.3. The effect of the shape of an input figure seems to increase by the use of GWDT.

The K-T method caused degeneration in Object 2, and could not extract the centerline satisfactorily in the branching part in Object 1 and Case1. The result was severely affected by shape noise in Case 3.

The T-F method extracted too many plane-like components, in particular in Case 1 and Case 3. This suggests that the method is affected relatively more by the rotation of a figure and by the shape noise.

Two branching parts were extracted for Object 1 by the S-T method. In the results for Object 2 and Case 1, the shapes of branching parts are unnatural. The effect of shape noise seems to be more severe compared to Algorithm 6.2 and 6.3 in Case 3.

Summarizing these experimental results for an artificial image, Algorithm 6.2 is affected by the density value distribution more than the shape of a figure. It works effectively in the way that density values are higher in the vicinity of ideal centerlines, but there is sensitivity to density noise.

A few algorithms have been developed to extract ridgelines of a 2D graytone image [Toriwaki75, Enomoto75, Enomoto76, Naruse77a]. By extending them to a 3D image, we will be able to derive algorithms with characteristics similar to Algorithm 6.2, although the topology of a figure is not always preserved. Algorithm 6.3 will provide a compromise between the centerline of a figure and a ridgeline of the density value distribution.

The followings is known from experimental results using a real CT image (Fig. 6.4, Object 3).

The core lines by Algorithm 6.2 and 6.3 are close to an ideal core line. On the other hand, the core lines by S-T method and K-T method are not smooth due to unevenness of the surface of regions used as an input figure in the experiment (= blood vessel regions), extracted automatically from 3D CT images.

The shape of a branching part is not suitable. Many plane-like components remain in the results when the T-F method is used. Algorithm 6.2 and 6.3

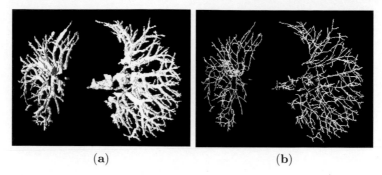

(a)   (b)

Fig. 6.4. Experimental results of Algorithm 6.2 (applied to real CT images): (**a**) Input image (blood vessels in a chest X-ray CT image); (**b**) the result of thinning.

were relatively better in the thinning of vessel region images used in this experiment. In fact, it is known from Fig. 6.4 that the core line obtained by Algorithm 6.2 preserves most of the important structure of vessel regions. More details are reported in [Yasue96].

6.4 Examples of algorithms – (2) ridgeline following

6.4.1 Meanings of a ridgeline

In order to extend the basic idea of ridgeline extraction of a 2D image (in (1) of Section 6.2.1) to a 3D image, we need to develop a procedure to extract a ridgeline of a hypersurface $u = f(x, y, z)$ representing a hypercurved surface of the density distribution in 3D space, that is, a hyper-curved surface in 4D space $u - f(x, y, z) = 0$. To achieve this, we first have to decide what conditions should be satisfied by points (voxels) on a *ridgeline*.

Let us consider a 2D image to find keys to a solution (Fig. 6.5). Our idea is to follow a point sequence to the direction of the minimum curvature from a local maximum (top) of density values. This means that we consider the direction of the minimum curvature coincides with the direction of a ridgeline. The minimum curvature means the minimum of principal curvature described in Section 3.4. However, it may not be correct to extract points with zero curvature because all parts that are locally flat may be extracted. If we exclude points of zero curvature, another inconvenience may be caused because any smooth top of a mountain that is differentiable is excluded.

So two different types of requirements are contained in the concept of *ridgeline* as follows.

(1) The state of the spatial distribution of density values in the neighborhood of each voxel is ridge-like. We call such a point a *ridge voxel*.
(2) Ridge voxels are arranged linearly.

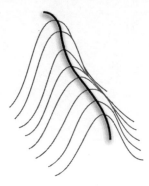

Fig. 6.5. A model of a ridgeline on a curved surface of density values distributed on 2D images.

The first requirement can be examined independently and point by point, although the procedure may not always be self-evident. To test the second requirement, we need to observe the local area of an image. From an analogy to a 3D surface, a point may look like a ridge point if the curvature is large in one direction and small in the direction perpendicular to it. We still need to select experimentally or by experience some ad hoc criterion regarding how large a curvature should be to be regarded as a ridge, because we do not have a known standard about the value of curvatures for a ridge point.

6.4.2 Algorithm

In spite of such complexity or ambiguity in the concept of a ridge point (ridge voxel) and a ridgeline, we will be able to derive algorithms to obtain a *ridgeline* by detecting ridge-like voxels and by following the sequence of such voxels. We will show an example of this type of algorithm as Algorithm 6.4 below.

[Definitions used in Algorithm 6.4]

Starting condition: Consider an arbitrary point (voxel) P of a 3D image, and we call two voxels Q_1 and Q_2 an *adjacent voxel pair* of a voxel P, if Q_1 and Q_2 are in the 26-neighborhood of P and their locations are symmetric with respect to P. A voxel P and its adjacent voxel pair Q_1 and Q_2 are said to satisfy the *starting point condition*, if the following inequality holds (Fig. 6.6).

Starting point condition: $[(f(\mathrm{P}) \geq f(Q_1)) \cap (f(\mathrm{P}) > f(Q_2))] \cup [(f(P) > f(Q_1)) \cap (f(\mathrm{P}) \geq f(Q_2))]$, where $f(\mathrm{P})$ means the density value of a voxel P.

Continuity condition: Let us represent by k_1, k_2, and k_3 three 4D principal curvatures at a current voxel P. Then the direction of the principal axis corresponding to the minimum of k_1, k_2, and k_3 is coincident to *the direc-*

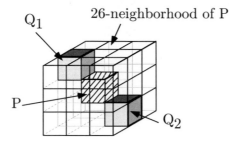

Fig. 6.6. The starting point condition of Algorithm 6.4.

tion of the tracing, and the sign and the amount of the curvature at the voxel P satisfy a given condition.

Algorithm 6.4 (Ridge line extraction tracing type).

[STEP 1] Scan the whole of an input image by the raster scan and start the procedure at the next voxel after the current voxel if it has not been traced yet.

Go to **[STEP 3]**, if all adjacent voxel pairs in the 26-neighborhood of a voxel P satisfy the starting condition.

Go to **[STEP 2]**, if 12 of 13 adjacent voxel pairs satisfy the starting condition.

Terminate tracing when the scan finishes.

[STEP 2] Select as tracing direction the direction toward one of the voxels of the adjacent voxel pair that does not fulfill the *starting point condition* from the trace starting point. Then start the actual tracing procedure.

Go to **[STEP 4]**, if the *tracing procedure* terminates.

[STEP 3] If there exists a voxel P′ that satisfies the continuity condition among voxels adjacent to a starting point, begin the *tracing procedure* in the direction connecting the above voxel P′ and the starting point.

Go to **[STEP 4]**, if the *tracing procedure* terminates.

Go to **[STEP 2]** unless the direction satisfying the *continuity condition* exists.

[STEP 4] Go back to the *starting point* and begin *tracing procedure* again, along the tracing direction rotated by *180* degrees (in the direction opposite to the previous one).

[*Tracing procedure*] Prepare an image F_W (work area; all voxels are initialized by *0*) of the same size as an input image.

[STEP I] Move a current voxel by one voxel in the direction of tracing. If the *continuity condition* is satisfied at the current voxel after the above one-voxel shift, then write value *1* into the voxel of the image F_W corresponding to the current voxel and repeat **[STEP I]**.

[STEP II] Move the current voxel by two voxels in the trace direction. If the *continuity condition* is satisfied at the current voxel after the above movement, then write value *1* into the corresponding voxel of the work image F_W and go to **[STEP I]**. Otherwise move the current voxel back to the previous position and go to **[STEP III]**.

[STEP III] Change the tracing direction into the direction connecting the current voxel and adjacent voxels and select such a direction that the amount of angle change is less than *90* degrees. Then move the current voxel by one voxel along the newly selected direction. If the *continuity condition* is satisfied at the current voxel after the movement, then write value *1* into the corresponding voxel of an image F_W and go to **[STEP I]**. Otherwise move the current voxel back to the starting point of the trace and terminate the tracing.

All directions traced in the past by the *tracing procedure* at all visited voxels should be recorded, and the *tracing procedure* is terminated if the direction of tracing in each step of the procedure is found to be the same as the one that was traced in the past. This is required in order to avoid the same voxel being traced more than once in the same direction.

Remark 6.4. The concrete content of *continuity condition* is not fixed here. As was stated in Chapter 3, however, only 20 cases occur in the size relation among three principal curvatures. The continuity condition will be fixed by giving which of those 20 cases are adopted as a ridge point. In the experiments presented in the text, for example, the following two cases:
(Set 1) Pattern 5, 6, 9, and 10 in Table 3.4
and
(Set 2) Two or more principal curvatures are positive, and only $|k_3|$ among $|k_1|$, $|k_2|$, and $|k_3|$ is not a local maximum
were tested.

The first set (Set 1) above was seen frequently on the centerline of an artificial image used here (Fig. 6.7). The centerline is really located along a line with the highest density value in this artificial figure, and is considered as a *ridgeline* intuitively. The second set (Set 2) above includes as the cases No. 1 $\sim$ 11 (excluding No. 4 and 8) of Table 3.4 and the case No. 19. Since (Set 2) contains (Set 1), the set of voxels extracted by using it includes the one extracted by (Set 1). In the mathematical analysis of a 3D curved surface, a curved surface such that $H < 0$ and $K < 0$ is sometimes called ridge surface, and the one such that $H < 0$ and $K = 0$ is called saddle ridge, where H and K represent the mean curvature and the Gaussian curvature, respectively (Table 3.4) [Haralick83]. By the analogy with this, the above (Set 2) will contain relatively more of patterns like the ridge surface and parts of saddle ridge of a 4D curved surface.

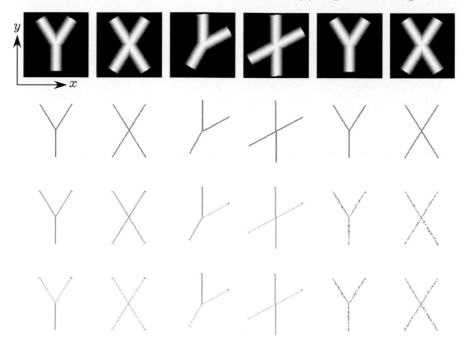

Fig. 6.7. Experimental results of Algorithm 6.4 applied to artificial images. From top to bottom, input images, ideal centerline, result (with the connectivity condition (Set 1)), and result (with (Set 2)).

6.4.3 Experiments

This algorithm was applied to an artificial image and a real CT image. Parts of results are presented in Fig. 6.7 and Fig. 6.8. For details, see [Hirano00].

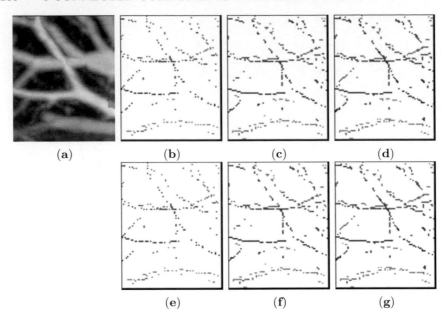

(a)   (b)   (c)   (d)

(e)   (f)   (g)

Fig. 6.8. Experimental results of Algorithm 6.4 applied to a real CT image: (a) Input image (by MIP (see 7.3.3)), (b) ~ (g) results by Algorithm 6.4 with different conditions as follows. (b) Connectivity condition (Set 1), division index $n = 1$, (c) (Set 1), $n = 2$, (d) (Set 1), $n = 3$, (e) (Set 2), $n = 1$, (f) (Set 2), $n = 2$, (g) (Set 2), $n = 3$. A parameter n (division index) denotes the spatial resolution of an input image. For details see [Hirano00, Hirano03].

7

VISUALIZATION OF 3D GRAY-TONE IMAGES

In this chapter we discuss the visualization of a 3D gray-tone image. Explained are tools for visualizing a 3D gray-tone image such as projection, surface rendering, and volume rendering. These topics belong to the field of computer graphics, and are discussed in detail in ordinary computer graphics textbooks. Here we will discuss only the topics that are used for the visualization of a 3D gray-tone image.

7.1 Formulation of visualization problem

Let us summarize briefly the meaning of visualization as presented in this chapter. The human eye is incapable of seeing a whole 3D gray-tone image $f(x, y, z)$. The reason is that in an image $f(x, y, z)$ a density value is assigned to every point (x, y, z) in 3D space, and we are unable to understand the whole 3D space from only looking at an object in the real world with our ordinary human vision. In order to solve this problem various methods have been developed by using computer graphics (CG) technologies. This problem also exists in data visualization and the development of methods for this. In this chapter we introduce the basics of displaying or visualizing a gray-tone 3D image.

Visualization means the presentation of the whole of a 3D image in such a way that a human observer can understand it when he or she looks at it. Therefore, the result (the output of the visualization process) should be drawn (or displayed) onto a 2D plane. In other words, visualization is a way of mapping, that is, to map the distribution of density values and forms of objects in a 3D (or higher dimensional) space onto a 2D plane. Therefore, it is unavoidable that part of the information contained in an original 3D image is lost except for in very specific cases. Intuitively the information concerning the depth (the information in the direction perpendicular to an image plane) will be lost, although some very complicated methods of compensation may be effective in few cases. In spite of this serious information loss problem, we have to use display on a 2D image plane (or mapping onto a 2D plane), because the human vision cannot observe the whole of the 3D image directly. This is the major premise in considering visualization discussed in this chapter.

We will add the following minor premises:

(i) The input to visualization procedure or the object data used to be visualized are voxel data representing a 3D gray-tone image.
(ii) Input data (an input 3D image) are given beforehand. They are usually obtained experimentally or as a result of observation or measurement. Mathematical descriptions and definitions of an explicit form are rarely available.

These facts stand in remarkable contrast to computer graphics in which most of the visualized objects are described by mathematical expressions or algorithms. More exactly, objects defined mathematically or by way of an algorithmic procedure will also be contained in a target of visualization. We need to treat the above types of data in visualization as well as well-formed data.

Remark 7.1. There are exceptional cases in which a 3D input image can be visualized on a 2D plane without losing any information:

(1) All 2D cross sections are presented as 2D images. This is a popular method in the medical diagnosis of X-ray CT images. It often takes a lot of work for human observers to do this due to large numbers of images that need examining. The 3D form of an object, in particular one featuring the spatial distribution of density values, is difficult to interpret.
(2) A 3D object consisting of a limited number of curved surfaces and polygons is drawn exactly by various methods of descriptive geometry such as a set of orthogonal projections in three directions which are perpendicular to each other. It is not easy for those unfamiliar with these drawing methods to intuitively understand 3D shapes.
(3) A polyhedron is specified by a net on a plane without any ambiguity.
(4) An "origami" is drawn on a 2D plane in the form of a net with folding lines. This is used mainly to explain the procedure generating individual work, and helps to visualize the procedure rather than the form. In fact we hardly can imagine a 3D shape of an "origami" work from its net.

Thus a result drawn using the above methods of Remark 7.1 is not always comprehensible. Sometimes a stereoscopic display can be useful in some kinds of applications, although these are not discussed here. In some computer graphics applications, we may be able to design a 3D image (or the structure of the 3D space) so that display results on a 2D plane are more effective for observers. In the visualization, however, the given 3D data cannot be changed in principle.

7.2 Voxel data and the polygon model

To begin with, let us clarify the form (it may be called *model* and *data struc-ture*) used to represent an image to be visualized.

We will discuss a 3D continuous gray-tone image and a 3D digitized gray-tone image. As explained in Chapter 2, these are represented by the notation $f(x, y, z)$ and $\boldsymbol{F} = \{f_{ijk}\}$, respectively. A digitized image is stored in a 3D array.

These data are called *voxel data*, or are named a *voxel model*. Another way to represent data, frequently used in visualization, is approximating the surface of an object to be visualized by polygons.This is called a *polygon model*. To simplify, a triangle is most frequently adopted to represent a polygon model. As a result the object surface is expressed by a set of many small triangular elements (called *triangular patches*).

To apply a polygon model to voxel data, we first segment an object from a 3D image, after which we approximate the object surface by a set of polygons, that is, we transform the object surface to a polygon representation. There are various methods to perform this procedure corresponding to different proper-ties of objects and the specific purpose. For digitized data, features specific to voxel data will be effectively used. It is important that each density value is put on the regular cubic lattice, and that an object itself is regarded as a set of cuboids. Let us discuss two examples.

7.2.1 Voxel surface representation

Here we regard each voxel as a small 3D continuous figure and render visible faces of cuboid voxels directly. In this case, all faces forming the object surface are squares of the same size. If we assume that the viewpoint is infinitely far, that is, if we adopt the orthogonal projection, only three kinds of faces appear around every vertex, looking to the same direction except for specific locations (Fig. 7.1). The spatial resolution of the imaging system used to obtain an original image is preserved, and shape deformation is not caused during the rendering procedure. These properties greatly contribute to the simplification of the visualization procedure.

On the other hand, artifacts are likely occur in rendering due to the fact that the surface is represented by only three kinds of parallelogram patches. Image quality of a visualization result may be not so good in such a resolution where individual voxels can be seen. The surface of a rendered figure lacks smoothness. The computation time is not always short compared with the computation time for triangular patches.

7.2.2 Marching cubes algorithm

Fitting triangular patches to the surface of an object is done by placing a triangular patch so that a set of patches makes a border surface between a set

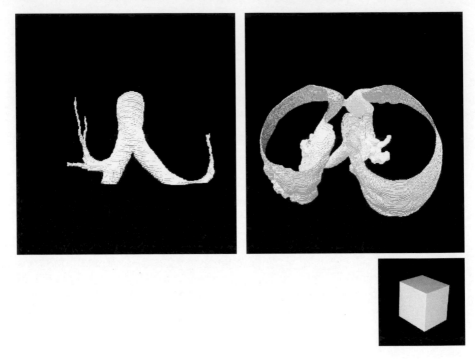

Fig. 7.1. Voxel surface representation.

of 1-voxels corresponding to an object and a set of 0-voxels corresponding to the background. Here we represent each voxel by a sample point at the center of a voxel.

Considering a set of $2 \times 2 \times 2$ voxels (sample points) and arranging the values 0 and 1 on them, there are 256 ($= 2^8$) possible patterns. However, by inverting 0 and 1 and taking into account the geometrical symmetry of patterns, it is found that only 14 patterns are essentially different from each other (Fig. 7.2). Therefore, it is sufficient to fix the locations before a triangular patch is inserted corresponding to each of these 14 patterns and store them in the computer memory. These $2 \times 2 \times 2$ local patterns do not exist independently, meaning that neighboring patterns strongly relate to each other according to some deterministic rules. By using this relation and the list of local patterns an effective algorithm was developed to generate triangular patches sequentially with raster scanning an image. This algorithm is called a *marching cubes algorithm* and is commonly used [Lorensen87, Watt98].

Remark 7.2. Strictly speaking, it is necessary to meet several additional conditions when using the algorithm. First, the inside and the outside relation should not contradict between adjacent patches. Second, a solid figure surrounded by a surface defined by a set of patches should have the same topo-

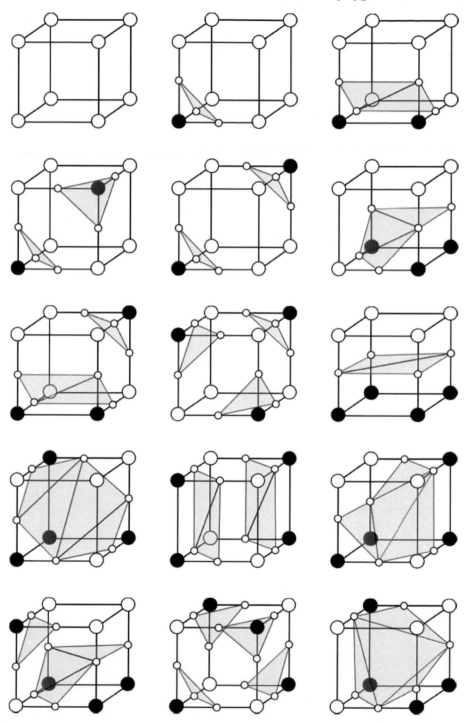

Fig. 7.2. Basic arrangements of $2 \times 2 \times 2$ voxels (marching cubes algorithm). Black circles indicate voxels of density values higher than a threshold t, while white ones indicate those lower than t. Equidensity surfaces of the density value t exist at the location shown in the figure.

logical properties as an original solid (this is the same for the polygon model mentioned previously).

Remark 7.3. Thresholding operations may be performed simultaneously to render the segmentation of a figure. This algorithm is also used for rendering an equidensity surface. The connectivity index (Chapter 4) may be used for testing the topology preservation.

7.3 Cross section, surface, and projection

7.3.1 Cross section

A cross section is a 2D gray-tone image presenting the surface plane of an object that appears when an object is cut by a plane. Most currently available CT systems generate many axial sections of the human body cut by parallel planes. The most basic way of visualization is to present these 2D sections directly. In fact, a clinical diagnosis in medicine is usually performed in this way, examining the set of cross-sectional images of the studied organs carefully. It is not difficult to generate a section in another direction if enough numbers of original sections are given with a small enough interval. A suitable 2D or 3D interpolation may become necessary to obtain a good quality of images if the direction of sections is different from the direction of rows and columns of initial voxels.

In many CT images, the spatial resolution on each cross-section image (or a *slice*) and the interval between section planes (or between slices) are different from each other. Usually the first is higher than the last. In recent CT machines the size of a voxel in each slice and the interval between slices (called *reconstruction pitch*) is chosen individually. These facts should be taken into consideration when obtaining good quality 3D images. Slices are often interpolated in order to create a given image more similar to a 3D image of cubic voxels when the slice interval is significantly larger than the voxel size in each slice.

A well-known simple method of interpolation is linear interpolation, as follows: Denote an arbitrary point on a cross section by P and assume that we need to determine the density of a point P (Fig. 7.3). Let us consider eight sample points $a, b, \cdots, h$ on original slices shown in Fig. 7.3. Then denoting the density values of those eight points by $f_a, f_b, \cdots, f_h$ the density value f_P of a point P is calculated as

$$f_P = w_a f_a + w_b f_b + \cdots + w_h f_h, \qquad (7.1)$$

where $w_a, w_b, \cdots, w_h$ are suitable weight coefficients.

More complicated interpolation (using splines and sampling functions, for example) also may be available. Significance, necessity, and effectiveness of such complicated methods still strongly depend on individual applications.

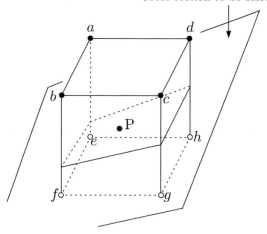

Cross section to be calculated

Fig. 7.3. Interpolation of a density value. A density value of an interpolated voxel P is calculated using density values of the nearest eight voxels.

The density value distribution along a curved surface is calculated in a similar way based on interpolation. Examples used in medical image processing include density value distribution along the surface of massive organs like liver, and on the inner walls of tubular or cavity organs such as the bronchus, colon, and stomach. To calculate density distributions along complicated surfaces is needed in applications such as virtual endoscopy, multiplanar reconstruction, and to unravel the colon [Harker00, Hayashi03, Oda06, Truong06, Wang98].

7.3.2 Surface

Rendering surfaces of solid objects is one of the major problems in computer graphics. Nowadays a variety of methods is available and explained in many computer graphics textbooks, in particular *surface rendering* [Foley84, Watt98, Bankman00]. This method is used primarily for rendering the shape of surface (a 3D curved surface) of a 3D solid object. If this surface is derived from a 3D gray-tone image by a suitable method, the surface rendering is useful also to visualize a 3D image. For example, if this surface represents an equidensity surface, a rendered result shows one of the characteristics of a density distribution in a 3D space.

Remark 7.4. Displaying a section of an image is regarded as rendering the gray value distribution patterns seen on a cutting plane. In this sense the visualization of a section is reduced to that of a surface. If we find a 3D coordinate value of a point drawn on a 2D image plane, then a density value for that point is derived directly from an original 3D image.

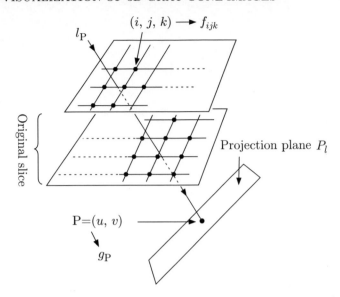

Fig. 7.4. Illustration of projection. A density value g_P of a point $\mathrm{P} = (u, v)$ on 2D projection plane P_l is obtained by adding density of values of voxels (i, j, k) in 3D space in the direction of a projection line l_P.

7.3.3 Projection

As was stated in Section 2.2.5, *projection* means the integration of a 3D image along a line l_p perpendicular to a plane P_L. In this chapter we extend the integration a little so that it includes a kind of mapping of a density value. Here a mapped value is calculated by various ways from the density values of a 3D image on the line l_p and is given to an intersection of the line l_p and the plane P_L. A result of projection is a 2D image and is presented on a display. There are several ways to calculate a mapped value. The following two types have been widely used in medical image processing (Fig. 7.4).

Denoting by g_P a density value of a point P on a plane P_l,

$$(i) \qquad g_\mathrm{P} = \int_{l_\mathrm{P}} w(x, y, z) f(x, y, z) ds \qquad (7.2)$$

where $\int_{l_\mathrm{P}}$ is the integration along the normal l_P of a projection plane P_l, and $w(x, y, z)$ is a suitable weight function.

$$(ii) \qquad g_\mathrm{P} = \max_{l_\mathrm{P}} \{w(x, y, z) f(x, y, z)\} \qquad (7.3)$$

where $\max_{l_\mathrm{P}}$ is the maximum density on the above line l_P and $w(x, y, z)$ is a suitable weight function.

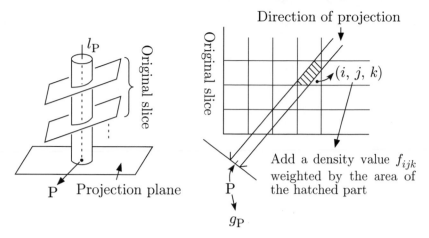

Fig. 7.5. Calculation of a density value in projection.

In the subsequent part we call the first case a *weighted sum projection*, and the second case *weighted maximum intensity projection*. They are simply referred to as the *accumulated sum projection* and *maximum intensity projection* (*MIP*), if $w(x, y, z) = 1$, $\forall(x, y, z)$.

Several additional problems should be taken into consideration when applying them to a digitized image. For example, there may be very few sample points or voxels on a projection line. One basic idea in this case is as follows. First, consider a normal line (a line perpendicular to the projection plane) at each sample point P on the projection plane. Then add density values of voxels within a predetermined distance from the normal one. A resultant value is given to the point P. A formal description will be given as follows (Fig. 7.5).

Let us denote by l_P a line perpendicular to the projection plane at a point $P = (u, v)$ on the projection plane and by f_{ijk} a density value at a voxel (i, j, k) of a 3D image. Then, a density value g_P of a point P on the projection plane is given by

$$g_P = \sum w(i, j, k; u, v) f_{ijk} \tag{7.4}$$

where $w(i, j, k; u, v)$ is a weight function determined by coordinate values (i, j, k) and (u, v). In many cases $w(i, j, k; u, v)$ is given as a function of the distance from a point (i, j, k) to a line passing a point P and is perpendicular to the projection plane. A linear interpolation given by Eq. 7.1 is also an example.

An alternative way is to assume a kind of beam of which the centerline is a line l_P with a constant thickness, and to calculate a weighted sum of density values of voxels intersecting the beam. A weight used here is determined based upon the area of the intersection of the beam and of each voxel (Fig. 7.5). The simplest case is the sum of density values of all voxels intersecting the line l_P without weighting.

The projection of a perpendicular plane to an original slice and a projection to a slant plane are reduced to the projection of a 2D image to a line. This is basically the same as the calculation of a section. The same type of method (and in particular the arithmetic method) is utilized in the reconstruction of a 2D section image from a CT projection.

In any of the mentioned methods, a high quality image is obtained only when an angle between a projection plane and a slice is relatively small. The calculation of projections and sections is one of the fundamental problems common to the display (or visualization) of 3D images and the reconstruction from projections. Special purpose hardware has been developed for obtaining sections and projections in a vertical direction. A method of rendering presented here is actually a good model showing what a 3D object and a 3D scene look like when we see them from a specific position in the real world. In a sense visualization is similar to painting a 3D scene or taking pictures. Considering this we often use words like a "viewpoint" and a "view direction" that are originally used for human image generating.

7.4 The concept of visualization based on ray casting – (1) projection of a point

The idea and methods presented here are basically the same as those in 3D computer graphics. We will explain them briefly considering the convenience of applying them to the visualization of a 3D gray-tone image.

For starters, let us imagine the 3D world containing a 3D image (object) to be rendered and an image plane (screen) for rendering. No other things exist in this world. We call this *imaginary (virtual) 3D space* and denote it by S_I. A light source and a ray in S_v are assumed only to be convenient tools for this visualization. They usually do not have any specific relation to those in the real world. This is one of the major differences from the generation of high-quality realistic images in photorealistic rendering in computer graphics.

In the subsequent part of this section we explain the case of a continuous image only for the sake of simplicity. It should be noted that digitization is performed in many steps like in the sampling on a ray as described before.

7.4.1 Displaying a point

Assume the coordinate system (x, y, z) in a 3D imaginary space S_I that is called the *world coordinate system* and the 2D coordinate system (X, Y) on a display plane H_p which we call the *image plane coordinate system*.

First of all we need to determine where an arbitrary point P $= (x, y, z)$ in space S_I should be mapped onto a display plane H_p, that is, which point on a plane H_p is the image of mapping. We call this mapping of a 3D point to a 2D plane *ray casting*. Positions of the plane H_p and a view point P_e are

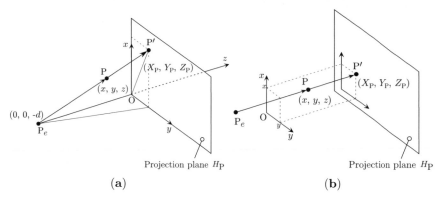

Fig. 7.6. Geometry of mapping of a point onto a plane: (**a**) Perspective projection; (**b**) parallel (orthogonal) projection.

selected arbitrarily. Here we assume that a viewpoint is at $Z = -d$ on the Z axis, that is, at $(0, 0, -d)$, and that an image plane is on the $x - y$ plane (Fig. 7.6).

Denoting by $P' = (X_P, Y_P, Z_P)$ a point on the image plane that corresponds to the point P, the following two kinds of projections are most frequently employed.

(1) *Orthogonal projection (parallel projection, normal projection)*

$$X_P = x, \ Y_P = y, \ Z_P = 0. \tag{7.5}$$

In this case, a point in 3D space is projected in parallel to the Z-axis of the world coordinate system. The position of P' does not depend on the viewpoint. In other words, the viewpoint is regarded to be infinitely far from an image plane.

(2) *Perspective projection (central projection)*

$$X_P = d \cdot x/(z + d), \ Y_P = d \cdot y/(z + d), \ Z_P = 0. \tag{7.6}$$

In this case, the point P' is located at the intersection of the image plane and a line connecting the point P and the viewpoint P_e (= the view direction).

By using these projections we can determine where on an image plane we should draw each point in the 3D space. In this space each voxel is drawn on an image plane and is determined in the same way, for example, by representing each voxel by its center point.

Since we are discussing the digitized space in practice, both a 3D image and a 2D image on a projected plane are digitized images. The coordinate value (x, y, z) in the above explanation is a center point of a voxel or a vertex of a voxel.

They are many different methods for mapping the shape of a 3D object onto a 2D plane in descriptive geometry, computer graphics, drawing, and painting. Details can be found in books in each field. The two methods that we discuss are sufficient to visualize a 3D image.

In the normal (parallel) projection, lines running parallel in a 3D space are drawn as parallel lines on a 2D plane. The length of a line segment and the area of a face that is parallel to a 2D image plane is coinciding with real values in the 3D space. The depth information is lost, however, and a drawn result lacks in perspective.

In the perspective projection, a group of lines running parallel in a 3D space and not parallel to an image plane are mapped to a group of lines intersecting at a common intersection point on a 2D image plane. This intersection point is called a *vanishing point*. The length of a line segment and the area of a face on a 2D image plane can be changed according to the distance in the depth direction, even if those lines and faces are parallel to an image plane. This is called a *perspective painting* and was a basic method of European painting after the Renaissance [Hockney01, Panofsky24].

Remark 7.5. In the wider sense, drawing perspective is the methodology for feelings of the 3D world on a 2D plane. For example, details of a far object are neglected without drawing, a distant view is drawn more bluish, a more distant scene is drawn in the upper part of an image and the scene in the foreground are in the lower area, a distant object is drawn vaguely and the foreground view is drawn clearly. All of those are part of a perspective drawing. More restrictive terms such as *linear perspective* may be used to represent the perspective projection in the narrow sense as defined above.

Remark 7.6. In practical display equipment, a point on a display screen is represented by its own coordinate system. The range of coordinate values is definite. Therefore, the image plane coordinate system used in Section 7.4.1 has to be transformed once more into this coordinate system for every type of display equipment. It is necessary to designate which part of an image plane (H_P in Fig. 7.6) in a virtual 3D space is displayed on a screen (window) on a certain type of display equipment. This is called *viewpoint transformation* in computer graphics (Fig. 7.7).

Remark 7.7. The whole of a 3D image that is to be visualized is not always mapped onto an image plane H_P in the mentioned imaginary 3D space. It is sufficient for the part that we want to observe to be rendered. An object that is to be rendered is simplified for easiness in observation and to reduce the computation time. Therefore, we frequently cut a 3D space by two planes parallel to an image plane, and render only the part of the 3D space situated between these two planes. In computer graphics this part of the 3D space that is rendered is called the *view volume*. The view volume is a prismoid in perspective projection and is in most cases a parallelepiped in the orthogonal projection (Fig. 7.7).

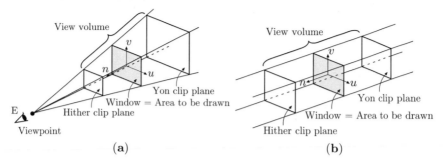

Fig. 7.7. Viewport transformation and view volume (clipping on 3D space): (**a**) Perspective projection; (**b**) parallel projection.

7.4.2 Displaying lines

A line (or a line segment) is determined automatically by fixing both of its end points. Thus there is no problem in the projection of a line segment except for in a few specific cases. For example, a part of a line segment in a 3D space may not be seen on a 2D image plane due to occlusion caused by other objects. This is an important problem that is widely known as a *hidden line problem* in computer graphics. We do not explain details of the hidden line problem here because they are discussed in many ordinary text books on graphics [Foley84, Watt98].

7.4.3 Displaying surfaces

A piece of a surface (= part of a plane in the finite area) is defined as an area surrounded by line segments (= edges) connecting vertexes. Therefore, the projection of a surface is obtained again by projecting vertexes (by the projection of points). However, additional considerations are required concerning at least two problems.

One problem is the question of which side of a borderline (usually a closed sequence of line segments or a polygon) is the surface that we are going to define. One possible assumption is that we regard the left-hand side of a border as the inside when we trace vertexes according to the order given beforehand, and that we consider the inside as the surface we want to define. The other is which surface is nearest to the viewpoint when more than one surface exist is the current 3D space.

The portion of a surface hidden by other surfaces must not be rendered on a 2D image plane. This is also called a *hidden surface problem* and has been studied extensively in computer graphics. Details can be found in computer graphics text books [Foley84, Watt98].

Displaying a surface is important also in the visualization of a 3D image of a voxel type, because the polygon model described in Section 7.2 is also employed frequently in practical applications.

Remark 7.8. The projection of a curved surface and a curve is discussed as follows:

(1) If they are defined by using mathematical expressions, those expressions are transformed mathematically into expressions for corresponding 2D curves and 2D figures.
(2) If curved surfaces or curves in a 3D space are represented by piecewise linear expressions, the methods explained here can be applied.

7.5 The concept of visualization based on ray casting – (2) manipulation of density values

The methods to determine where an arbitrary point (or voxel) in a 3D space should be mapped onto a 2D image plane was explained in the previous section. The next step to consider is what density value should be given to a point projected on a 2D image plane by methods presented in previous sections. The following methods have been developed for this problem:

(1) Suitable light and dark shades are added when rendering surfaces in a 3D space so that the shape of a surface may be perceived easily. This process is called *shading*.
(2) Appropriate values reflecting density values of corresponding points (or voxels) in 3D spaces are given to each point on a 2D image plane. By doing this, we aim to visualize information of the spacial distribution of density values in a 3D space on a 2D image plane.
(3) We can effectively use colors in the second method as described above. Colors are usually represented by three numerical values corresponding to the three color components, red (R), green (G), and blue (B). We call this the triplet *color code*. A few different definitions have been proposed for the physical meanings of the color code.

These three methods are important topics in computer graphics. Here we only explain the minimum needed for visualizing a 3D gray-tone image. Let us note that our objective here is to provide images that assist us to understand the contents of 3D images. We do not intend to generate images with a high reality level.

7.6 Rendering surfaces based on ray casting – surface rendering

The existence of a surface in a 3D space is not perceived until each point on a surface is given density values (or it is shaded suitably) in such a way that it is compatible with the shape and other properties of a surface.

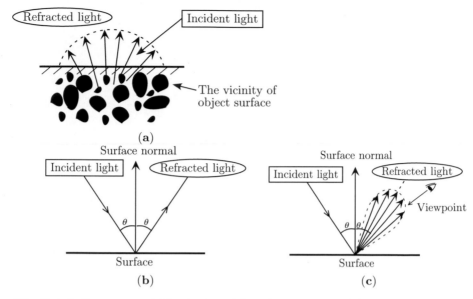

Fig. 7.8. Reflectance model for shading: (**a**) Diffuse reflection; (**b**) specular reflection (smooth surface); (**c**) specular reflection (uneven surface).

To do this we first assume a virtual light source in the above virtual 3D space and consider light and darkness of a surface by this virtual light source. Brightness at each point P on the surface determined by this light source is calculated using a suitable model of reflection by surface. This value of brightness depends on both the position of the point P on the surface and the position of the viewpoint set in 3D virtual space. The brightness value of the point P' on an image plane, which is a projection of a point P onto an image plane H_P, is determined by giving the above brightness value of P to P'. That is, the density value at a point P' on an image plane H_P (= a 2D image rendered on H_P) is equal to the brightness value of P in 3D space when it was observed from the direction connecting P and the viewpoint. Using physical analogy, the amount of the brightness at a point P' on an image plane H_P is considered to be the amount of energy radiated from a point P toward the viewpoint passing through a point P'.

7.6.1 Calculation of the brightness of a surface

Properties concerning the reflectance of a surface are suitably assumed. The following examples are adopted frequently (Fig. 7.8).

(a) Diffuse reflection

Incident light is reflected with equal intensity in all directions. This kind of reflection is called *diffuse reflection*.

(a-1) *Irradiation by parallel rays*: When a light source is located infinitely far away like the sun, all rays radiated from the source are regarded as parallel. In this case, the intensity of the reflected light is given by

$$I = kI_i \cos \alpha \qquad (7.7)$$

where

I_i = intensity of incident light,

I = intensity of reflected light,

α angle between the normal of a surface and the direction of the incident light at a point P (= incident angle),

k = reflectance (index of reflection) of a surface in diffuse reflection.

(a-2) *Irradiation from a point source*: If a light source Q is at a definite distance from an object and its physical size is small enough compared to an object, the source is regarded as a *point source*. Then, the intensity of the reflected light I is given by

$$I = kI_q \cos \alpha / r^2, \qquad (7.8)$$

where

I_q = amount of luminous intensity of a light source Q (= brightness of a light source),

I = intensity of the reflected light at a point P,

α = angle between the surface normal and the direction of a light source PQ,

k = reflectance (reflection index) of a surface in diffuse reflection,

r = distance between a point P and light source Q.

(b) Specular reflection

Specular reflection is intuitively known as a phenomenon that reflected light from a surface is concentrated in a particular direction. This is observed typically in the reflection by an ideal mirror. The well-known law of the incident and reflected light holds here. That is, the angle of incidence is equal to the angle of reflection (Fig. 7.8 (**b**)). Actually reflected light expands to some extent around the direction of the specular reflection. We will introduce here a typical model by Eq. 7.9 (Fig. 7.8 (**c**))

$$I = I_i k_\alpha \cos^n \delta, \qquad (7.9)$$

where

I = intensity of reflected light at a point P,

I_i = intensity of incident light at a point P,

δ = angle between the direction of reflection and the direction to a viewpoint,

α = angle of incidence,

k_α = specular reflection index at a point P (function of α),

n = parameter representing the extent of expansion of reflected light around the exact reflection direction.

In either (1) and (2), a density value (brightness) at a point P' on a 2D image plane H_P is determined by the intensity of reflected light given above. This process of giving light and dark appropriately to a surface is called *shading*. The shading in the context of this chapter is simply a tool for rendering an object surface in such a way that the 3D shape of an object is perceived easily. Parameters in equations given above are suitably selected in consideration of easiness in understanding the shape of an object.

In computer graphics, in particular in photorealistic rendering, we intend to generate an image that looks like real objects or real scenes or an image that gives as an impression as similar to the real phenomena as possible. Models and parameters are selected considering physical properties of real light and material. We shall leave details of such sophisticated rendering techniques to other books on graphics [Foley84, Watt98].

It should be noticed that the intensity of light reflected by a surface at a point P' on a 2D image strongly depends on the normal vector at a point P on a surface of a 3D object. This suggests that the brightness of a 2D image may be calculated using Eqs. 7.7 ~ 7.9 if the surface normal is given at each point, even if details of an object are not described exactly.

7.6.2 Smooth shading

The following problems may occur in applying methods explained above to surfaces of objects generated by a polygon model.

(i) Normal vectors are not defined uniquely on a vertex and on an edge.

(ii) Normal vectors change rapidly on both sides of an edge. As a result, an abrupt change in brightness levels arises in the vicinity of edges. Spurious edges or artifacts that look like fold lines may be seen even on a smooth plane surface. On a rendered image, a border or an edge between two adjacent faces of a polygon is enhanced too much. The Mach effect of the human vision system emphasizes this phenomenon furthermore, and as a result the image quality deteriorates significantly.

These problems are overcome by interpolating brightness values or only normal vectors appropriately and smoothing changes in them. This is called *smooth shading*. We will introduce examples below (Fig. 7.9).

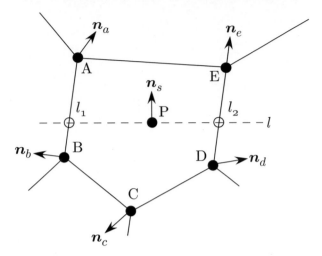

○ Surface normal n_a—→ calculating the whole of a surface (without smoothing)
○ Normal vectors at vertexes are calculated from the definition of a curved surface
  —→Normal vectors at points on an edge are determined by interpolating normal vectors of vertexes
  —→Surface normal at an arbitrary point on a plane is calculated by interpolating those of points on edges [Phong75]
○ Density values at vertexes are determined by the definition of surface, practical measurement, etc.
  —→Density values of points on an edge are determined from density values of vertexes by interpolation
  —→Density values an arbitrary points on a surface are determined by the interpolation of both end points of the scan line (l_1, l_2 in the figure) [Gouraud71]

Fig. 7.9. Smooth shading.

(a) Gouraud shading [Gouraud71, Watt98]

(1) Calculate a normal vector at each vertex from results of measurement or definitions of curved surfaces.
(2) Calculate the intensity (brightness) on a displayed image H_P of reflected light at each vertex.
(3) Calculate brightness values at points on an edge by the linear interpolation from those values at both end points (vertexes) of the edge.
(4) Determine a brightness value at a point P inside a face (polygon) by interpolating brightness values at crossings of edges and the horizontal line (scan line of a display image plane) passing the point P.

(b) Phong shading [Phong75, Watt98]

In step (2) and subsequent steps in the above procedure, determine normal vectors of each point by the linear interpolation and calculate brightness values of each point using those normal vectors.

7.6.3 Depth coding

A simpler method of shading so that a brighter value is given to a plane or point nearer to an image plane H_P (or nearer to the viewpoint) is available for rendering a plane surface. That is,

$$I = I_i/(k_1 + k_2 d), \qquad (7.10)$$

where

I = brightness value at a point P' on a display image plane H_P (= density value of a 2D projection image),

I_i = brightness value (density value of an image on H_P) given to the point P' of H_P corresponding to the point nearest to an image plane H_P in 3D space,

d = distance to an arbitrary point P in virtual 3D space from an image plane H_P,

k_1, k_2 = parameters.

This method is called *depth coding*. Although this procedure is not always a direct analogy of the optical phenomenon, it is frequently used because the computation is simple and is performed relatively easily, and still can give perspective to a resultant image.

7.6.4 Ray tracing

Drawing a scene in the 3D world viewed from a suitably selected viewpoint is regarded as putting a plane corresponding to a 2D image plane between a viewpoint V_E and an object and projecting 3D space and the object with which we have interest onto the image plane. The projection here is performed by generating a line toward a point P from the viewpoint V_E and extending the line to find a point Q, where the line intersects an object nearest to the viewpoint V_E. We call a line from the viewpoint to an object a *ray* and generation of a ray *ray casting* (Fig. 7.10).

After a ray meets the first object at Q_1, a ray is reflected to the direction determined by the law of reflection peculiar to the object. The reflected ray is extended in the direction of reflection. If the ray reaches a light source, we may find that a ray from the light source is reflected by an object at a point Q_1, and reaches to a point P on an image plane. Then we paint a color with the intensity (brightness) both determined by properties of the light source and the characteristics of colors and reflection of the object.

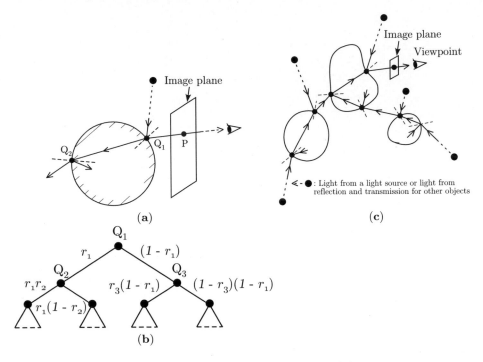

Fig. 7.10. Ray casting and ray tracing: (**a**) Single object; (**b**) tree structure representing the ray tracing procedure. Q_1, Q_2, Q_3 are crossing points among a ray and an object, and r_1, r_2, and r_3 mean the index of reflection at each crossing point; (**c**) multiple objects.

If a ray reflected at Q_1 meets the surface of another object at Q_2 before it reaches a light source, we can find that a point Q_1 is in the shadow of an object including a point Q_2. Then we give a point P a density value representing the shadow (black, for example) instead of a color of a light source. We alternatively may extend a ray further using a model of reflection by the surface of an object at Q_2 instead of giving a color of shadow to P immediately.

Then a ray may reach another light source. As a result, a density value at a point P is determined by the light reflected at Q_2 after the reflection at Q_1. In this way we can render an image of an object reflected on the surface of another object (*reflected image*). If a ray is extended infinitely without meeting any light source, we give a color of the background (ambient light) to a point P.

If an object is transparent or translucent, part of a ray proceeds reflectively into the inside of an object and the other part is reflected on the outside of an object. Directions and intensities of refracted and reflected light are determined by properties concerning refraction and reflection of materials existing in the both sides of a surface. The same procedure is repeated if more

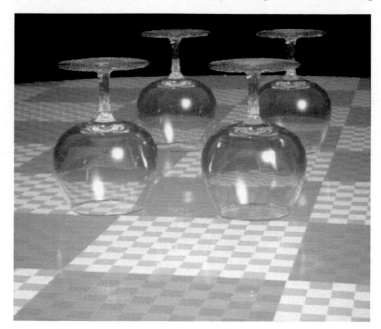

Fig. 7.11. Wine glasses generated by ray tracing. Part of checkerboard pattern seen through a glass in distorted by refraction. A brighter part on the top of a glass is generated by direct reflection of a virtual light source. Images of parts of other glasses are observed on a surface ("reflection image") and on the floor of the glass. This shows a typical example of photorealistic rendering in early 1980s [Horiuchi87, Kurashige86].

than one object exists in 3D space. By using this method, we can render an image of objects reflected on the surface of other objects and objects behind other transparent object.

As explained above, this procedure is implemented by tracing light paths inversely from the viewpoint toward an object and a light source. Note that real light radiates from a light source toward objects and repeats reflection and/or refraction before reaching our eyes. The above procedure is called *ray tracing* [Whitted80, Watt98]. This is a type of simulation of an optical phenomenon in the neighborhood of a surface of an object and a border between adjacent objects. Really photorealistic rendering has become possible by this method. It contributed much to raise the evaluation of computer graphics. A large number of papers have been published on improvement of the ray tracing and its applications. An example of its application is shown in Fig. 7.11. However, the ray tracing explained above is not always suitable as a main topic for this chapter.

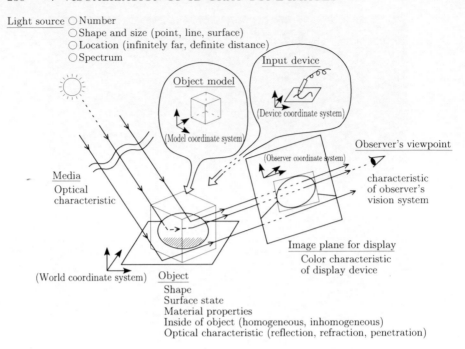

Fig. 7.12. General frame of computer graphics.

7.7 Photorealistic rendering and rendering for visualization

Mathematical models presented in Sections 7.4 ~ 7.6 were developed to generate images that arouse feelings similar to the ones we have when we see the scene in the real world. In this sense, they are tools of what we call *photorealistic rendering*, or tools for designing industrial products utilized in the real world. The whole of a basic idea common to them is presented in Fig. 7.12.

Light is irradiated by a light source and shines on objects. Then part of a light reflected by objects or passed through objects reaches *the position of eye* located at a *viewpoint*. An image plane that corresponds to a screen of a display device exists somewhere on the way of this light path. The above model for rendering is a modeling that realizes all such phenomena concerning the image generation process within acceptable image quality and computation cost.

Major factors in image generation by this model are a light source, a space through which light propagates, interaction among light and objects, positional relation among an image plane, a viewpoint and an object, and optical properties of objects. All of them and many other factors relating to image generation have been studied extensively in the field of computer graphics. Ray tracing and radiosity methods following this remarkably contributed to the progress of this field [Nishita85, Cohen85, Cohen88]. For details, see books on technical computer graphics [Watt98].

However, a different kind of rendering has attracted much attention in these years, and this rendering is called *nonphotorealistic rendering*. This technique aims at generating a freer style of images such as pictures that look like classical European style paintings, those similar to India-ink paintings, and those similar to other fine arts produced by human artists.

We stress that visualization is different from any of those. The most important feature of this is using rendering as a tool to understand the characteristics of given data (a 3D gray-tone image). We must consider that a 3D image that is to be visualized is put at the position of an object in Fig. 7.12, and a viewpoint and an image plane are the same as in that figure. All other factors such as a light source and the interaction of objects and light itself are simply tools for *perceiving* the data structure with the human vision. There do not always have to be meanings related to real optical and other physical phenomena. The process of volume rendering described in the next section is regarded as a method developed for visualization of a 3D gray-tone image with a rough analogy of optical phenomena.

7.8 Displaying density values based on ray casting – volume rendering

7.8.1 The algorithm of volume rendering

Consider a 3D image in which each point has a density value (3D gray-tone image). Using the same scheme of ray casting as in the previous section, a point P in 3D space (virtual space) is projected to a point P' on an image plane H_P (Fig. 7.13). Then all points on a line segment connecting a viewpoint V_e and a point P' (we call this line a *ray*, too) are projected to the same point P'. This means that all points on this ray in 3D space are seen, overlapping each other at the position P'. The problem to be solved here is how to visualize information of density values at these points. One basic idea employed here is to accumulate in some ways information stored at points on the ray. A color or brightness value of a point P' on an image plane is determined by a result of this accumulation. This method is called *volume rendering* [Levoy88, Drebin88]. Below we present a procedure to perform this processing (Fig. 7.13).

First let us assume that a brightness value b_i is stored at a point P_i in a 3D image, and that an intermediate result of accumulation $I_{in}(i)$ has been sent to P_i. Then a brightness value $I_{out}(i)$ given below is output to be sent to the next point.

$$I_{out}(i) = I_{in}(i) \cdot (1 - \alpha_i) + b_i \cdot \alpha_i \qquad (7.11)$$

Here a letter i represents the sequential number given to a sample point (voxel) selected along a current ray, which is smaller at a point further from a view-

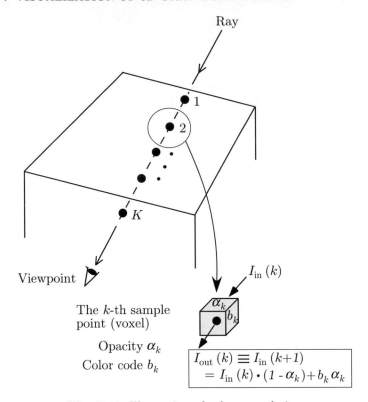

Fig. 7.13. Illustration of volume rendering.

point. The α_0 is assumed to be *1*, and b_0 is a suitably selected constant that corresponds to a parameter called *ambient light* in computer graphics. A parameter α_i is called *opacity* and b_i is often called *color value* in volume rendering. From physical analogy, a larger value of brightness looks clearer (looks darker). See Remark 7.9, too.

Equation 7.11 is applied recursively along a ray by regarding an output value of the k-th sample point $I_{\text{out}}(k)$ as an input brightness value to the $(k + 1)$-th sample point $I_{\text{in}}(k + 1)$. As a result, the following equation is obtained which gives an output brightness value $I_{\text{out}}(K)$ of the K-th sample point from the background.

$$I_{\text{out}}(K) = \sum_{k=0}^{K}\{b_k \cdot \alpha_k \cdot \prod_{p=k+1}^{K}(1 - \alpha_p)\}. \qquad (7.12)$$

In actual rendering, parameters α_k and b_k are also given appropriately. This method has a large degree of freedom for a user because such large numbers of free parameters are contained. This also means that the usage is complicated and much experience is required to use it effectively. We will present examples produced by volume rendering in Fig. 7.14.

7.8.2 Selection of parameters

Let us present several examples of ideas concerning parameters in Eq. 7.12 [Drebin88]. Parameters are roughly divided into two groups $\{b_k\}$ and $\{\alpha_k\}$.

(a) Selection of $\{b_k\}$

Values of parameters $\{b_k\}$ determine the basic color tone in rendering and are called *color codes* or *color values*. They are usually fixed by giving relative ratios of three components R, G, and B in color codes. We may select different arbitrary values so that they correspond to different objects or different physical phenomena. Examples are shown below.

(i) Color values are changed corresponding to the range of density values in an original image or a histogram of density values of an original image. In a medical CT image, for example, the range of CT values varies corresponding to each organ. Thus we will be able to distinguish organs by color in a rendered image. If some abnormal shadows are distinguishable by CT values, their existence may be noticed easily by changing colors of voxels having CT values to which attention should be paid in diagnosing a rendered image.

(ii) Colors may be changed by a position in 3D space. This makes it easy to observe the state of the density value distribution in a region of interest and its vicinity.

Both methods are used to mark a place to be noticed. The name *color code* comes from this type of usage. In other words, this is regarded as performing a kind of clustering of voxels beforehand and then utilizing resultant clusters of voxels for the following processing.

(b) Selection of $\{\alpha_k\}$

Usually we set this group of parameters so that the special distribution of density values in a 3D image may be observed clearly as well as possible. Basically a value of α_k is selected to be nearer to 1 at a point satisfying a condition that we want to see on a rendered 2D image. In other cases we select values of $\{\alpha_k\}$ empirically with observing resulting 2D images. As an example, if any one of $\alpha_{k+1}, \alpha_{k+2}, \cdots, \alpha_k, \alpha_u \simeq 1$, for example, then $1 - \alpha_u \simeq 0$. Therefore, $\beta_k \simeq (1 - \alpha_k)(1 - \alpha_{k-1}) \cdots (1 - \alpha_{k+1})(1 - \alpha_k) \simeq 0$. This means that the value of b_k does not contribute to $I_{\text{out}}(K)$ significantly. That is, the value of b_k does not reach a displayed image plane. This corresponds to the case that opaque material exists at a point P_u on the way from a point P_k to a display image plane.

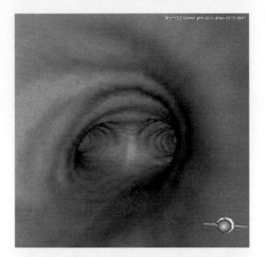

-600 ~ -400	[H.U.]	1.0 ~ 1.0
-400 ~ -100	[H.U.]	1.0 ~ 1.0
-100 ~ 100	[H.U.]	1.0 ~ 1.0
100 ~	[H.U.]	1.0 ~ 1.0

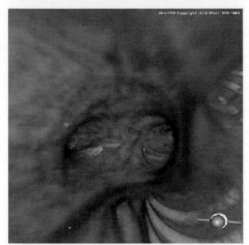

-600 ~ -400	[H.U.]	0.0 ~ 0.1
-400 ~ -100	[H.U.]	0.1 ~ 0.1
-100 ~ 100	[H.U.]	0.1 ~ 0.3
100 ~	[H.U.]	1.0 ~ 1.0

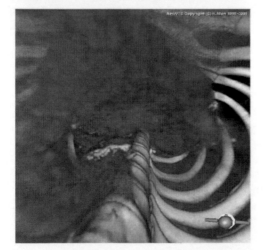

-600 ~ -400	[H.U.]	0.0 ~ 0.0
-400 ~ -100	[H.U.]	0.0 ~ 0.01
-100 ~ 100	[H.U.]	0.01 ~ 0.05
100 ~	[H.U.]	1.0 ~ 1.0

Fig. 7.14. Examples of volume rendering generated from a 3D X-ray CT image of a human body. H.U.: Hounsfield Unit. Numbers show values of opacity.

Alternatively, if $\alpha_u \simeq 0$, for all u such that $u = K, K-1, \cdots, k, 1-\alpha_u \simeq 1$. Therefore, $\beta_k \simeq 1$. This means that the amount α_k in b_k contributes to a density value of a displayed image with little loss. This corresponds to the case that material between a point P_u and P_k is almost transparent.

(c) Visualization of equidensity surface of a density value f^*

Assign suitably an opacity value α^* to a density value f^*, and then give a value near to α^* to a point having a density value similar to f^*. Using the gradient, for instance,

$$
\alpha_i = \begin{cases} 1, \text{ if } |\nabla f_i| = 0, \text{ and } f_i = f^* \\ 1 - (1/r) \cdot (f_i - f^*)/|\nabla f_i|, \\ \quad \text{ if } |\nabla f_i| > 0, \text{ and } f_i - r|\nabla f_i| \le f^* \le f_i + r|\nabla f_i| \\ 0, \text{ if otherwise} \end{cases} \tag{7.13}
$$

where f_i is a density value at a voxel P_i, ∇f_i is the gradient at a point P_i, and r is an appropriately given constant [Drebin88].

(d) The visualization of a border surface in a 3D image

If it is known beforehand that typical density values are $f_n^*, n = 1, 2, \cdots, N$, where $f_1^* < f_2^* < \cdots < f_N^*$ then opacities α_k^* that are proportional to density values f_k^* are employed. If a density value f_i of a voxel P_i takes an intermediate value among them, a value of α_i corresponding to it is given as follows.

$$
\alpha_i = \begin{cases} 1, \text{ if } |\nabla f_i| \times \alpha_{n+1}[(f_i - f_n^*)/(f_{n+1}^* - f_n^*)] \\ \quad + \alpha_n[(f_{n+1}^* - f_i)/(f_{n+1}^* - f_n^*)], \\ \quad \text{ if } f_n^* \le f_i \le f_{n+1}^* \\ 0, \text{ if otherwise} \\ \qquad\qquad (i = 1, 2, \ldots, N - 1) \end{cases} \tag{7.14}
$$

As is known from these examples, the volume rendering also intends to visualize a surface that may exist in a 3D gray-tone image. A surface to be visualized (or displayed) is determined by only the spatial distribution of density values in 3D space. In examples presented above, the existence of a surface is detected mainly by the gradient. Larger values of the opacity are assigned to the part of small gradient values in the case of visualizing equidensity surfaces and to the part having larger gradient values in the case of visualizing a border surface, so that those surfaces may become more noticeable.

7.8.3 Front-to-back algorithm

Let us introduce another procedure to perform the volume rendering that is called *front-to-back algorithm* [ERTL00].

A brightness value $I_{\text{out}}(i)$ to be output at a point P_i along a ray is given by the following equation.

$$I_{\text{out}}(i) = I_{\text{out}}(i-1) + \beta_i \cdot b_i,$$

$$\beta_i = \alpha_i \cdot \prod_{k=1}^{i-1}(1 - \alpha_k), \tag{7.15}$$

where

α_i = opacity value at a point P_i,
b_i = brightness value at a point P_i.

The number i is given in the increasing order starting at a sample point nearest to a viewpoint on a ray. The β_i in Eq. 7.15 is called *accumulated opacity*. The calculation is iterated on each ray until a point is reached that is regarded as having no significant effect on density values of a rendered image. A resulting value of $I_{\text{out}}(i)$ (accumulated brightness value) is given to a corresponding pixel on a 2D image on an image plane.

This procedure is intuitively interpreted as follows. Let us assume first that the i-th point P_i has the brightness value b_i and opacity α_i. Then we consider that there is a light source of the power $\alpha_i \cdot b_i$. The light reaches a viewpoint (or an image plane) after passing through points $P_{i-1}, P_{i-2}, \ldots, P_i$. The fraction $(1 - \alpha_i) \cdot \alpha_i \cdot b_i$ incident to P_{i-1} passes through point P_{i-1} and comes to the next point. Total sum of contribution from all of K sample points on a ray to a viewpoint is given to a corresponding pixel on an image plane as its density value (color value). In fact, $I_{\text{out}}(i)$ of Eq. 7.15 is expressed as follows considering all contributions from the K-th sample point to the first sample point.

$$I_{\text{out}}(K) = I_{\text{out}}(0) + b_1\alpha_1 + \sum_{k=2}^{K}\left\{b_k\alpha_k \prod_{n=1}^{k-1}(1 - \alpha_n)\right\}. \tag{7.16}$$

Each term in the summation $\sum$ in the right-hand side of this equation corresponds to the term interpreted as was explained above.

7.8.4 Properties of volume rendering and surface rendering

Let us summarize properties of volume rendering compared with surface rendering.

(a) Volume rendering

(1) Volume rendering can be applied without extracting surfaces to be visualized beforehand. In this sense, volume rendering is a tool to visualize or to observe the structure of a 3D gray-tone image that has not been structurized yet. It does not require any preprocessing such as segmentation and

border extraction. A surface to be visualized is determined substantially (and implicitly) by setting parameters $\{\alpha_i\}$ (opacity).

(2) The essential part of volume rendering is in calculating the mixture of the information that has been accumulated and propagated to a current point along a ray and the information given by a density value of a current point. The ratio of two types of information is determined in fusing them and controlled by a value of the opacity α_i in each point. A resulting mixture is sent to the next point along a ray. If $\alpha_i = 1$, for example, only a density value at a sample point P_i propagates, and brightness values accumulated along a ray in the past disappear there and do not contribute to a density (brightness) value on a rendered image at all. This corresponds to a completely opaque medium. Alternatively, if $\alpha_i = 0$, the effect of a density value of a point P_i disappears there. This means that the medium is completely transparent.

(3) By utilizing the above property, we can extract component patterns by thresholding density values or similar processing. This is considered as inserting the segmentation procedure into the procedure of rendering. This also means that we cannot always avoid the problem of parameter selection completely since selection of $\{\alpha_i\}$ relates to selection of threshold values substantially.

(4) Even if a surface seems to be extracted correctly, it is not always guaranteed that a surface or a border is extracted exactly from the viewpoint of the shape. This is because the rendering is based on the opacity parameter $\{\alpha_i\}$ and is performed only by a density value of each point, and any information concerning shapes is not considered.

(5) Results are sensitive to random noise. Inappropriate settings of $\{\alpha_i\}$ may cause apparently unexpected artifacts.

(6) We need not take care of the failures in border surface extractions. From the beginning border extraction algorithms are not required.

(7) Even if a border surface is perceived visually in a rendered image, the location of the surface cannot be determined exactly. This is because the border extraction is not actually performed in volume rendering. The surface is visible in a rendered image only by human vision. We cannot designate an object using a border surface that can be seen in a rendered image. Neither can we obtain quantitative measurements from a border surface that is seen in an image drawn by volume rendering.

(8) The computation time is likely to be longer in the volume rendering than in surface rendering, because the volume rendering procedure contains an accumulation of density values along a ray. This problem is being overcome in newer computers with a graphic engine.

(9) Although objects existing on the same ray overlap, it should be avoided that an object in the back of another object is completely invisible (occurrence of occlusion). Exact results of rendering depend on setting of parameters $\{\alpha_i\}$.

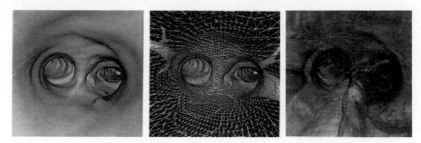

Fig. 7.15. Surface rendering and volume rendering applied to the same object. Left: Surface rendering with smooth shading. Center: Polygon model used in generation of the left image. Right: Volume rendering.

(b) Surface rendering

Surface rendering, on the other hand, has the following properties that are in strong contrast to those mentioned above.

(1) We can designate each object or obtain quantitative measurements of features interactively on a rendered 2D image, since a border surface is determined strictly beforehand.
(2) Computation time tends to be shorter because the accumulation of density values along a ray is not necessary.
(3) The detection and extraction of border surfaces satisfying geometrical constraints is possible, if a border extraction algorithm works well. The description of a 3D image structure is also possible by using those results. Results may be affected strongly by the failure of those algorithms. Border detection or segmentation is required before rendering.
(4) Algorithms to extract border surfaces of each object have to be prepared before rendering.
(5) After rendering a surface of one object, other objects behind them become invisible unless some particular methods are employed.

Examples of applications of both methods on the same object are presented in Fig. 7.15.

Remark 7.9. Before application of the volume rendering, the density values of a 3D image to be visualized are replaced by parameter values $\{\alpha_0\}$ and $\{b_i\}$ given in Eqs. 7.11 $\sim$ 7.16. Such parameter values are stored beforehand in a 3D array or the replacement of density values by $\{\alpha_i\}$ is performed in the procedure of rendering. In the first case an extra 3D array is needed. It is desirable that these values are calculated at sample points selected with equal intervals on a line representing a ray. They are calculated by suitably interpolating voxel values of the 3D image to be visualized. It is worth noticing that this digitization along a ray might cause errors in feature measurements on a displayed image or on unexpected artifacts. Additionally, the following should be taken into consideration. It is not an original image itself but the spatial distribution of the opacity that is visualized. Therefore, improper settings of opacity parameters $\{\alpha_i\}$ also may cause artifacts.

Remark 7.10. A 3D image (which is a set of density values filling 3D space) is compared to a 3D space filled with dirty water or is seen as a foggy world in which the density varies from place to place. Volume rendering is compared to looking though such a space. A borderline or a border surface that we can perceive on a 2D image rendered on an image plane can be seen as a result of looking through such a world in a certain direction. It cannot be recognized in its vicinity like a border of clouds in the sky. An object that is seen vaguely at a distant place could be a solid wall of a building. The suitable setting of opacities makes it possible to visualize an example such as the latter one.

Remark 7.11. If we project the simple sum of density values along a ray to a point P without designating a particular value for $\{\alpha_i\}$, the result is approximately equivalent to the projection mentioned in Section 7.3.3. If a viewpoint is infinitely far, the projection method reduces to the orthogonal projection in Section 7.4 and the result coincides with the projection mentioned in Section 7.3. The density values on a projected image may be a little different from each other due to different approximations employed in the projection performed in the digitized space. This type of projection is regarded as a type of simulation in an imaging process. For example, in the visualization of a 3D image obtained by X-ray CT, the above projection for visualization is regarded as the simulation of taking an X-ray image of the human body, in which an X-ray source is at the position of a viewpoint and an X-ray film is put on a projection plane. This is an ideal imaging situation in which an X-ray source is a point source and no scattering occurs by an object. An X-ray source can be put at an arbitrary place in the human body in this simulation. From this viewpoint, it might be possible to generate interesting images.

Remark 7.12. The volume rendering explained above is a tool of visualization and does not always relate exactly to real physical phenomena. Some other methods of rendering have been developed that intend to simulate optical phenomena occurring along a ray propagating through continuous media such as air and water. Effects of optical phenomena such as reflection, refraction, scattering, and absorption are accumulated along a path of light and utilized to render a scene irradiated by various light sources. Those methods are sometimes named *volume rendering*, too. Examples of applications include rendering of cloud, fog, flare, smoke, and gemstones including impurity. This kind of method originated from [Kajiya82, Kajiya84] and has been studied actively in the field of computer graphics [Yokoi86, Nishita85, Horiuchi87, Kurashige86, SIGGRPH88], etc. The expression such as "rendering volume densities" was used in their papers. The term of volume rendering seems to be first used in [Levoy88] among journal papers and appeared in several conference proceedings about the same time.

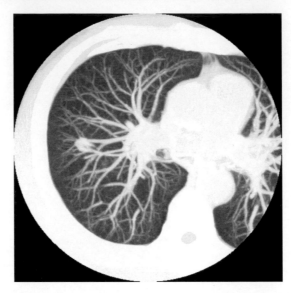

Fig. 7.16. Example of rendering by the MIP method (chest X-ray CT image of the human body).

Remark 7.13. The maximum value of densities on a ray may be projected instead of accumulation along a ray. This is called the *maximum intensity projection* (*MIP*) and is used frequently in the visualization of CT images (Fig. 7.16).

7.8.5 Gradient shading

The methods of rendering explained in Sections 7.5 and 7.6, and in particular the surface rendering method, are necessary for the normal vector of a surface to be rendered. However, voxel data obtained by binarizing a gray-tone CT image, e.g., a binary image in which a value *1* corresponds to the skull, do not have enough information to uniquely determine the normal vector of the object surface. One method to obtain the normal vector in such a case is to fit a plane to each voxel and its neighborhood and to use the normal plane. An alternative method is to utilize the gradient vector of the density value distribution in the neighborhood of a surface and to regard the gradient as the surface normal [Hoehne86].

Let us discuss this briefly. Consider the coordinate system as in Fig. 7.17. We consider an image plane L and a pixel $P' = (i', j')$ on L. The directions i and j are assumed to be coincident to the row and the column directions (i and j) of the 3D space including a point P' and a 3D image (or a 3D object) to be visualized. The surface including a point (i, j, k) to be rendered is assumed at the distance k from a point P' on the image plane in the direction

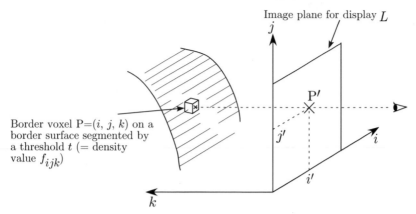

In rendering a border surface for a threshold t, a density value $g_{i'j'}$ of a pixel
$P' = (i', j')$ of a rendered 2D image is given by

$$g_{i'j'} = A \cos[\ (f_{i,j+1,k} - f_{i,j-1,k})\ /\ B\ ]\ ,$$

$$A, B : \text{suitable constant}$$

Here we assume that a voxel $P=(i, j, k)$ of a 3D image is projected to pixel P'

Fig. 7.17. Illustration of gradient shading [Hoehne86].

perpendicular to the image plane L. Then a density $g_{i'j'k'}$ of a point $P' =
(i', j')$ on the image plane L is given as follows.

$$g_{i'j'k'} = A \cos\{(f_{i,j+1,k} - f_{ijk})/B\}, \qquad (7.17)$$

where

$f_{i'j'k'}$ = a density value of a 3D gray-tone image before binalization,
A, B = suitable constants.

This method is called *gradient shading* [Hoehne86]. This enables us to
render a 3D gray-tone image by treating it as if light reflected by some surface
has a virtually normal vector. This method is frequently used in combination
with the volume rendering for visualization of medical CT images.

Remark 7.14. In the virtualization methods discussed here, a viewpoint and
view direction are selected arbitrarily. Therefore, we can select a physically
unrealizable viewpoint inside the human body. Furthermore, by generating a
sequence of images while viewing an object from continuously moving viewpoints, we can present a moving image looking as if it is flying through the
inside of a 3D solid object. This technique has recently gained popularity
when observing 3D CT images in medicine. This is called *virtual endoscopy*,
because it is regarded as a simulation of an endoscope. Sometimes it is called
by the name of a target organ to which it is applied, like virtual colonoscopy
and virtual bronchoscopy [Rogalla01].

Remark 7.15. Virtual endoscopy was first reported in 1993 [Vining93]. The method employed volume rendering and the editing of video images. It took 8 hours to generate the first fly-through image [Vining03]. Authors reported interactively generated moving images (2.2 frames/sec on the average by Silicon Graphics IRIS) of virtual bronchoscopy in 1994, using surface rendering of bronchus branches automatically extracted from chest CT images [Mori94b]. These days images obtained by surface rendering are generated much faster than volume rendering by using graphic engines in workstations. Nowadays, virtual endoscopy has become one of the important tools in medical diagnosis and the quality of presented images has greatly improved. Most of them seem to employ volume rendering, and a viewpoint and a view direction are freely controlled interactively (9.1 frames/sec on the average by conventional PCs (CPU: Intel; Xeon 3.2GHz × 2)) [Hong97, Hayashi03, Mori03, Dachman03, Rogalla01, Bankman00].

References

[Amarunnishad90] T.M.Amarunnishad and P.P.Das : Estimation of length for digitized straight lines in three dimensions, Pattern Recognition Letters, vol.11, pp.207–213 (1990)

[Arce87] G.R.Arce and M.P.McLoughlin : Theoretical analysis of the max/median filter, IEEE Trans. on ASSP, vol.35, no.1, pp.60–69 (1987)

[Arcelli92] C.Arcelli and G.S. di BajaA : Ridge points in Euclidean distance maps, Pattern Recognition Letters, vol.13, pp.237–243 (1992)

[Artzy85] E.Artzy, G.Frieder, and G.T.Herman : The theory, design, implementation, and evaluation of a three-dimensional boundary detection algorithm, Computer Graphics and Image Processing, vol.29, pp.196–215 (1985)

[Bertrand94a] G.Bertrand : Simple points, topological numbers and geodesic neighborhoods in cubic grids, Pattern Recognition Letters, vol.15, pp.1003–1011 (1994)

[Bertrand94b] G.Bertrand and G.Malandain : A new characterization of three-dimensional simple points, Pattern Recognition Letters, vol.15, pp.169–175 (1994)

[Bertrand95] G.Bertrand : A parallel thinning algoritm for medial surfaces, Pattern Recognition Letters, vol.16, pp.979–986 (1995)

[Bertrand96] G.Bertrand : A Boolean characterization of three-dimensional simple points, Pattern Recognition Letters, vol.17, pp.115–124 (1996)

[Bitter01] I.Bitter, A.E.Kaufman, and M.Sato : Penalized-distance volumetric skeleton algorithm, IEEE Trans. on Visualization and Computer Graphics, vol.7, no.3, pp.195–206 (2001)

[Blezek99] D.J.Blezek and R.A.Robb : Centerline algorithm for virtual endoscopy based on chamfer distance transform and Dijkstra's single source shortest path algorithm, Proc. of SPIE, vol.3660, pp.225–233 (1999)

[Blinn77] J.F.Blinn : Models of light reflection for computer synthesized pictures, Computer Graphics, vol.11, no.2, pp.192–198 (1977)

[Borgefors84] G.Borgefors : Distance transformations in arbitrary dimensions, Computer Vision, Graphics, and Image Processing, vol.27, pp.321–345 (1984)

[Borgefors86a] G.Borgefors : Distance transformations in digital images, Computer Vision, Graphics, and Image Processing, vol.34, pp.344–371 (1986)

[Borgefors86b] G.Borgefors : A new distance transformation aproximating the Eucledean distance, Proc. 8th ICPR, pp.336–339 (1986)

[Borgefors97] G.Borgefors and I.I.Nystrom : Efficient shape representation by mini-
    mizing the set of centres of maximal discs/spheres, Pattern Recognition Letters,
    vol.18, pp.465–472 (1997)

[Borgefors99] G.Borgefors, I.I.Nystrom, and G. Sanniti Di Baja : Computing skele-
    tons in three dimensions, Pattern Recognition, vol.32, pp.1225–1236 (1999)

[Bovik83] A.C.Bovik, T.S.Huang, and D.C.Munson Jr. : A generalization of median
    filtering using linear combinations of order statistics, IEEE Trans. on ASSP,
    vol.31, no.6, pp.1342–1350 (1983)

[Brechbuhler95] Ch.Brechbuhler, G.Gerig, and O.Kubler : Parametrization of closed
    surfaces for 3-D shape description, Computer Vision and Image Understanding,
    vol.61, no.2, pp.154–170 (1995)

[Bribiesca92] E.Bribiesca : A geometric structure for two-dimensional shapes and
    three-dimensional surfaces, Pattern Recognition, vol.25, no.5, pp.483–496
    (1992)

[Brejl00] M.Brejl and M.Sonka : Directional 3D edge detection in anisotropic data:
    detector design and performance assenssment, Computer Vision and Image
    Understanding, vol.77, pp.84–110 (2000)

[Bsel86] P.J.Besl and R.C.Jain : Invariant surface characteristics for 3D object
    recognition in range images, Computer Vision, Graphics and Image Processing,
    vol.33, pp.33–80 (1986)

[Bykov99] A.I.Bykov, L.G.Zerkalov, and M.A.Rodriguez Pineda : Index of a point of
    3-D digital binary image and algorithm for computing its Euler charactersistic,
    Pattern Recognition, vol.32, pp.845–850 (1999)

[Carlsson85] K.Carlsson, P.E.Danielsson, R.Lenz, A.ALiljeborg, L.Majl, and
    N.Aslund : Three-dimensional microscopy using a confocal laser scanning mi-
    croscope, J. Optical Soc. of America, vol.10, pp.53–55 (1985.1)

[Chattopadhyay92] S.Chattopadhyay and P.P.Das, Estimation of the original length
    of a straight line segment from its digitization in three dimensions, Pattern
    Recognition, vol.25, pp.787–798 (1992)

[Coquin95] D.Coquin and Ph.Bolon : Discrete distance operator on rectangular
    grids, Pattern Recognition Letters, vol.16, pp.911–923 (1995)

[Cohen85] M.F.Cohen and D.P.Greenberg : The hemi-cube: a radiosity solution for
    complex environment, Computer Graphics, vol.19, no.3, pp.31–40 (1985)

[Cohen88] M.F.Cohen, S.E.Chen, J.R.Wallace, and D.P.Greenberg : A progres-
    sive refinement approach to fast radiosity image generation, Proc. of SIG-
    GRAPH'88, pp.75–84 (1988)

[Danielsson80] P.E.Danielsson : Euclidean distance mapping, Computer Graphics
    and Image Processing, vol.14, pp.227–248 (1980)

[Danielsson90] P-E.Danielsson and O.Seger : Generalaized and separable Sobel op-
    erators, Machine Vision for Three Dimensional Scenes, Academic Press, pp.347–
    379 (1990)

[Dohi00] T.Dohi : Sugical robotics and three dimensional display for computer aided
    surgery, Proc. of CARS 2000, pp.715–719 (2000)

[Drebin88] R.A.Drebin, L.Caepenter, and P.Hanrahan : Volume rendering, Com-
    puter Graphics, vol.22, no.3, pp.65–74 (1988)

[Dror91] Dror Bar-Natan : Random-dot stereograms, The Mathematica Journal,
    vol.1, issue3, pp.69–75 (1991)

[Edelsbrunner94] H.Edelsbrunner : A three-dimenisonal alpha shapes, ACM Trans.
    on Graphics, vol.13, no.1, pp.43–72 (1994)

[Englmeier00] K.-H. Englmeier, M.Siebert, G.-F. Rust, U.J.Shoepf, and M.Reiser : Immersive visualization and intuitive interaction of virtual endoscopy, Proc. of CARS 2000, pp.79–84 (2000)

[Enomoto75] H.Enomoto and T.Katayama : Structual lines of images, Proc. of 2nd USA-Japan Computer Conf., pp.470–474 (1975)

[Enomoto76] H.Enomoto and T.Katayama: Structual lines of images, Proc. of 3rd IJCPR, pp.811–815 (1976)

[ERTL00] T.Ertl : 6.Volume visualization, in B.Girod, G.Greines, and H.Niemann eds : Principles of 3D Image Analysis and Synthesis, pp.243–278, Kluwer Academic Publishers, Boston, U.S.A. (2000)

[Fritsch94] D.S.Fritsch, S.M.Pizer, B.S.Morse, D.H.Eberly, and A.Liu : The multi-scale medial axis and its applications in image registration, Pattern Recognition Letters, vol.15, pp.445–452 (1994)

[Gagvan99] N.Gagvani and D.Silver : Parameter-controlled volume thinning, Graphical Models and Image Processing , vol.61, pp.149–164 (1999)

[Geissler99] P.Geissler and T.Dierig : Depth-from-focus, in B.Jahne, H.Haussecker, and P.Geissler eds. : Handbook of Computer Vision and Application, vol.2, pp.591–626, Academic Press, New York (1999)

[Gelder94] A.V.Gelder, and J.Wilhelms : Topological considerations in isosurface generation, ACM Transactions on Graphics, vol.13, no.4, pp.337–375 (1994)

[Gouraud71] H.Gouraud: Continuous shading of curved surfaces. IEEE Trans. on Computers, vol.C-20, no.6, pp.623–628 (1971)

[Greenberg 98] D.Greenberg, K.Torrance, and P.Shirly : A framework for realistic image synthesis, Proc. of SIGGRAPH'97, pp.477–494 (1997)

[Gong90] W. Gong, and G. Bertrand : A simple parallel 3D thinning algorithm, Proc.10th ICPR, vol.1, pp.188–190 (1990)

[Gray71] S.B.Gray : Local properties of binary images in two dimensions, IEEE Trans. on C, vol.C-20, no.5, pp.551–561 (1971)

[Haralick83] R.M.Haralick : Ridges and valleys on digital images, Computer Vision, Graphics and Image Processing, vol.22, pp.28–38 (1983)

[Haralick81] R,M.Haralick and L.Watson : A facet model for image data, Computer Graphics and Image Processing, vol.15, pp.113–129 (1981)

[Haralick87] R.M.Haralick, S.R.Sternberg, and X.Shuang : Image analysis using mathematical morphology, IEEE Trans. on PAMI, vol.9, no.4, pp.532–550 (1987)

[Hafford84] K.J.Hafford and K.Preston, Jr. : Three-dimensional skeletonization of elongated solids, Computer Vision, Graphics and Image Processing, vol.27, pp.78–91 (1984)

[Hardin00] R.W.Hardin : Researhers use computed tomography for auto-parts, Image Processing Europe, July / August issue, pp.15–22 (2000)

[Harker00] S.Harker, S.Angenent, A.Tannenbaum, and R.Kikinis : Nondistorting flattening maps and the 3D visualization of colon CT images, IEEE Trans. Medical Imaging, vol.19, pp.665–670 (2000)

[Hayashi00] Y.Hayashi, K.Mori, T.Saito, J.Hasegawa, and J.Toriwaki : Advanced navigation diagnosis with automated fly-through path generation and presentation of unobserved regions in the virtualized endoscope system, Proc. of MIRU2000, pp.331–336 (2000) (in Japanese)

[Hayashi03] Y.Hayashi, K.Mori, Y.Suenaga, J.Hasegawa, and J.Toriwaki : A method for detecting undisplayed regions in virtual colonoscopy and its application to quantitative evaluation of fly-through methods, Academic Radiology, vol.10, no.12, pp.1380–1391 (2003)

[Herman78] G.T.Herman and H.K.Liu : Dynamic boundary surface detection, Computer Graphics and Image Processing, vol.7, pp.130–138 (1978)

[Herman90] G.T.Herman : On topology as applied to image analysis, Computer Vision, Graphics and Image Processing, vol.52, pp.409–415 (1990)

[Herman93] G.T.Herman : Oriented surfaces in digital spaces, Graphical Models and Image Processing, vol.55, no.5, pp.381–396 (1993)

[Hilditch69] J.C.Hilditch : Linear skeletons from square cupboards, in B.Meltzer and D.Michie, eds. Machine Intelligence IV, Edinburgh Univ. Press, Edinburgh, pp.403–420 (1969)

[Hirano00] Y.Hirano, A.Shimizu, J.Hasegawa, and J.Toriwaki : A tracking algorithm to extract ridge lines for three dimensional gray images using curvature of hypersurface, Trans. on IEICE D-II, vol.J83-D-II, no.1, pp.126–136 (2000) (in Japanese)

[Hirano03] Y.Hirano, K.Kunimitsu, J.Hasegawa, and J.Toriwaki : A region growing method using hypersurface curvature and its application to extraction of blood vessel region from chest X-ray CT Images, Journal of the Computer-Aided Diagnosis of Medical Images (CADM Journal), vol.7, no.3, pp.1–10 (2003) (in Japanese)

[Hirata96] T.Hirata : A unified linear time algorithm for computing distance maps, Information processing Letters, vol.43, pp.129–133 (1996)

[Hoehne86] K.H.Hohhne and R.Bernstein : Shading 3D-images from CT using gray-lever gradients, IEEE Trans. on Medical Imaging, vol.5, no.1, pp.45–47 (1986)

[Hong97] L.Hong, S.Muraki, A.Kaufman, D.Bartz, and T.He : Virtual voyage: Interactive navigation in the human colon, Computer Graphics (Proc. of Siggraph '97), pp.27–34 (1997)

[Horiuchi87] K.Horiuchi, S.Yokoi, and J.Toriwaki : Method for rendering transparent solid of revolution by using ray tracing and smooth shading, Journal of Information Processing Society of Japan, vol.28, no.8, pp.870–877 (1987) (in Japanese)

[Ichikawa94] Y.Ichikawa and J.Toriwaki : A digital ULSI inspection method using parallel scanning confocal microscope, Proceedings of IAPR Workshop on Machine Vision Applications (MVA'94), pp.568–570 (1994)

[Ichikawa95] Y.Ichikawa and J.Toriwaki : ULSI inspection system using digital scanning confocal microscopy with applications to PZT film, Proc. International Symp. on Semiconductor Manufacturing, pp.110–113 (1995)

[Ichikawa96] Y.Ichikawa and J.Toriwaki: Confocal microscope 3D visualizing method for fine surface characterization of microstructures, International Sym. on Optical Science, Engineering, and Instrumentation, SPIE Annual Meeting, SPIE (1996)

[Idesawa91a] M.Idesawa : Perception of 3-D transpararent illusory surface in binocular fusion, Japanese Journal of Applied Physics vol.30, no.7B, pp.L1289–L1292 (1991)

[Idesawa91b] M.Idesawa : Perception of 3-D illusory surface with binocular viewing, Japanese Journal of Applied Physics vol.30, no.4B, pp.L751–L754 (1991)

[Imiya99] A.Imiya and U.Eckhardt : The Euler charactersitics of discrete objects and discrete quasiobjects, Computer Vision and Image Understanding, vol.75, no.3, pp.307–318 (1999)

[Ishii99] M.Ishii : On a general method to calculate vertices of N-dimensional product-regular polytopes, FORMA, vol.14, no.3, pp.221–237 (1999)

[Johnston75] E.G.Johnston and A.Rosenfeld : Digital detection of pits, peaks, ridges and ravines, IEEE Trans. on SMC, vol.5, pp.472–480 (1975)

[Jonas97] A.Jonas and N.Kiryate : Digital representation scheme for 3D curves, Pattern Recognition, vol.30, no.1, pp.1803–1816 (1997)

[Jones90] V.F.R.Jones : Knot theory and statistical mechanics, Scientific American, vol.266, no.11, pp.52–57 (1990)

[Jones06] M.W.Jones, J.A.Baerentzen, and M.Sramek : 3D distance fields: a survey of techniques and applications, IEEE Trans. on Visualization and Computer Graphics, vol.12, pp.581–599 (2006)

[Julesz62] B.Julesz and J.E.Miller : Automatic stereoscopic presentation of functions of two variables, Bell System Technical J., vol.41, pp.663–676 (1962)

[Kajiya82] J.Kajiya : Ray tracing parametric patches, Computer Graphics, vol.16, no.3, pp.245–254 (1982)

[Kajiya84] J.T.Kajiya and B.P.V.B.Herzen : Ray tracing volume densities, Computer Graphics, vol.18, pp.165–174 (1984)

[Kato95] T.Kato, T.Hirata, T.Saito, and K.Kise : An efficient algorithm for the Euclidean distance transformation, Trans. of IEICE, Japan, DII, vol.J78-D-II, no.12, pp.1750–1757 (1995) (in Japanese)

[Kawase85] Y.Kawase, S.Yokoi, J.Toriwaki, and T.Fukumura : A thinning algorithm for three-dimensional binary images, Trans. on IEICE, Japan, vol.J68-D, no.4, pp.481–488 (1985)

[Kenmochi98] Y.Kenmochi, A.Imiya, and A.Ichikawa : Boundary extraction of discrete objects, Computer Vision and Image Understanding, vol.71, no.3, pp.281–293 (1998)

[Kenmochi98a] Y.Kenmochi and A.Imiya : Deformation of discrete surfaces, in R.Klette, A.Rosenfeld, and F.Sloboda, eds., Advances in Digital and Computational Geometry, Chapter 9, pp.285–316, Springer (1998)

[Kenmochi98b] Y.Kenmochi, A.Imiya, and A.Ichikawa : Boundary extraction of discrete objets, Computer Vision and Image Understanding, vol.71, no.3, pp.281–293 (1998)

[Kim82a] C.E.Kim and A.Rosenfeld : Digital straight lines and covexity of digital regions, IEEE Trans. Pattern Analysis Mach. Intell., vol.4, pp.149–153 (1982)

[Kim82b] C.E.Kim : On cellular straight line segments, Computer Graphics and Image Processing, vol.18, pp.369–381 (1982)

[Kim83] C.E.Kim : Three-dimensional digital segments, IEEE Trans. Pattern analysis Mach. Intell., vol.5, pp.231–234 (1983)

[Kim84] C.E.Kim : Three-dimensional digital planes, IEEE Trans. Pattern Analysis Mach. Intell., vol.6, pp.639–645 (1984)

[Kiryati95] N.Kiryati and O.Kubler : On chain code probabilities and length estimators for digitized three-dimensional curves, Pattern Recognition, vol.28, pp.361–372 (1995)

[Kitasaka02a] T.Kitasaka, K.Mori, J.Hasegawa, J.Toriwaki, and K.Katada : Recognition of aorta and pulmonary artery in the mediastinum using medial-line models from 3D CT images without contrast material, Medical Imaging Technology, vol.20, no.5, pp.572–583 (2002)

[Kitasaka02b] T.Kitasaka, K.Mori, J.Hasegawa, and J.Toriwaki : A method for extraction of bronchus regions from 3D chest X-ray CT images by analyzing structural features of the bronchus, FORMA, vol.17, no.4, pp.321–338 (2002)

[Klette85] R.Klette : The m-dimensional grid point space, Computer Vision, Graphics and Image Processing, vol.30, pp.1–12 (1985)

[Kong85] T.Y.Kong and A.W.Roscee : A theory of binary digital pictures, Computer Vision, Graphics and Image Processing, vol.48, pp.357–393 (1989)

[Kong89] T.Y.Kong and A.Rosenfeld : Digital topology: introduction and survey, Computer Vision, Graphics and Image Processing, vol.32, pp.221–243 (1989)

[Kurashige86] S.Yokoi, K.Kurashige, and J.Toriwaki : Rendering gems with asterism and chatoyancy, Visual Computer, vol.2, no.5, pp.307–312 (1986)

[Kuwabara82] E.Kuwabara, S.Yokoi, J.Toriwaki, and T.Fukumura : Distance function and distance transformation on 3D digital image data, Trans. on IECE, vol.J65-D, no.8, pp.195–202 (1982) (in Japanese)

[Lee91] C-N.Lee, T.Poston, and A.Rosenfeld : Winding and Euler numbers for 2D and 3D digital images, CVGIP: Graphical Models and Image Processing, vol.53, no.6, pp.522–537 (1991)

[Lee93] C-N.Lee, T.Poston, and A.Rosenfeld : Holes and genus of 2D and 3D digital images, CVGIP: Graphical Models And Image Processing, vol.55, no.1, pp.20–47 (1993)

[Lee94] Ta-Chih Lee, R.L.Kashyap, and C.-N.Chu : Building skeleton models via 3-D medial surface/axis thinning algorithms, CVGIP: Graphical Models and Image Processing, vol.56, no.6, pp.462–478 (1994)

[Levoy88] M.Levoy : Display of surface from volume data, IEEE Computer Graphics and Applications, vol.8, no.3, pp29–37 (1988)

[Liu77] H.K.Liu : Two- and three-dimensional boundary detection, Computer Graphics and Image Processing, vol.6, pp.123–134 (1977)

[Lobregt80] S.Lobregt, P.W.Verbeek and F.C.A.Groen : Three-dimensional skeletonization : Principle and algorithm, IEEE Transactions on Pattern Analysis and Machine Intelligence, vol.2, no.1, pp.75–77 (1980)

[Lorensen87] W.E.Lorensen and H.E.Cline : Marching cubes : a high resolution 3D surface construction algorithm, Computer Graphics (Proc. ACM SIGGRAPH'87), vol.21, no.4, pp.163–169 (1987)

[Ma95] C.M.Ma : A 3D fully parallel thinning algorithm for generating medial faces, Pattern Recognition Letters, vol.16, pp.83–87 (1995)

[Ma96] C.M.Ma and M.Sonka : A 3D fully parallel 3D thinning algorithm and its application, Computer Vision and Image Understanding, vol.64, pp.420–433 (1996)

[Mase81] K.Mase, J.Toriwaki, and T.Fukumura : Modified digital Voronoi diagram and its applications to image processing, Trans.of IECE, vol.J64-D, no.11, pp.1029–1036 (1981)

[Matsumoto84] T.Matsumoto, J.Toriwaki, S.Yokoi, and T.Fukumura : A border-following algorithm of three dimensional digitized binary pictures, Trans. of IECE., vol.J67-D, no.10, pp.1250–1257 (1984) (n Japanese)

[Matsumoto85] T.Matsumoto, J.Toriwaki, S.Yokoi, and T.Fukumura : A border following algorithm of three dimensional digitized binary pictures, Systems and Computers in Japan, vol.16, no.4, pp.57–65 (1985) (English version of [Matsumoto84])

[McAndrew97] A.McAndrew and C.Osborne : The Euler charactersitic on the face-centred cubic lattice, Pattern Recognition Letters, vol.18, pp.229–237 (1997)

[Maragos87a] P.Maragos and R.W.Schafer : Morphological filters - Part I: Their analysis and relations to linear shift-invariant filters, IEEE Trans. on ASSP, vol.35, no.8, pp.1153–1169 (1987)

[Maragos87b] P.Maragos and R.W.Schafer : Morphological filters - Part II: Their relations to median, order-statistics, and stack filters, IEEE Trans. on ASSP, vol.35, no.8, pp.1170–1184 (1987)

[McLoughlin87] M.P.McLoughlin and G.R.Arce : Determination properties of the recursive separable median filter, IEEE Trans. of ASSP, vol.35, no.1, pp.98–106 (1987)

[Miyazawa06] M.Miyazawa, P.Zeng, N.Iso and T.Hirata : A systolic algorithm for Euclidean distance transformation, IEEE Trans. on PAMI, vol.26, no.7, pp.1127–1134 (2006)

[Molgouyres99] R.Malgouyres and G.Bertrand : A new local property of strong n-surfaces, Pattern Recognition Letters, vol.20, pp.417–428 (1999)

[Molgouyres00] R.Malgouyres and A.Lenoir : Topology preservation within digital surfaces, CVGIP: Graphical Models, vol.62, pp.71–84 (2000)

[Monga91] O.Monga, R.Deriche, and J-M. Rocchisani : 3D edge detection using recursive filtering: application to scanner images, CVGIP: Image Understanding, vol.53, no.1, pp.78-87 (1991)

[Monga95] O.Monga and S.Benayoun : Using partial derivatives of 3D images to extract typical surface features, Computer Vision and Image Understanding, vol.61, no.2, pp.171–189 (1995)

[Montanari68] U.Montanari : A method for obtaining skeletons using a quasi-Euclidean distance, J. Assoc. Comput. Mach., vol.15, no.4, pp.600–624 (1968)

[Mori94a] K.Mori, J.Hasegawa, J.Toriwaki, Y.Anno, and K.Katada : A procedure with position-variant thresholding and distance transformation for automated detection of lung cancer lesions from 3-D chest X-ray CT images, Medical Imaging Technology, vol.12, no.3, pp.216–223 (1994)

[Mori94b] K.Mori, J.Hasegawa, J.Toriwaki, Y.Anno, and K.Katada : A method to extract pipe structured components in three dimensional medical images and simulation of bronchus endoscope images, Proc. of 3D image Conference '94, pp.269-274 (1994) (in Japanese)

[Mori03] K.Mori, Y.Suenaga, and J.Toriwaki : Fast software-based volume rendering using multimedia instructions on PC platforms and its application to virtual endoscopy, Proc. of SPIE, vol.5031, pp.111–122 (2003)

[Mukherjee89] J.Mukherjee and B.N.Chatterji : Thinning of 3-D images using the safe point thinning algorithm, Pattern Recognition Letters, vol.10, pp.167–173 (1989)

[Mukherjee90a] J.Mukherjee and B.N.Chatterji : Segmentation of three-dimensional surfaces, Pattern Recognition Letters, vol.11, pp.215–223 (1990)

[Mukherjee90b] J.Mukherjee, P.P.Das, and B.N.Chatterji : An algorithm for the extraction of the wire frame structure of a three-dimensional object, Pattern Recognition, vol.23, no.9, pp.999–1010 (1990)

[Nackman82] L.R.Nackman : Curvature relations in three-dimensional aymmetric axes, Computer Graphics and Image Processing, vol.20, pp.43–57 (1982)

[Nackman85] L.R.Nackman and S.M.Pizer : Three-dimensional shape description using the symmetric axis transform I: Theory, IEEE Trans. PAMI, vol.7, no.2, pp.187–202 (1985)

[Nakajima00] S.Nakajima, S.Prita, K.Masamune, I.Sakuma, T.Dohi, and K.Nakamura : Real 3-D display system for use in medical applications, Proc. of CARS 2000, pp.613–618 (2000)

[Nakamura00] A.Nakamura and A.Rosenfeld : Digital knots, Pattern Recognition, vol.33, pp.1541–1553 (2000)

[Naruse77a] T.Naruse, J.Toriwaki, and T.Fukmumura : Comparative study of thinning algorithms for grey pictures, Trans. of IECE, vol.J60-D, no.12, pp.1093–1100 (1977)

[Naruse77b] T.Naruse, J.Toriwaki, and T.Fukmumura : Fundamental properties of the grey weighted distance transformation, Trans of IECE, vol.J60-D, no.12, pp.1101–1108 (1977)

[Niblack92] C.W.Niblack, P.B.Gibbons, and D.W.Capson : Generating skeltons and centerlines from the distance transform, CVGIP: Graphical Models and Image Processing, vol.54, no.5, pp.420–437 (1992)

[Nilsson97] F.Nilsson and P.E.Danielsson : Finding the ninimal set of maximum disks for binary objects, Graphical Models and Image Processing, vol.59, no.1, pp.55–60 (1997)

[Nishita85] T.Nishita and E.Nakamae : Continuous tone representation of three-dimensional objects taking into account of shadows and interreflection, Computer Graphics, vol.19, no.3, pp.23–30 (1985)

[Nishita90] .Nishita, T.Sederberg, and M.Kakimoto : Ray tracing trimmed rational surface patches, Computer Graphics, vol.24, no.4, pp.337–345 (1990)

[Nodes82] T.A.Nodes and N.C.Gallagher, Jr. : Median filters: some modifications and their properties, IEEE Trans. on ASSP, vol.30, no.5, pp.739–746 (1982)

[O'Callaghan84] J.F.O'Callaghan and D.M.Mark : The extraction of drainage networks from digital elevation data, CGIP, vol.28, pp.323–344 (1984)

[Oda06] M.Oda, Y.Hayashi, T.Kitasaka, K.Mori, and Y.Suenaga : A method for generating virtual unfolded view of colon using spring model, Proceedings of SPIE, Vol.6143, pp.61431C-1–12 (2006)

[Okabe83a] N.Okabe, J.Toriwaki, and T.Fukumura : Fundamental properties of distance functions on the three-dimensional digitized image data, Transactions of the IECE, Japan, J66-D, vol.3, pp.259-266 (1983)

[Okabe83b] N.Okabe, J.Toriwaki, and T.Fukumura : Paths and distance function on three-dimensional digitized pictures, Pattern Recognition Letters, vol.1, pp.205–212 (1983)

[Pai94] T.W.Pai and John H.L.Hansen : Boundary-constrained morphological skeleton minimization and skeleton reconstruction, IEEE Trans. Pattern Analysis and Machine Intell., vol.16, no.2, pp.201–208 (1994)

[Palagyi99] K.Palagyi and A.Kuba : A parallel 3D 12-subiteration thinning algorithm, Graphical Models and Image Processing, vol.61, pp.199–221 (1999)

[Park71] C.H.Park and A.Rosenfeld : Connectivity and genus in three dimensions, Univ.of Maryland, Computer Science Center, Techinical Report TR-156 (1971)

[Peucker75] T.K.Peucker and D.H.Douglas : Detection of surface specific points by local parallel processing of discrete terrain elevation data, CGIP, vol.4, pp.375–387 (1975)

[Phong75] B.T.Phong : Illumination for computer generated pictures, Communications of the ACM, vol.18, no.6, pp.311–317 (1975)

[Preston79] K.Preston, Jr., M.J.B.Duff, S.Levialdi, P.E.Norgren, and J.Toriwaki : Basics of cellular logic with some applications in medical image processing, Proc. IEEE, vol.67, no.5, pp.826–856 (1979)

[Preston80] K.Preston, Jr. : The crossing number of a three-dimenisonal dode-camino, J. of Combinatorics, vol.5, no.4, pp.281–286 (1980)

[Preston84] K.J.Hafford and K.Preston, Jr. : Three-dimensional skeletonization of elongated solids, Computer Vision, Graphics, and Image Processing, vol.27, no.1, pp.78–91 (1984)

[Ragnemalm90] I.Ragnemalm : Generation of Euclidean distance maps, Linkoping Studies in Science and Technology Thesis, No.206, Linkoping, Sweden (1990)

[Ritman03] E.L.Ritman : Evolution of medical tomographic imaging - as seen from a Darwinian perspective, Proc. IEEE, vol.91, no.10, pp.1483–1491 (2003)

[Rosenfeld67] A.Rosenfeld and J.L.Pfaltz : Sequential operations in digital picture processing, J. Assoc. Comput. Mach., vol.13, no.4, pp.471–494 (1967)

[Rosenfeld74] A.Rosenfeld : Digital straight line segments, IEEE Trans. on C, vol.23, pp.1264–1269 (1974)

[Saha94] P.K.Saha and B.B.Chaudhuri : Detection of 3-D simple points for topology preserving transformations with application to thinning, IEEE Trans. on PAMI, vol.16, no.10, pp.1028–1032 (1994)

[Saha95] P.K.Saha and B.B.Chaudhuri : A new approach to computing the Euler characteristic, Pattern Recognition, vol.28, no.12, pp.1955–1963 (1995)

[Saha97] P.K.Saha, B.B.Chaudhuri, and D.D.Majumder : A new shape-preserving parallel thinning algorithm for 3D digital images, Pattern Recognition, vol.30, pp.1939–1955 (1997)

[Saito90] T.Saito, S.Yokoi, and J.Toriwaki : Topology of the 3D digital line figure - an analysis of knot, Paper of Professional Group of Pattern Recognition and Understanding, IECE, Japan, PRU90-83, vol.90, no.38, pp.15–22 (1980) (in Japanese)

[Saito92] T.Saito and J.Toriwaki : Algorithms of three dimensional Euclidean distance transformation and extended digital Voronoi diagram, and analysis of human liver section images, J. of the Institute of Image Electornics, Japan, vol.21, no.5, pp.468-474 (1992)

[Saito93] T.Saito and J.Toriwaki : Fast algorithms for n-dimensional Euclidean distance transformation, Proc. of the 8th SCIA-93 (Scandinavian Conf. on Image Analysis), pp.747–754 (1993)

[Saito94a] T.Saito and J.Toriwaki : New algorithms for n-dimensional Euclidean distance transformation, Pattern Recognition, vol.27, no.11, pp.1551–1565 (1994)

[Saito94b] T.Saito and J.Toriwaki: Reverse distance transformation and skeletons based upon the Euclidean metric for n-dimensional digital binary pictures, IEICE Trans. INF & SYST, Japan, vol.E77-D, no.9, pp.1005–1016 (1994)

[Saito95] T.Saito and J.Toriwaki : A sequential thinning algorithm for three dimensional digital pictures using the Euclidean distance transformation, Proc. 9th SCIA (Scandinavian Conf. on Image Analysis), pp.507–516 (1995)

[Saito96] T.Saito, K.Mori, and J.Toriwaki : A sequential thinning algorithm for three dimensional digital pictures using the Euclidean distance transformation and its properties, Tran. of IEICE, Japan, vol.J79-D-II, no.10, pp.1675–1685 (1996) (in Japanese)

[Saito00] T.Saito, K.Mori, Y.Suenaga, J.Toriwaki, and K.Katada : A method for specifying three dimensional interested regions on volume rendered images and its evaluation for virtual endoscopy system, Proc. of CARS 2000, pp.91–96 (2000)

[Saito01] T.Saito, S.Banjou, and J.Toriwaki : An improvement of three dimensional thinning method using a skeleton based on the Euclidean distance transformation - A method to control spurious branches, Trans. of IEICE, Japan, vol.J84-DII, no.8, pp.1628–1635 (2001) (in Japanese)

[Salari84] E.Salari and P.Siy : The ridge-seeking method for obtaining the skeleton of digital images, IEEE Trans. SMC, vol.14, no.3, pp.524–528 (1984)

[Sander90] P.T.Sander and S.W.Zucker : Inferring surface trace and differential structure from 3-D images, IEEE Trans. on PAMI, vol.12, no.9, pp.833–854 (1990)

[Shimizu93] A.Shimizu, J.Hasegawa, and J.Toriwaki : Minimum directional difference filter for extraction of circumscribed shadows in chest X-ray images and its characteristics, Trans. of IEICE, Japan, vol.J76D-II, no.2, pp.241–249 (1993) (in Japanese)

[Shimizu95a] A.Shimizu, J.Hasegawa, and J.Toriwaki : Characteristics of rotatory second order difference filter for computer aided diagnosis of medical images, Trans. of IEICE, Japan, vol.J78-D-II, no.1, pp.29–39 (1995) (In Japanese)

[Shimizu95b] A.Shimizu, M.Hakai, J.Hasegawa, and J.Toriwaki : Performance evaluation of 3-D enhancement filters for detection of lung cancer from 3-D chest X-ray CT images, Medical Imaging Technology, vol.13, no.6, pp.853–864 (1995)

[SIGGRPH88] Siggraph, Conference Proceedings, Computer Graphics, vol.22, no.4 (1988) 15th Annual Conference on Computer Graphics and Interactive Techniques. The same preceedings have been published since 1974

[Stefanelli71] R.Stefanelli and A.Rosenfeld : Some parallel thinning algorithms for digtal pictures, J. ACM, vol.8, no.2, pp.255–264 (1971)

[Suzuki83] S.Suzuki and K.Abe : Max-type distance transformation for digitized binary pictures and its applications, Trns. IECE, Japan, vol.E-66, no.2, pp.94–101 (1983)

[Suzuki85] H.Suzuki, H.Shinyashiki, and J.Toriwaki : Structural analysis of line patterns using distance transformation (DTLP), Trans. of IECE, Japan, vol.J68-D, no.2, pp.145–152 (1985) (in Japanese)

[Tamura78] H.Tamura : A comparison of line thinning algorithms from digital geometry viewpoint, Proc. of 4th Joint Conf. of Pattern Recognition, pp.715–719 (1978)

[Tamura83] H.Tamura : Multidisciplinary image proceeing and its software support system, Researchs of the Electrotechnical Laboratory, No.835 (1983) (in Japanese with English abstract)

[Taylor96] R.H.Taylor, S.Lavallee, G.C.Burdea and R.Mosges eds. : Computer-integrated Surgery: Technology and Clinical Applications, The MIT Press, Cambridge, Massachusetts, U.S.A. (1996)

[Thimblely94] H.W.Thimblely, S.Inglis, and I.H.Witter : Displaying 3D images: algorithms for single-image random-dot stereograms, IEEE Computer, vol.27, no.10, pp.38–48 (1994)

[Thirion95] J-P.Thirion and A.Gourdon : Computing the differential characteristics of isointensity surfaces, Computer Vision and Image Understanding, vol.61, no.2, pp.190–202 (1995)

[Tomasi98] C.Tomasi and R.Manduchi : Bilateral filtering techniques for gray and color images, Proc. of 1998 Int. Conf. on Computer Vision, pp.839–846 (1998)

[Toriwaki75] J.Toriwaki and T.Fukumura : Extraction of structual information from gray pictures, Comp. Graphics and Image Processing, vol.4, pp.375–387 (1975)

[Toriwaki79] J.Toriwaki, N.Kato, and T.Fukumura : Parallel local operations for a new distance transformation of a line pattern and their applications, IEEE Trans. SMC, vol.9, no.10, pp.628–643 (1979)

[Toriwaki81] J.Toriwaki and S.Yokoi : Distance transformations and skeletons of digitized pictures with applications, in A.Rosenfeld and L.Kanal, eds., : Progress in Pattern Recognition, vol.1, pp.187–264, North-Holland, Amsterdam, N.Y (1981)

[Toriwaki82a] J.Toriwaki, M.Tanaka, and T.Fukumura : A generalized distance transformation of a line pattern with grey values and its applications, Computer Graphics and Image Processing, vol.20, no.4, pp.319–346 (1982)

[Toriwaki82b] J.Toriwaki, K.Mase, Y.Yashima, and T.Fukumura : Modified digital Voronoi diagram and relative neighbors on a digitized picture and their applications to tissue image analysis, Proc. the First International Symposium on Medical Imaging and Image Interpretation, pp.362–367 (1982)

[Toriwaki83] J.Toriwaki and S.Yokoi : Algorithms for skeletonizing three-dimensional digitized binary pictures, Proceeding of the SPIE Architecture and Algorithms for Digital Image Processing, vol.435, pp.2–9 (1983)

[Toriwaki84] J.Toriwaki, Y.Yashima, and S.Yokoi : Adjacency graphs on a digitized figure set and their applications to texture analysis, Proc. the 7th. ICPR, pp.1216–1218 (1984)

[Toriwaki85a] J.Toriwaki and S.Yokoi : Basics of algorithms for processing three-dimensional digitized pictures, Journal of IECE, in Japan, vol.J68-D, no.4, pp.426–432 (1985) (in Japanese)

[Toriwaki85b] J.Toriwaki, H.Ohshita, and T.Saito : Understanding forms by man and computer using computer graphics and image processing, in S.Ishizaka, ed., Proceedings of the Second International Symposium for Science on Form, pp.219–231 (1990)

[Toriwaki88] J.Toriwaki and S.Yokoi : Voronoi and related neighbors on digitized two-dimensional space with applications to texture analysis, in G.T.Toussaint, ed., Computational Morphology, pp.207–228, North-Holland, The Netherlands (1988)

[Toriwaki92] J.Toriwaki, M.Okada, and T.Saito : Distance transformation and skeletons for shape feature analysis, Visual Form : Analysis and Recognition (Proc. of the International Workshop on Visual Form, 1991.5.27-30), pp.547–563, Plenum Press, New York (1992)

[Toriwaki00] J.Toriwaki : Trends and future problem in computer aided diagnosis of X-ray images, Trans. of IEICE, Japan, vol.J83D-II, no.1, pp.3–26 (2000) (in Japanese)

[Toriwaki01] J.Toriwaki and K.Mori : Distance transformation and skeletonization of 3D pictures and their applications to medical images, in G.Bertrand, A.Imiya, and R.Klette, eds., Digital and Image Geometry, Advanced Lectures, LNCS(Lecture Notes in Computer Science), vol.2243, pp.412–428, Springer Verlarg (2001)

[Toriwaki02a] J.Toriwaki and T.Yonekura : Euler number and connectivity indexes of a three-dimensional digital picture, FORMA, vol.17, no.3, pp.173–209 (2002)

[Toriwaki02b] J.Toriwaki and T.Yonekura : Local patterns and connectivity indexes in a three dimensional digital picture, FORMA, vol.17, no.4, pp.275–291 (2002)

[Toriwaki04] J.Toriwaki, K.Mori, and J.Hasegawa : Recent Progress in Medical Image Processing, in K.Aizawa, K.Sakaue, Y.Suenaga, eds., Image Processing Technologies, Algorithms, Sensors, and Applications, Marcel Dekker, Inc., N.Y., pp.233–357 (2004)

[Truong06] T.D.Truong, T.Kitasaka, K.Mori, and Y.Suenaga : Simulation of Stomach Specimens Generation Based on Deformation of Preoperative CT Images, Proc. of ISBMS 2006, LNCS 4072, pp.178–187 (2006)

[Tsao81] Y.F.Tsao and K.S.Fu : A parallel thinning algorithm for 3-D pictures, Computer Graphics and Image Processing, vol.17, pp.315–331 (1981)

[Tsao82a] Y.Tsao and K.S.Fu : A 3D parallel skeletonwise thinning algorithm, IEEE, pp.678–683 (1982)

[Tsao82b] Y.F.Tsao and K.S.Fu : A general scheme for constructing skeleton models, Information Science, vol.27, pp.53–87 (1982)

[Tyler90] C.W.Tyler and M.B.Clark : The autostereogram, SPIE Stereoscopic Display and Applications, vol.1, 258, pp.182–196 (1962)

[Udupa94] J.Udupa : Multidimensional digital boundaries, CVGIP: Graphical Models and Image Processing, vol.56, no.4, pp.311–323 (1994)

[Verwer91] B.J.H.Verwer : Local distances for distance transformations in two and three dimensions, Pattern Recognition Letters, vol.12, pp.671–682 (1991)

[Vining93] D.J.Vining, A.R.Padhani, S.Wood, E.A.Zerhouni, E.K.Fishman, and J.E.Kuhlman : Virtual bronchoscopy: A new perspective for viewing the tracheobronchial tree, Radiology, vol.189(P), p.438 (1993)

[Vining03] D.J.Vinig : 1 Virtual colonoscopy: The inside story, in A.H.Dachman, ed., Atlas of Virtual Colonoscopy, Springer-Verlag, Berlin, New York, Heidelberg, pp.3-4 (2003)

[Vitria96] J.Vitria and J.Llacer : Reconstructing 3D light microscope images using the EM algorithm, Pattern Recognition Letters, vol.17, pp.1491–1498 (1996)

[Voxel95] Voxel Man : The novel hypermedia, system for UNIX work-stations, Catalogue of Springer (1995)

[Wang98] G.Wang, E.G.McFrland, B.P.Brown, and M.W.Vannier : GI tract unraveling with curves cross sections, IEEE Medical Imaging, vol.17, pp.318–322 (1998)

[Watanabe86] Y.Watanabe : Structural features of three-dimensional image, Science on Form : Proceedings of the First International Symposium for Science on Form, S.Ishizaka, gen. ed., Y.Kato, R.Takaki, and J.Toriwaki, eds., pp.247–254 (1986)

[Whitted80] T.Whitted : An improved illumination model for shaded display, Communications of the ACM, vol.23, no.6, pp.343–349 (1980)

[Wong04] W.C.K.Wong, A.C.S.Chung and S.C.H.Yu : Trilateral filtering for biomedical images, Proc. of 2004 IEEE Int. Symp. on Biomedical Images, pp.820–823 (2004)

[Workshop99] Proc. of the Third International Workshop on Cooperative Distributed Vision (CDV-WS99), Nov. 19-20, Kyoto, Japan (1999)

[Yamada84] H.Yamada : Complete Euclidean distance transformation by parallel operation, Proc. of 7th Int. Conf. on Pattern Recognition, pp.69–71 (1984)

[Yamashita83] M.Yamashita, Y.Inagaki, and N.Honda : The relation between parallel and sequential transformations on digital images, Trans. of IECE, Japan, vol.J66-D, no.4, pp.429–436 (1983) (in Japanese)

[Yamashita84] M.Yamashita and N.Honda : Distance functions defined by variable neighborhood sequences, Pattern Recognition, vol.17, no.5, pp.509–513 (1984)

[Yamashita86] M.Yamashita and T.Ibaraki : Distances defined by neighborhood sequences, Pattern Recognition, vol.19, no.3, pp.237–246 (1986)

[Yang89] W-J. Yang : Hndibook of Flow Visualization, Hemisphere Pbulishing, Co., New York (1989)

[Yashima83] Y.Yashima, S.Yokoi, J.Toriwaki and T.Fukumura : Adjacency graphs on a digitized picture and their applications, Trans. on IECE, Japan, vol.J66-D, no.10, pp.1099–1106 (1983) (in Japanese)

[Yasue96] M.Yasue, K.Mori, T.Saito, J.Hasegawa, and J.Toriwaki : Thinning algorithms for three-dimensional gray images and their application to medical images with comparative evaluation of performance, Trans. of IEICE, Japan, vol.J79-D-II, no.10, pp.1664–1674 (1996) (in Japanese)

[Yokoi75] S.Yokoi, J.Toriwaki, and T.Fukumura : An analysis of topological properties of digitized binary pictures using local features, Computer Graphics and Image Processing, vol.4, no.1, pp.63–73 (1975)

[Yokoi79] S.Yokoi, J.Toriwaki, and T.Fukumura : A sequential algorithm for shrinking binary pictures, Trans. IECE, Japan, vol.62-D, no.8, pp.537–542 (1979) (in Japanese)

[Yokoi81] S.Yokoi, J.Toriwaki, and T.Fukumura : On generalized distance transformation of digitized pictures, IEEE Trnas. PAMI, vol.3, no.4, pp.424–443 (1981)

[Yokoi86] S.Yokoi, K.Kurashige, and J.Toriwaki : Rendering gems with asterism and chatoyancy, Visual Computer, vol.2, no.5, pp.307–312 (1986)

[Yokoyama03] K.Yokoyama, T.Kitasaka, K.Mori, Y.Mekada, J.Hasegawa, and J.Toriwaki : Liver region extraction from 3D abdominal X-ray CT images using distribution features of abdominal organs, Journal of Japan Society of Computer-Aided Diagnosis of Medical Images, vol.7, no.4-3, pp.1–11 (2003)

[Yonker94] P.P.Yonker and A.Vossepoel : Connectivity in high dimensional images, Proc. of IAPR Workshop on Machine Vision Applications (MVA'94), pp.30–32 (1994)

[Yu90] S.S.Yu and W.H.Tsai : A new thinning algorithm for gray-scale images by the relation technique, Pattern Recognition, vol.23, no.10, pp.1067–1076 (1990)

[Yonekura80a] T.Yonekura, J.Toriwaki, T.Fukumura, and S.Yokoi : Topological properties of three-dimensional digitized pictuture data (1) - connectivity and Euler umber, PRL80-1 (1980)

[Yonekura80b] T.Yonekura, J.Toriwaki, T.Fukumura, and S.Yokoi : Topological properties of three-dimensional digitized picture data (2) - connectivity number and deletability, PRL80-30 (1980)

[Yonekura80c] T.Yonekura, J.Toriwaki, T.Fukumura, and S.Yokoi : Topological properties of three-dimensional digitized picture data (3) - shrinking algorithm for three dimensional digitized picutres, PRL80-31 (1980)

[Yonekura82a] T.Yonekura, S.Yokoi, and J.Toriwaki : Connectivity and Euler number of figures in the digitized three-dimensional space, Trans. of IEICE, Japan, vol.J65-D, no.1, pp.80–87 (1982) (in Japanese)

[Yonekura82b] T.Yonekura, S.Yokoi, J.Toriwaki, and T.Fukumura : Connectivity number and deletability of a three-dimensional digitized binary picture, Trans. of IEICE, Japan, vol.J65-D, no.5, pp.652–659 (1982) (in Japanese)

[Yonekura82c] T.Yonekura, J.Toriwaki, S.Yokoi, and T.Fukumura : Deletability of 1-voxels and a shrinking algorithm for 3-dimensional digitized pictures, Trans. of IEICE, Japan, vol.J65-D, no.12, pp.1543–1550 (1982) (in Japanese)

[Yonekura82d] T.Yonekura, T.Fukumura, J.Toriwaki, and S.Yokoi : Connectivity number and deletability of a three-dimensional digitized binary picture, Systems Computers Controls, vol.13, pp.40–48 (1982)

[Zucker79] S.W.Zucker and R.A.Hummel : A three-dimensional edge operator, Proc. of PRIP'79, pp.162–168 (1979)

[Zucker81] S.W.Zucker and R.A.Hummel : A three-dimensional edge operator, IEEE Trans. of PAMI, vol.3, no.3, pp.324–331 (1981)

[Zhan94] S.Zhan and R.Mehrota : A zero-crossing-based optimal three-dimensional edge detector, CVGIP: Image Understanding, vol.59, no.2, pp.242–253 (1994)

[Zhou00] K.Zhou, T.Hamada, A.Shimizu, J.Hasegawa, and J.Toriwaki : Comparative performance evaluation of three dimensional image processing expert systems 3D-IMPRESS and 3D-IMPRESS-Pro, J. of Computer-Aided Diagnosis of Medical Images, vol.4, no.2, pp.1–9 (2000)

– Supplementary list 3D surface/axis thinning –

[Bertrand95] [Bitter01] [Borgefors99] [Gagvan99] [Gong90] [Hafford84] [Lee94] [Lobregt80] [Ma95] [Ma96] [Mukherjee89] [Mukherjee90b] [Nackman82] [Nackman85] [Palagyi99] [Preston84] [Saha94] [Saha97] [Saito95] [Saito96] [Saito01] [Toriwaki83] [Toriwaki85a] [Toriwaki01] [Tsao81] [Tsao82a] [Tsao82b]

– Books for reference: monographs, handbooks, and textbooks –

[Bankman00] I.N.Bankman, ed. : Handbook of Medical Imaging, Academic Press, 2000
[Berg97] M. de Berg and M. van Kreveld : Computational Geometry Algorithms and Applications, Springer-Verlag, 1997
[Bertland01] G.Bertland, A.Imiya, and R.Klette, eds. : Digital and Image Geometry, Advanced Lectures, LNCS, 2243, Springer, 2001
[Block89] J.R.Block and H.Yuker : Can you believe your eyes ? Gardner Press, Inc., U.S.A., 1989
[Borik00] A.Borik, ed. : Handbook of Image and Video Processing, Academic Press, 2000
[Carmo76] M.P.de Carmo : Differential Geometry of Curves and Surfaces, Prentice Hall Inc., Englewood Cliffs, N.J., 1976
[Corrochano05] E.B.Corrochano : Handbook of Geometric Computing, Springer-Verlag, Berlin, Heidelberg, Germany, 2005
[Cromwell97] P.R.Cromwell : Polyhedra, Cambridge University Press, 1997
[Dachman03] A.H.Dachman, ed. : Atlas of Virtual Colonoscopy, Springer-Verlag, Berlin, New York, Heidelberg, 2003
[Duda01] R.O.Duda, P.E.Hart, and D.G.Stork : Pattern Classification, 2nd ed., John Wiley & Sons, Inc., 2001
[Fano61] R.M.Fano : Transmission of Information - a Statistical Theory of Communication, M.I.T.Press, U.S.A., 1961
[Foley84] J.D.Foley and A.Van Dam : Fundamentals of Interactive Computer Graphics, Addison-Wesley, 1982
[Forsyth03] D.A.Forsyth and J.Ponce : Computer Vision: A Modern Approach, Prentice Hall, New York, 2003
[Girod00] B.Girod, G.Greines, and H.Niemann, eds : Principles of 3D Image Analysis and Synthesis, Kluwer Academic Publishers, Boston, U.S.A., 2000
[Goodman04] J.E.Goodman and J.O'Rourke, eds. : Handbook of Discrete and Computational Geometry, 2nd ed., Chapman & Hall/Crc, London, 2004
[Hall79] E.L.Hall : Computer Image Processnig and Recognition, Academic Press, 1979
[Herman98] G.T.Herman : Geometry of Digital Spaces, Birkhauser, Boston, 1998
[Hockney01] D.Hockney : Secret Knowledge Rediscovering the Lost Techniques of the Old Masters, Thames & Hudson Ltd., 2001
[Horn86] B.K.P.Horn : Robot Vision, the MIT Press, U.S.A, 1986
[Jahne99] B.Jahne, H.Haussecker, and P.Geissler : Handbook of Computer Vision and Application, vol.1, 2, 3, Academic Press, 1999

[Johnson06] C.Johnson, R.Moorhead, T.Muzner, H.Pfister, P.Rheingans, and
T.S.Yoo : NIH/HSF Visualization Research Challenges Report, IEEE, 2006

[Julesz71] B.Julesz : Foundations of Cyclopian Perception, Univ. of Chicago Press,
Chicago, Illinois, 1971

[Kanatani90] K.Kamatani : Group-theoretic Methods in Image Understanding,
Springer-Verlag, 1990

[Kauffman87] L.H.Kauffman : On Knots, Princeton Univ. Press, U.S.A., 1987

[Kaufman91] A.Kaufman : Volume Visualization, IEEE Computer Society Press,
1991

[Klette98] R.Klette, A.Rosenfeld, and F.Sloboda, eds. : Advances in Digital and
Computational Geometry, Springer, 1998

[Matheron75] G.Matheron : Random Sets and Integral Geometry, John Wiley &
Sons., 1975

[Nikolaridis01] N.Nikolaridis : 3-D Image Processing Algorithms, John Wiley &
Sons., N.Y., 2001

[Ohta99] Y.Ohta and H.Tamura : Mixed Reality -Merging Real and Virtual Worlds,
Ohmsha, 1999

[Panofsky24] E.Panofsky : Die Perspektive als "symbolische Form," Vortrage der
Bibliotek Warburg, 1924–1925

[Rogalla01] P.Rogalla, J.T.van Scheltinga, and B.Hamm : Virtual Endoscopy and
Related 3D Techniques, Springer, 2001

[Rosenfeld82] A.Rosenfeld and A.C.Kak : Digital Picture Processing, 2nd. ed., vols.1
and 2, Academic Press, 1982

[Pratt78] W.K.Pratt : Digital Image Processing, Wiley, N.Y., 1978

[Russ92] J.C.Russ : The Image Processing Handbook, CRC Press, 1992

[Russ95] J.C.Russ : The Image Processing Handbook, 2nd ed., CRCPress, 1995

[Serra82] J.Serra : Image Analysis and Mathematical Morphology, Academic Press,
1982

[Toth72] L.F.Toth : Laerungen in der Ebene auf der Kugel und im Raum, Springer-
Verlag, Heidelberg, 1972

[Toriwaki78] J.Toriwaki : Digital Image Processing for Image Understanding (I) and
(II), Shokodo, Tokyo, Japan, 1978, 1979 (in Japanese)

[Watt98] A.Watt and F.Policarpo : The Computer Image, Addison Welsey, 1998

[Weibel79] E.R.Weibel : Stereological Methods, vol.I, Academic Press, 1979

[Weng93] J.Weng, T.S.Huang, and N.Ahuj'a : Motion and Structure from Image
Sequences, Springer-Verlag, 1993

– Surveys and bibliographies –

[Rosenfeld69] A.Rosenfeld : Picture processing by computer, Comput. Survey, 1,
pp.147–176 (1969)

[Rosenfeld73] A.Rosenfeld : Progress in picture processing : 1969-1971, Comput.
Surv., 5, pp.81–108 (1973)

[Rosenfeld72] A.Rosenfeld : Picture processing : 1972, Comput. Graphics Image
Process., 1, pp.394–416 (1972)

[Rosenfeld74] A.Rosenfeld : Picture processing : 1973, Comput. Graphics Image
Process., 3, pp.178–194 (1974)

[Rosenfeld75] A.Rosenfeld : Picture processing : 1974, Comput. Graphics Image
Process., 4, pp.133–155 (1975)

258   References

[Rosenfeld76] A.Rosenfeld : Picture processing : 1975, Comput. Graphics Image
    Process., 5, pp.215–237 (1976)
[Rosenfeld77] A.Rosenfeld : Picture processing : 1976, Comput. Graphics Image
    Process., 6, pp.157–183 (1977)
[Rosenfeld78] A.Rosenfeld : Picture processing : 1977, Comput. Graphics Image
    Process., 7, pp.211–242 (1978)
[Rosenfeld79] A.Rosenfeld : Picture processing : 1978, Comput. Graphics Image
    Process., 9, pp.354–393 (1979)
[Rosenfeld80] A.Rosenfeld : Picture processing : 1979, Comput. Graphics Image
    Process., 13, pp.46–79 (1980)
[Rosenfeld81] A.Rosenfeld : Picture processing : 1980, Comput. Graphics Image
    Process., 16, pp.52–89 (1981)
[Rosenfeld82] A.Rosenfeld : Picture processing : 1981, Comput. Graphics Image
    Process., 19, pp.35–75 (1982)
[Rosenfeld83] A.Rosenfeld : Picture processing : 1982, Comput Vision, Graphics,
    Image Process., 22, pp.339–387 (1983)
[Rosenfeld84] A.Rosenfeld : Picture processing : 1983, Comput. Vision, Graphics,
    Image Process., 26, pp.347–393 (1984)
[Rosenfeld85] A.Rosenfeld : Picture processing : 1984, Comput. Vision, Graphics,
    Image Process., 30, pp.189–242 (1985)
[Rosenfeld86] A.Rosenfeld : Picture processing : 1985, Comput. Vision, Graphics,
    Image Process., 34, pp.204–251 (1986)
[Rosenfeld87] A.Rosenfeld : Picture processing : 1986, Comput. Vision, Graphics,
    Image Process., 38, pp.147–225 (1987)
[Rosenfeld88] A.Rosenfeld : Image analysis and computer vision : 1987, Comput.
    Vision, Graphics, Image Process., 42, pp.234–293 (1988)
[Rosenfeld89] A.Rosenfeld : Image analysis and computer vision : 1988, Comput.
    Vision, Graphics, Image Process., 46, pp.196–264 (1989)
[Rosenfeld90] A.Rosenfeld : Image analysis and computer vision : 1989, Comput.
    Vision, Graphics, Image Process., 50, pp.188–240 (1990)
[Rosenfeld91] A.Rosenfeld : Image analysis and computer vision : 1990, Image Un-
    derstanding, 53, pp.322–365 (1991)
[Rosenfeld92] A.Rosenfeld : Image analysis and computer vision : 1991, Image Un-
    derstanding, 55, pp.349–380 (1992)
[Rosenfeld93] A.Rosenfeld : Image analysis and computer vision : 1992, Image Un-
    derstanding, 58, pp.85–135 (1993)
[Rosenfeld94] A.Rosenfeld : Image analysis and computer vision : 1993, Image Un-
    derstanding, 59, pp.367–404 (1994)
[Rosenfeld95] A.Rosenfeld : Image analysis and computer vision : 1994, Comput.
    Vision and Image Understanding, 62, pp.90–143 (1995)
[Rosenfeld96] A.Rosenfeld : Image analysis and computer vision : 1995, Comput.
    Vision and Image Understanding, 63, pp.568–612 (1996)
[Rosenfeld97] A.Rosenfeld : Image analysis and computer vision : 1996, Comput.
    Vision and Image Understanding, 66, pp.33–93 (1997)
[Rosenfeld98] A.Rosenfeld : Image analysis and computer vision : 1997, Comput.
    Vision and Image Understanding, 70, pp.239–284 (1998)
[Rosenfeld99] A.Rosenfeld : Image analysis and computer vision : 1998, Comput.
    Vision and Image Understanding, 74, pp.36–95 (1999)
[Rosenfeld00a] A.Rosenfeld : Image analysis and computer vision : 1999, Comput.
    Vision and Image Understanding, 78, pp.222–302 (2000)

[Price] K.Price : Annotated Computer Vision Bibliography, available at http://iris.usc.edu/Vision-Notes/bibliography/contents.html

[Rosenfeld00b] A.Rosenfeld : Classifying the literature related to computer vision and image analysis, Computer Vision and Image Understanding, 79, pp.308–323 (2000)

[Katsuri91a] R.Katsuri and R.C.Jain : Computer Vision : Principles, IEEE Computer Soc. Press, U.S.A., 1991

[Katsuri91b] R.Katsuri and R.C.Jain : Computer Vision, Advances and Applications, IEEE Computer Soc. Press, U.S.A., 1991

[Chellappa85a] R.C.Chellappa and A.Sawchuk : Digital Image Processing and Analysis : Volume 1 : Digital Image Processing, IEEE Computer Society Press, 1985

[Chellappa85b] R.C.Chellappa and A.Sawchuk : Digital Image Processing and Analysis : Volume 2 : Digital Image Analysis, IEEE Computer Society Press, 1985

[Chellappa92] R.C.Chellappa and A.Sawchuk : Digital Image Processing, IEEE Computer Society Press, 1992

[IEEE00] Special issues on 20th Anniversary of PAMI, IEEE Trans. on PAMI, 22, 1, 2000

[IEEE99] Special issue on Medical Graphics, IEEE Computer Graphics and Applications, 19, 3, 1999

[IEEE98] Special issue on Virtual and Augmented Reality in Medicine, Proc.IEEE, vol.86, no.3, 1998

[IEEE96a] Theme section : Virtual Reality, IEEE Engineering in Medicine and Biology Magazine, 15, 2, 1996

[IEEE96b] Special issue on Applications in Surgery and Therapy, IEEE Computer Graphics and Applications, 16, 1, 1996

[IEEE95a] Special issue on Computer Applications in Surgery, IEEE Computer, 29, 1, 1996

[IEEE95b] Special issue on Virtual Reality, IEEE Computer Graphics and Applications, 15, 5, 1995

[IEEE95c] Special issue on Scientific Visualization, IEEE Trans. on Visualization and Computer Graphics, 1, 2, 1995

[IEEE95d] Special issue on Virtual Environment, IEEE Computer, 28, 6, 1995

[TIME95] Special issue on Welcome to Cyberspace, Time, 145, 19, 1995

[IEEE95e] Special issue on Virtural Reality for Medicine, IEEE Computers in Biology and Medicine, 25, 2, 1995

Index